Digital Cardiac Imaging

Digital Cardiac Imaging

edited by

ANDREW J. BUDA, M.D.
Department of Internal Medicine,
Cardiology Division,
University of Michigan Medical School,
Ann Arbor, Michigan, U.S.A.

and

EDWARD J. DELP, Ph.D.
School of Electrical Engineering,
Purdue University,
West Lafayette, Indiana, U.S.A.

1985 **MARTINUS NIJHOFF PUBLISHERS**
A MEMBER OF THE KLUWER ACADEMIC PUBLISHERS GROUP
BOSTON / DORDRECHT / LANCASTER

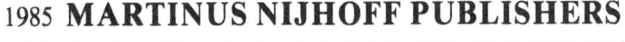

Distributors

for the United States and Canada: Kluwer Academic Publishers, 190 Old Derby Street, Hingham, MA 02043, USA

for the UK and Ireland: Kluwer Academic Publishers, MTP Press Limited, Falcon House, Queen Square, Lancaster LA1 1RN, UK

for all other countries: Kluwer Academic Publishers Group, Distribution Center, P.O. Box 322, 3300 AH Dordrecht, The Netherlands

Library of Congress Cataloging in Publication Data

```
Digital cardiac imaging.

    Includes index.
    1. Heart--Diseases--Diagnosis.  2. Imaging systems
in medicine.  3. Image processing--Digital techniques.
I. Buda, Andrew J.  II. Delp, Edward J.  [DNLM:
1. Computers.  2. Heart--radiography.  3. Heart--radio-
nuclide imaging.  4. Echocardiography.  5. Tomography,
X-Ray Computed.  WG 141 D574]
RC683.D53  1985       616.1'2075       84-22712
```
ISBN-13: 978-94-010-8712-4   e-ISBN-13: 978-94-009-4996-6
DOI: 10.1007/978-94-009-4996-6

Copyright

To the memory of our fathers,
Joseph Buda and Edward J. Delp, Jr.,
who inspired us to strive for excellence.

Preface

It is 1984, a year immortalized by George Orwell some 35 year ago. In 1949, he prophesized a world dominated by television images and electronic communications. Orwell's vision of an incredible technologic revolution is the reality of the 1980's. Over the past three decades, this technical explosion has impacted on all levels of society, including the practice of Medicine.

In 1949, the cardiologist had available to him only his stethoscope, the chest roentgenogram, the electrocardiogram, and his clinical astuteness. In 1984, the cardiologist still requires great clinical skills, but also has available to him echo-cardiography, radionuclide perfusion and functional tests, digital radiography, computed tomography, positron emission tomography, and nuclear magnetic resonance imaging. These imaging modalities are the result of the development of the digital computer, and the explosive advances in microelectronics. Cardiac imaging has rapidly evolved into a specialized area of interest shared by cardiologists, radiologists, engineers, physicists, and statisticians. Our book, *Digital Cardiac Imaging,* provides a multidisciplinary approach to this rapidly developing field and presents an overview of the technical issues and clinical applications of the many sophisticated procedures currently in use. The various modalities explored are often complementary in providing information regarding cardiac physiology and pathophysiology in animal models and in man. They have un-doubtedly expanded our knowledge concerning the heart and the investigation and management of heart disease. Cardiac imaging is a field that is expanding quickly as evidenced by the introduction of new instrumentation on a three to six monthly cycle. It is clear that these computerized tools will become the foundations of Cardiology in the years to come. Better understanding of their design, applications, and limitations will contribute to our successful use of them in patient care.

Our book consists of two parts: basic considerations (Chapters 2–6) and clinical applications (Chapters 7–16). The chapters related to basic considerations lead the reader through various basic principles related to digital image processing and physical principles of imaging modalities. These chapters provide the technical

VIII

and basic foundation necessary to appreciate the usefulness and limitations of the various cardiac imaging modalities presented in subsequent chapters. The chapters related to clinical applications review the many imaging modalities that are presently available. More recent advances are emphasized, and each chapter is well referenced to guide the interested reader to other literature.

The editing of this book has been an enjoyable experience for us. We have learned that an interdisciplinary approach is critical to research related to or employing digital cardiac imaging approaches, just as it is becoming increasingly necessary in most other endeavors in Cardiology. We wish to acknowledge the support of our colleagues and collaborators, many of whom are contributors to this text. We wish to thank Mr. Boudewijn F. Commandeur of Martinus Nijhoff Publishers for giving us the opportunity to edit this text. Mr. Commandeur has been gracious and always a pleasure to work with. We are grateful to Mrs. Sharon Haglund for her editorial and secretarial assistance in coordinating this effort. Finally, we wish to thank our wives, Heather J. Buda and Maureen Delp, for their constant support and understanding.

Although Orwell prophesized a grim picture of 1984, it is obvious that our technologic revolution has contributed positively to our society and to the practice of Cardiology. The many advances of digital cardiac imaging promise to further improve our understanding and treatment of cardiovascular diseases over many future years.

Ann Arbor, Michigan
June, 1984

Andrew J. Buda, M.D.
Edward J. Delp, Ph.D.

Contents

X

List of contributors

Aisen, Alex M., M.D.
Assistant Professor of Radiology, Department of Radiology, University of Michigan Medical School, Ann Arbor, Michigan.

Bookstein, Fred L., Ph.D.
Research Scientist, Center for Human Growth and Development, and Program in Developmental and Reproductive Biology, University of Michigan, Ann Arbor, Michigan.

Brundage, Bruce H., M.D.
Professor of Medicine, Chief, Cardiology Section, University of Illinois at Chicago Medical School, Chicago, Illinois.

Buda, Andrew J., M.D.
Associate Professor of Internal Medicine, Cardiology Division, Department of Internal Medicine, University of Michigan Medical School, Ann Arbor, Michigan.

Delp, Edward J., Ph.D.
Associate Professor of Electrical Engineering, School of Electrical Engineering, Purdue University, West Lafayette, Indiana.

Gallagher, Kim P., Ph.D.
Assistant Professor of Physiology and Surgery, Departments of Physiology and Surgery (Thoracic Section), University of Michigan Medical School, Ann Arbor, Michigan.

Grover, Maleah, M.D.
Post Doctoral Scholar, Division of Nuclear Medicine, University of California at Los Angeles School of Medicine, Los Angeles, California.

Juni, Jack E., M.D.
Assistant Professor of Internal Medicine, Division of Nuclear Medicine, Department of Internal Medicine, University of Michigan Medical School, Ann Arbor, Michigan.

Higgins, Charles B., M.D.
Professor of Radiology, Department of Radiology, University of California, San Francisco School of Medicine, San Francisco, California.

Laufer, Nathan, M.D.
Instructor of Internal Medicine, Cardiology Division, Department of Internal Medicine, University of Michigan Medical School, Ann Arbor, Michigan.

Mancini, G.B. John, M.D.
Assistant Professor of Internal Medicine, Cardiology Division, Department of Internal Medicine, University of Michigan Medical School, Ann Arbor, Michigan.

Meyer, Charles R., Ph.D.
Assistant Professor of Radiology, Department of Radiology, University of Michigan Medical School, Ann Arbor, Michigan.

Pitt, Bertram, M.D.
Professor of Internal Medicine, Director, Cardiology Division, Department of Internal Medicine, University of Michigan Medical School, Ann Arbor, Michigan.

Schelbert, Heinrich R., M.D.
Professor of Radiological Sciences, Division of Nuclear Medicine, University of California at Los Angeles School of Medicine, Los Angeles, California.

Snider, A. Rebecca, M.D.
Associate Professor of Pediatrics, Division of Pediatric Cardiology, Department of Pediatrics, University of Michigan Medical School, Ann Arbor, Michigan.

Vogel, Robert A., M.D.
Associate Professor of Internal Medicine, Department of Internal Medicine, University of Michigan Medical School; Chief, Cardiology Section, Veterans Administration Hospital, Ann Arbor, Michigan.

1. Myocardial imaging: The promise and challenge of digital image processing

BERTRAM PITT

Digital image processing has led to the rapid development and application of myocardial imaging techniques for the diagnosis and evaluation of patients with cardiovascular disease. One of the first major applications of digital imaging processing techniques to myocardial imaging was the development of multiple gated acquisition radionuclide ventriculography. Radionuclide ventriculography had been shown to be of value in determining ventricular ejection fraction and regional myocardial wall motion [1, 2]. Although clinically useful the widespread application of this technique did not occur until computer processing allowed the acquisition and analysis of multiple images for determination of the ventricular time activity curve [3, 4]. Subsequent studies have shown that digital processing of radionuclide ventriculographic images is useful in determining: ejection fraction; ventricular volumes; rates of ventricular emptying and filling, both at rest and during exercise; as well as in determining the extent of valvular regurgitation and cardiac shunting [5]. Radionuclide ventriculography with computer acquisition and processing has found wide application for the diagnosis of myocardial disease and in the evaluation of therapeutic interventions to improve cardiac function. The resting left ventricular ejection fraction as determined by radionuclide ventriculography in the post-infarction period has been found to be an important prognostic indicator. These studies and those showing that the change in ejection fraction from rest to exercise in patients with significant anatomic coronary artery disease is a better predictor of subsequent cardiovascular events and success of coronary artery bypass graft surgery than the extent of anatomic coronary artery narrowing as determined at angiography [6] promises to further increase the utility and application of this technique over the comming years.

Digital image processing of myocardial thallium-201 images improves the diagnostic accuracy of this technique in detecting patients with ischemic heart disease. In conjunction with tomographic imaging techniques digital processing of myocardial thallium-201 images can provide accurate information on the mass of infarcted, ischemic, and normal myocardium [7, 8]. These measurements should prove to be important predictors of subsequent cardiac events. The application of digital image processing techniques to echocardiography although still in its relative early stages of development shows promise of providing accurate, easily quantifiable information on ventricular function [9]. The further development of digital echocardiography should allow rapid evaluation of the effectiveness of therapeutic interventions in improving ventricular function as well as providing an improved means of detecting and evaluating patients with ischemic heart disease. Digital image processing of computerized axial tomography (CAT) images, positron emission tomography (PET) images, and nuclear magnetic resonance (NMR) images promise even greater insight into pathophysiology. Determination of regional myocardial blood flow, function, and metabolism by these techniques should provide new information in patients with cardiomyopathy, ischemic, and valvular heart disease.

Experience with these new 'non-invasive' myocardial imaging techniques has led to a re-assessment of the 'gold standard' of myocardial imaging – cardiac catheterization with contrast ventriculography and coronary arteriography. Determination of ventricular volumes by radionuclide ventriculography appears to be more accurate than that determined by standard contrast left ventriculography. Coronary artery anatomy as determined from selective contrast angiography does not appear to be accurate 'gold standard' against which we can evaluate the new non-invasive myocardial imaging techniques. It is increasingly recognized that the visual interpretation of the coronary angiogram is highly subjective and poorly reproducible. New digital processing techniques have shown that one can reproducibly determine the extent of anatomic cross-sectional coronary artery narrowing [10]. The direct measurement of residual coronary artery lumen in millimeters is a better indicator of the extent of coronary artery atherosclerosis than determination of percent narrowing. Even with new digital imaging processing techniques it is, however, evident that the contrast angiographic technique is limited in its ability to determine the true extent of coronary atherosclerotic involvement. This has led to the development of new digital image processing techniques to determine the functional implications of a given coronary arterial narrowing [11]. New techniques to measure myocardial blood flow and flow reserve using digital coronary arteriography show promise of more reliably selecting coronary vessels for angioplasty or bypass graft surgery and in assessing the success of these interventions. New 'gold standards' based upon functional rather than anatomic information should provide better insight into the diagnostic accuracy of existing non-invasive techniques as well as providing new prognostic indicators for selecting subsets of patients with coronary artery disease who are at high and low risk of subsequent cardiac events.

The developments in myocardial imaging detailed in this book although remarkable when compared to our knowledge prior to the application of digital image processing techniques almost a decade ago will undoubtedly be supplanted by even more rapid and remarkable progress over the next decade. Application of new computer chips with the ability to quickly and cheaply process and store vast amounts of data combined with new advances in computer language, programs, and networking promises to provide the clinician both in major academic centers and in remote practice settings with a powerful tool for detecting and evaluating cardiovascular disease. The fulfillment of this promise of improved diagnosis, evaluation, and prognosis of cardiovascular disease may not however be as easy to attain as one would expect from the rapid technical progress we have recently experienced in this area.

Although the technical achievements in digital image processing have been truly remarkable, we have failed to make equal progress in our understanding as to how to most efficiently apply these new techniques in the clinical setting. Interdisciplinary rivalry between specialties and sub-specialties has in many instances kept us from the most efficient utilization of these new techniques and impeded further development and application of these techniques in clinical decision making. There is insufficient data as to the relative merits of one or the other of these techniques or their combination in a given clinical circumstance. There is relatively little information on cost-effectiveness of these new myocardial imaging techniques as related to clinical decision making and clinical outcome. If we are to reap the benefits provided by digital image processing for improved cardiovascular diagnosis, evaluation, and prognosis, we will have to make equal if not greater progress in the organization of medical care. New training programs are required to provide physicians with the broad technical background necessary not only to continue the technical revolution currently underway but to understand the most cost-effective way to apply these new techniques. It is no longer acceptable in a patient with suspected acute myocardial infarction to obtain serial electrocardiograms, serial serum enzymes, radionuclide ventriculography, infarct avid imaging, thallium-201 myocardial imaging, echocardiography, PET scanning, CAT scanning, and NMR scanning, without a clear indication of the impact of any one or combination of these procedures on clinical decision making, outcome, or cost-effectiveness. The challenge to industry and the clinical investigator to develop new image processing techniques is great. The challenge to the clinician to use these techniques is an intelligent and cost-effective manner is of equal or greater magnitude. If the challenge to the clinican cannot be met,, the exciting technicological progress outlined in this book will come to a halt. The coming decade with its emphasis on cost containment needs to generate the same innovation and brillance in clinical application of myocardial imaging techniques as has been evident during 'the last decade in the development of new imaging and digital processing techniques.

References

1. Strauss HW, Zaret BL, Hurley PJ, Natarajan TK, Pitt B: A scintiphotographic method for measuring left ventricular ejection fraction in man without cardiac catheterization. Am J Cardiol 28: 575–580, 1971.

4

2. Zaret BL, Strauss HW, Hurley PJ, Natarajan TK, Pitt B: A non-invasive scintiphotographic method for detection of regional dysfunction in man. N Engl J Med 284: 1165–1170, 1971.

3. Bachrach SC, Green MV, Borer JS, Douglas MA, Ostrow HG, Johnston GS: A real time system for multi-image gated cardiac studies. J Nucl Med 18: 79, 1977.

4. Burow R, Strauss HW, Singleton R, Pond M, Rehn T, Bailey IK, Griffith LSC, Nickoloff E: Analysis of left ventricular function from multiple gated acquisition (MUGA) cardiac blood pool imaging: comparison to contrast angiography. Circulation 56: 1024–1028, 1977.

5. Pitt B, Strauss HW: Current concepts: evaluation of ventricular function by radioisotopes. N Engl J Med 296: 1097–1099, 1977.

6. Jones RH, Floyd RD, Austin EH, Sabiston DC Jr: The role of radionuclide angiocardiography in the preoperative prediction of pain relief and prolonged survival following coronary artery bypass grafting. Ann Surg 197: 743–754, 1983.

7. Keyes JW Jr, Leonard PF, Brody SL, Svetkoff DJ, Rogers WL, Lucchesi BR: Myocardial infarct quantification in the dog by single photon emission computed tomography. Circulation 58: 227–232, 1978.

8. Weiss RJ, Buda AJ, Pasyk S, O'Neill WW, Keyes JW Jr, Pitt B: Noninvasive quantification of jeopardized myocardial mass in dogs using 2-dimensional echocardiography and thallium-201 tomography. Am J Cardiol 52: 1340–1344, 1983.

9. Buda AJ, Delp EJ, Meyer CR, Jenkins JM, Smith DN, Bookstein FL, Pitt B: Automatic computer processing of digital 2-dimensional echocardiograms. Am J Cardiol 52: 384–389, 1983.

10. Smith DN, Colfer H, Brymer JD, Pitt B, Kliman SH: A semiautomatic computer technique for processing coronary angiograms. IEEE Computers in Cardiol 325–328, 1981.

11. Vogel R, LeFree M, Bates E, O'Neill W, Foster R, Kirlin P, Smith D, Pitt B: Application of digital techniques to selective coronary arteriography: use of myocardial contrast appearance time to measure coronary flow reserve. Am Heart J 107: 153–164, 1984.

2. Digital image processing

EDWARD J. DELP and ANDREW J. BUDA

Introduction and historical perspective

What is a digital image? What is digital image processing? Why does the use of computers to process pictures seem to be everywhere? The space program, robots, and even people with personal computers are using digital image processing techniques. The use of computer methods in image processing with respect to cardiac imaging is over 15 years old and increasing everyday. In this chapter we shall describe what a digital image is, how one obtains digital images, what the problems with digital images are (yes they are not trouble-free), and finally how these images are used by computers. A discussion of processing digital images is presented later in the chapter. At the end of this chapter is an extensive list of references of recent digital image processing books and journal articles.

The use of computers to process pictures is about 25 years old. While some work was done over 50 years ago [46], the year 1960 is usually the accepted date when serious work was started in areas such as optical character recognition, image coding, and the space program [12]. NASAs Ranger moon mission was one of the first programs to return digital images from space. The Jet Propulsion Laboratory (JPL) established one of the early general purpose image processing facilities using second generation computer technology. JPL was also among the first research centers to apply this technology to medical images.

The early attempts at digital image processing were hampered due to the relatively slow computers used, e.g. the IBM 7094, the fact that computer time itself was expensive, and that image digitizers had to be built by the research centers. It was not until the late 1960s that image processing hardware was generally available (although expensive). Today it is possible to put together a small laboratory system for less than $ 60 000; a system based on a popular home computer can be assembled for about $ 8 000. As the cost of computer hardware decreases, more uses of digital image processing will appear in all facets of life. Some people have predicted that by the turn of the century at least 50% of the images we handle in our private and professional lives will have been processed on a computer.

What is a digital image?

A digital image is nothing more than a matrix of numbers. The question is how does this matrix represent a real image that one sees in the laboratory or clinic?

Like all imaging processes, whether they are analog or digital, one first starts with a sensor (or transducer) that converts the original imaging energy into an electrical signal. These sensors, for instance, could be the photomultiplier tubes used in an X-ray digital subtraction angiography system that converts the X-ray energy into *a known* electrical voltage. The transducer system used in 2-D echocardiography is another example where sound pressure is converted to electrical energy. A simple TV camera is perhaps the most ubiquitous example. An important fact to note is that the process of conversion from one energy form to an electrical signal is not necessarily a *linear* process. In other words, a proportional charge in the input energy to the sensor will not always cause the same proportional charge in the output electrical signal. In many cases calibration data is obtained in the laboratory or clinic (sometimes daily) so that the relationship between the input energy and output electrical signal is known. This data is necessary because some transducer performance characteristics change with age and other usage factors [4].

The sensor is not the only thing needed to from an image in an imaging system. The sensor must have some spatial extent before an image is formed. By spatial extent one means that the sensor must not be a simple point source examining only one location of energy output. To explain this further, let us examine two types of imaging sensors used in cardiac imaging: the Anger camera used in nuclear medicine and the ultrasound transducer used in echocardiography [4].

In nuclear medicine the Anger camera consists of an *array* of photomultiplier tubes. The image is formed by examining the output of each photomultiplier tube in a preset order for a finite time. The electronics of the system then forms an electrical signal very similar to a television signal which produces an image that is shown on a cathode-ray tube (CRT) display. The image is formed because there is an array of sensors, each one examines only one spatial location of the region to be sensed (in this case for gamma rays).

The process of sampling the output of the sensor array in a particular order is known as *scanning*. Scanning is the typical way used to convert a two-dimensional energy signal or image to a one-dimensional electrical signal that can be handled by the computer. (An image can be thought of as an energy field with spatial extent.) Another form of scanning is used in two-dimensional echocardiography. In this application there is *only one* sensor instead of an array of sensors. The ultrasound transducer is moved or steered (either mechanically or electrically) to various spatial locations on the patient's chest. As the sensor is moved to each location the output electrical signal of the sensor is sampled and the electronics of the system then form a television-like signal which is displayed. Nearly all the transducers used in medical imaging form an image by either using an array of sensors or a single sensor that is moved to each spatial location. A simple television camera is an example of an array sensor.

One immediately observes that both of the approaches discussed above are equivalent in that the energy is sensed at various spatial locations of the object to be imaged. This energy is then converted to an electrical signal by the transducer. The image formation processes described above are classical analog image formation with the distance between the sensor locations limiting the spatial resolution in the system. In the array sensors, resolution is determined by how close the sensors are located in the array. In the single sensor approach the spatial resolution is limited by how far the sensor is moved. In an actual system spatial resolution is also determined by performance characteristics of the sensor. We are assuming for our purposes here 'perfect' sensors.

In digital image formation one is concerned about two processes: *spatial sampling* and *quantization*. Sampling is very similar to scanning in analog image formation. The second process is known as *quantization* or *analog-to-digital conversion* whereby at each spatial location a *number* is assigned to the amount of energy the transducer observes at that location. This number is usually proportional to the electrical signal at the output of the transducer. The overall process of sampling and quantization is known as *digitization*. Sometimes the digitization process is just referred to as analog-to-digital conversion or A/D conversion; however, the reader should remember that digitization also includes spatial-sampling.

The digital image formulation process is summarized in Figure 1. The spatial sampling process can be considered as overlaying a grid on the object with the sensor examining the energy output from each grid box and converting it to an electrical signal. The quantization process then assigns a number to the electrical signal; the result, which is a *matrix* of numbers, is the digital representation of the image. Each spatial location in the image (or grid) to which a number is assigned is known as a *picture element* or *pixel* (or pel). The size of the sampling grid is usually given by the number of pixels on each side of the grid, i.e. 256×256, 512×512, 488×380, etc.

The quantization process is necessary because all information to be processed using computers must be represented by numbers. The quantization process can be thought of as one where the input energy to the transducer is represented by a finite number of energy values. If the energy at a particular pixel location does not take on one of the finite energy values it is assigned to the closest value. For instance, suppose that we assume a priori that only energy values of 10, 20, 50, 110, will be represented (the units are of no concern in this example). Suppose at one pixel an energy of 23.5 was observed by the transducer. The A/D converter would then assign this pixel the energy value of 20 (the closest one). Notice that the quantization process makes mistakes; this error in assignment is known as *quantization error* or *quantization noise*.

In our example above, each pixel is represented by one of four possible values.

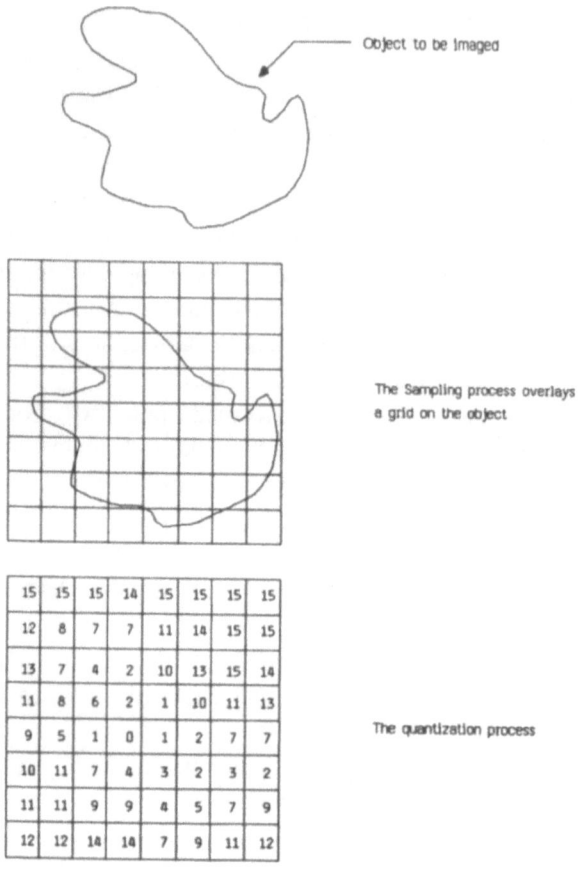

Object to be imaged

The Sampling process overlays
a grid on the object

The quantization process

15	15	15	14	15	15	15	15
12	8	7	7	11	14	15	15
13	7	4	2	10	13	15	14
11	8	6	2	1	10	11	13
9	5	1	0	1	2	7	7
10	11	7	4	3	2	3	2
11	11	9	9	4	5	7	9
12	12	14	14	7	9	11	12

Figure 1. Digital image formation sampling and quantization.

For ease of representation of the data, it would be simpler to assign the value to each pixel the number 0, 1, 2, 3, instead of 10, 20, 50, 110. In fact, this is typically done by the quantization process. One needs a simple table to know that a pixel assigned the value 2 corresponds to an energy of 50. Also the number of possible energy levels is typically some integer power of two to also aid in ease of representation. This power is known as the number of *bits* needed to represent the energy of each pixel. In our example above each pixel is represented by two bits.

One question that immediately arises is how accurate is the digital representation of the image when one compares the digital image with a corresponding analog image. It should first be pointed out that after the digital image is obtained one requires special hardware to convert the matrix of pixels back to an image that can be viewed on a CRT display. If one prints out the digital image on a typical computer output device, such as a terminal or printer, all one would observe is just the pixel numbers. The process of converting the digital image back to an image that can be viewed is known as *digital-to-analog conversion* or *D/A conversion*.

The quality of representation of the image is determined by how close spatially the pixels are located and how many levels or numbers are used in the quantization, i.e. how coarse or fine is the quantization. The sampling accuracy is usually measured in how many pixels there are in a given area and is cited in pixels/unit length, e.g. pixels/cm. This is know as the *spatial sampling rate*. One would desire to use the lowest rate possible to minimize the number of pixels needed to represent the object. If the sampling rate is too low then obviously some details of the object to be imaged will not be represented very well. In fact, there is a mathematical theorem which determines the lowest sampling rate possible to preserve details in the object. This rate is known as the *Nyquist* sampling rate (named after the late Bell Laboratories engineer Harry Nyquist). The theorem states that the sampling rate must be *twice* the highest possible detail one expects to image in the object. If the object has details closer than, say 1 mm, one must take at least 2 pixels/mm. (The Nyquist theorem actually says more than this but a discussion of the entire theorem is beyond the scope of this book. The reader should see reference [1] for more details.) If we sample at a lower rate than the theoretical lowest limit, the resulting digital representation of the object will be distorted. This type of distortion or sampling error is known as *aliasing* error [1]. Aliasing errors usually manifest themselves in the image as Moire patterns (Figure 2). The important point to remember is that there is a *lower limit* to the spatial sampling rate such that object detail can be maintained. The sampling rate can also be stated as the total number of pixels needed to represent the digital image, i.e. the matrix size (or grid size). One often sees these sampling rates cited as 256×256, 512×512, and so on. If the same object is imaged with a large matrix size, the sampling rate has obviously increased. Typically, cardiac images are sampled on 64×64, 128×128, 256×256, or 512×512 grids depending on the application and type of modality. One immediately observes an important issue in digital representation of images: that of the large number of pixels needed to represent the image. A 256×256 image has 65 536 pixels and a 512×512 image has 262 144 pixels! We shall return to this point later when we discuss processing or storage of these images.

The quality of the representation of the digital image is also determined by the number of levels or shades of gray that are used in the quantization. If one has more levels, then fewer mistakes will be made in assigning values at the output of the transducer. Figure 3 demonstrates how the number of gray levels affects the digital representation of an artery. When a small number of levels are used the quantization is coarse and the quantization error is large. The quantization error usually manifests itself in the digital image by the appearance of 'false contouring' in the picture. One usually needs at least 6 bits or 64 gray levels to represent an image adequately [1]. Higher quality imaging systems use 8 bits (256 levels) or

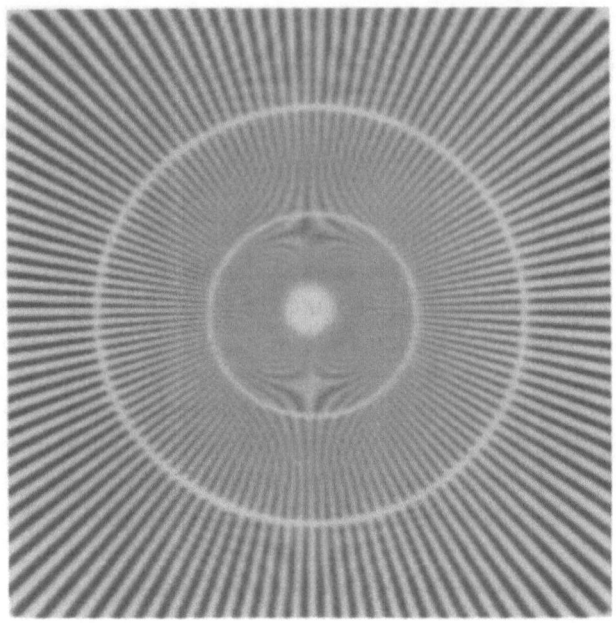

Figure 2. This image shows the effects of aliasing errors due to sampling the image at a too low rate. The image should be straight lines converging at a point. Due to undersampling, it appears as if there are patterns in the lines at various angles. These are known as Moire patterns.

even as high as 10 bits (1024 levels) per pixel. In most applications, the human observer cannot distinguish quantization error when there are more than 256 levels. (Many times the number of gray levels are cited in bytes. One byte is 8 bits, e.g. high quality digital imaging systems use one byte per pixel.)

One of the problems briefly mentioned above is the large number of pixels needed to represent an image which translates into a large amount of digital data needed for the representation. A 512 × 512 image with 8 bits/pixel (1 byte/pixel) of gray level representation requires 2097152 bits of computer data to describe it. A typical computer file that contains 1000 words usually requires only about 56000 bits to describe it. The 512 × 512 image is 37 times larger! (A picture is truly worth more than 1000 words.) This data requirement is one of the major problems with using digital imaging given that the storage of digital images in a computer file system is expensive. Perhaps another example will demonstrate this problem. Many computers and word processing systems have the capability of transmitting information over telephone lines to other systems at data rates of 30 characters/s (300 baud). At this speed it would require over 2 h to transmit the 512 × 512 image! Moving objects, such as the heart, are imaged digitally by taking 'digital snapshots' of them. True digital imaging would acquire about 30 images/s to capture all the important motion of the heart. At 30 images/s with each image sampled at 512 × 512 and with 8 bits/pixel, the system must handle 62914560

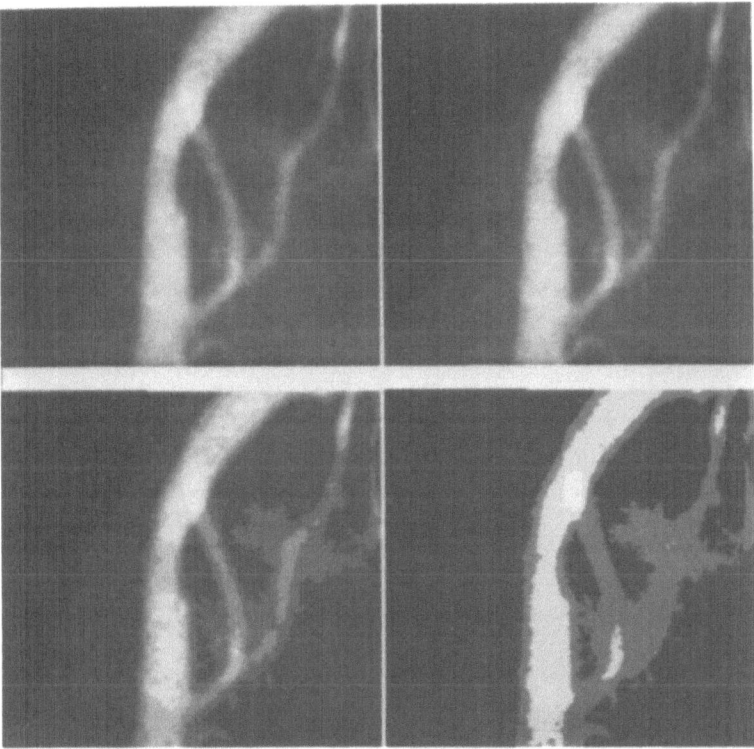

Figure 3. This image demonstrates the effects of quantization error. The upper left image is an coronary artery image with 8 bits (256 levels of shades of gray) per pixel. The upper right image has 4 bits/pixel (16 levels). The lower left image has 3 bits/pixel (8 levels). The lower right image has 2 bits/pixel (4 levels). Note the 'false contouring' in the images as the number of possible levels in the pixel representation is reduced. This 'false contouring' is the quantization error and as the number of levels increases the quantization error decreases because fewer mistakes are being made in the representation.

bits/s. Only very expensive acquisition systems are capable of handling these large data rates. Most systems can only acquire data at this rate for only a few (less than ten) cardiac cycles.

Despite these problems of digital representation there are advantages to digital images. Digital images do not degrade with age like film or videotape. While a computer magnetic tape will age and it is possible that digital images stored on the tape can be damaged this, however, is a rare process. Special procedures known as 'error-correction' can alleviate most types of problems if the image has been stored with reasonable care. One of the authors (EJD) has used digital images stored on magnetic tape for over ten years with no problems.

The best advantage of digital images is that they can be processed on a computer. Any type of operation that one can do on a computer, can be done to a digital image. Recall that a digital image is just a (huge) matrix of numbers.

Digital image processing is the process of using a computer to extract useful information from this matrix. Processing that cannot be done optically or with analog systems (such as early video systems) can be easily done on computers. The disadvantage is that a large amount of data needs to be processed and on some small computer systems this can take a long time (hours). Computer engineers use image processing as an example of 'number crunching'. We shall examine image processing in more detail in the next section and discuss some of the computer hardware issues in a later chapter.

Point operations

Perhaps, the simplest image processing operation is that of modifying the values of individual pixels in an image. These operations are commonly known as *point operations* [11]. An example of a point operation is shown in Figure 4 where the gray-levels of the image were inverted. This operation is performed by (assuming 8 bits/pixel) assigning a pixel with value 255 to 0, a pixel with value 254 to 1 and so on until all are inverted.[1] The effect is that the new image is the negative of the old image (as shown in Figure 4).

A point operation might be used to highlight certain regions in an image. Suppose one wished to know where all the pixels in a certain gray-level region were *spatially* located in the image. One would modify all those pixels values to 0 (black) or 255 (white) such that the observer could see where they were located. This is also shown in Figure 4 where all the pixels having values between 160–255 were set equal to 255. In the resultant image these regions are displayed as full white regions. Point operations are sometimes implemented in the computer hardware that converts a digital image back to an analog signal that can be examined on a CRT display. These operations are performed in something known as a *lookup table*. This is a device that maps all the pixels in an image that have a particular gray value to another gray value.

Another example of a point operation is *contrast enhancement* or *contrast stretching*. The pixel values in a particular image may occupy only a small region of gray level distribution. For instance, the pixels in an image may only take on values between 0–63 when they could nominally take on values between 0–255. This is sometimes caused by the way the image was digitized and/or by the type of transducer used. When this image is examined on a CRT display the contrast looks washed out.[2] A simple point operation that multiplies each pixel value in the image by four will increase the apparent contrast in the image, the new image

---

[1] In this chapter we shall assume that pixels having the value 0 are 'black' and pixels having the value 255 are 'white'.

[2] We shall define the contrast of a digital image to be the difference between the maximum pixel value and the minimum pixel value in the image.

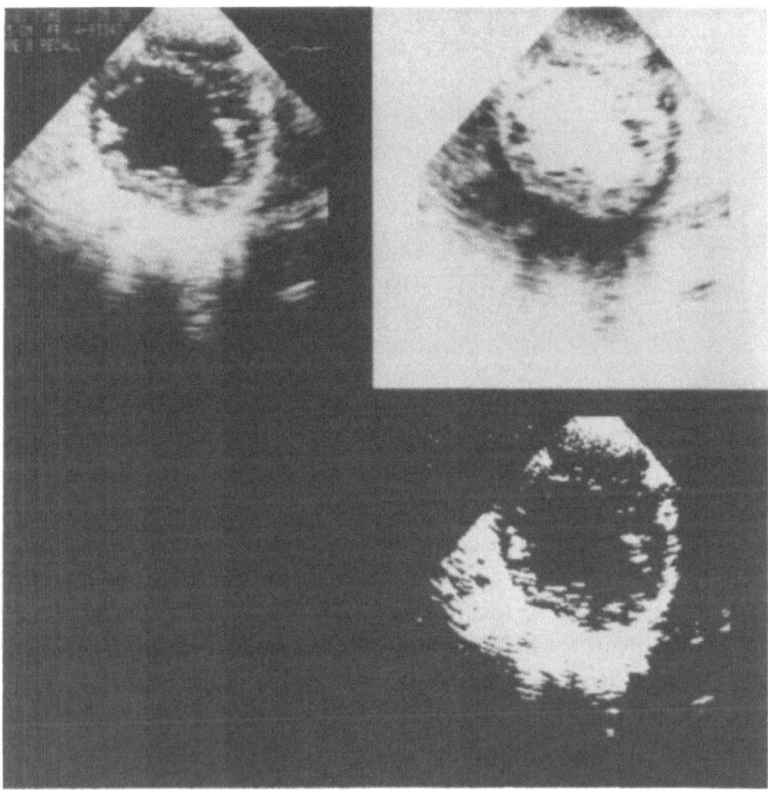

Figure 4. Simple point operations. The upper left image is an echocardiographic image. The upper right image is the same picture with the gray levels inverted using a simple point operation (as described in the text). The lower right image depicts the spatial location of the pixels that have gray values between 160 and 255.

now has gray values between 0–252. This operation is shown in Figure 5. Possibly the most widely used point operation in medical imaging is *pseudo-coloring* [3]. In this point operation all the pixels in the image with a particular gray value are assigned a *color*. Various schemes have been proposed for appropriate pseudo-color tables that assign the gray values to colors [2, 3]. It should be mentioned that point operations are often cascaded, e.g. an image undergoes contrast enhancement and then pseudo-coloring.

The operations described above can be thought of as operations (or *algorithms*) that modify the range of the gray levels of the pixels. An important feature that describes a great deal about an image is the *histogram* of the pixel values. A histogram is a table that lists how many pixels in an image take on a particular gray value. This data is often plotted as a function of the gray value. A typical histogram is shown in Figure 6. Point operations are also known as *histogram*

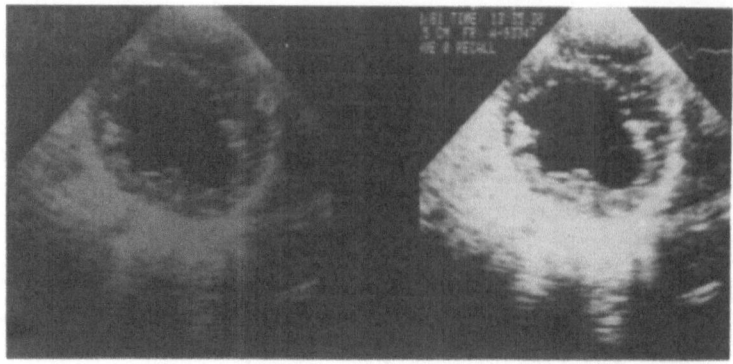

Figure 5. Contrast stretching. The image on the right has gray values between 0 and 63 causing the contrast to look washed out. The image on the right has been contrast enhanced by multiplying the gray levels by four.

modification or *histogram stretching*. The contrast enhancement operation shown in Figure 5 modifies the histogram of the resultant image by stretching the gray values from a range of 0–63 to a range of 0–252. Some point operations are such that the resulting histogram of the processed image has a particular shape [3]. A popular form of histogram modification is known as histogram equalization whereby the pixels are modified such that the histogram of the processed image is almost flat, i.e. all the pixel values occur equally [3].

It is impossible to list all possible types of point operations; however, the important thing to remember is that these operations process one pixel at a time by modifying the pixel based *only* on its gray level value and *not* where it is distributed spatially (i.e. location in the pixel matrix). These operations are performed to enhance the image, make it easier to see certain structures or regions in the image, or to force a particular shape to the histogram of the image. They are also used as initial operations in a more complicated image processing algorithm.

Image enhancement

Image enhancement is the use of of image processing algorithms to remove certain types of distortion in an image. The image is enhanced by removing noise, making the edge structures in the image stand-out, or any other operation that makes the image 'look' better.[3] Point operations discussed in the preceding

---

[3] Image enhancement is often confused with *image restoration*. Image enhancement is the ad hoc application of various processing algorithms to enhance the appearance of the image. Image restoration is the application of algorithms that use knowledge of the degradation process to enhance or restore the image, e.g. deconvolution algorithms used to remove the effect of the aperture point spread function in echocardiography. A discussion of image restoration is beyond the scope of this book. The reader should see [1, 16] for an excellent presentation of the subject.

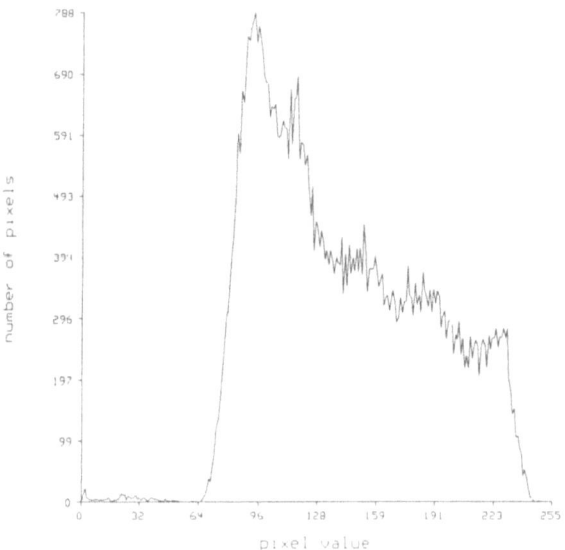

Figure 6. A typical histogram of a digital image.

section are generally considered to be enhancement operations. Enhancement also includes operations that use groups of pixels and the spatial location of the pixels in the image.

The most widely used algorithms for enhancement are based on pixel functions that are known as *window operations*. A window operation performed on an image is nothing more than the process of examining the pixels in a certain region of the image, called the window region, and computing some type of mathematical function derived from the pixels in the window. In most cases the windows are square or rectangle, although other shapes have been used [1]. After the operation is performed, the result of the computation is placed in the center pixel of the window. This is shown in Figure 7 where a 3 × 3 pixel window has been extracted from the image. The values of the pixels in the window, labeled $\alpha_1, \alpha_2, \ldots \alpha_9$, are used to compute a new pixel value which replaces the value of α_5, then the window is moved to a new center location until all the pixels in the original image have been processed. As an example of a window operation, suppose we computed the average value of the pixels in the window. This operation is know as *smoothing* and will tend to reduce noise in the image, but unfortunately it will also tend to blur edge structures in the image (see Figure 8).

Another window operation often used is the computation of a linear weighted sum of the pixel values. Let α_5' be the new pixel value that will replace α_5 in the original image. We then form

$$\alpha_5' = \sum_{i=1}^{9} \alpha_i \cdot \alpha_i \tag{1}$$

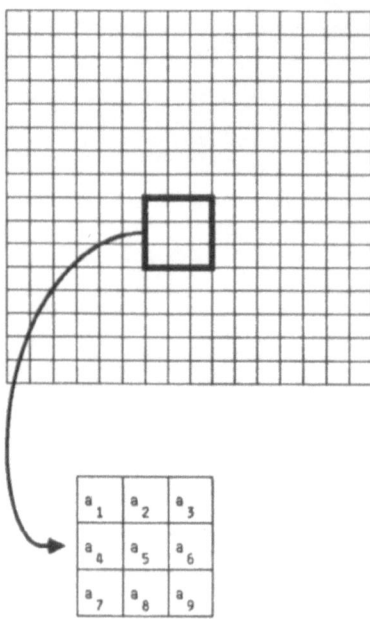

Figure 7. A small 3 × 3 window extracted from a larger digital image.

where the a_i's are any real numbers. For the simple smoothing operation described above we set $a_i = 1/9$ for all i. Usually one lists the coefficients a_i by placing them in a 3 × 3 matrix as shown in Figure 9. These matrices of coefficients are also known as *templates* or *masks* [1]. By changing the values of the a_i weights one can perform different types of enhancement operations to an image. Any window operation that can be described by equation (1) is known as a *linear window operation* or *convolution operator.*[4] If some of the a_i coefficients take on negative values one can enhance the appearance of edge structures in the image. An example of this is shown in Figures 8 and 10 with the masks used for the operations of Figure 10 shown in Figure 11. In fact, two masks were used to create the image shown in Figure 10, the results of each operation was then combined non-linearly to create the image shown in Figure 10. This particular operation is known as the *Sobel operator* [3].

It is possible to compute a non-linear function of the pixels in the window. One of the more powerful non-linear window operations is that of *median filtering* [1]. In this operation all the pixels in the window are listed in descending magnitude and the middle or *median* pixel is obtained. The median pixel then is used to replace a_5. The median filter is used to remove noise from an image and at the same time preserve the edge structure in the image.

---

[4] Many books and journal articles often state that any window operation can be considered to be convolution. This is incorrect, *only linear* operations are convolution operators.

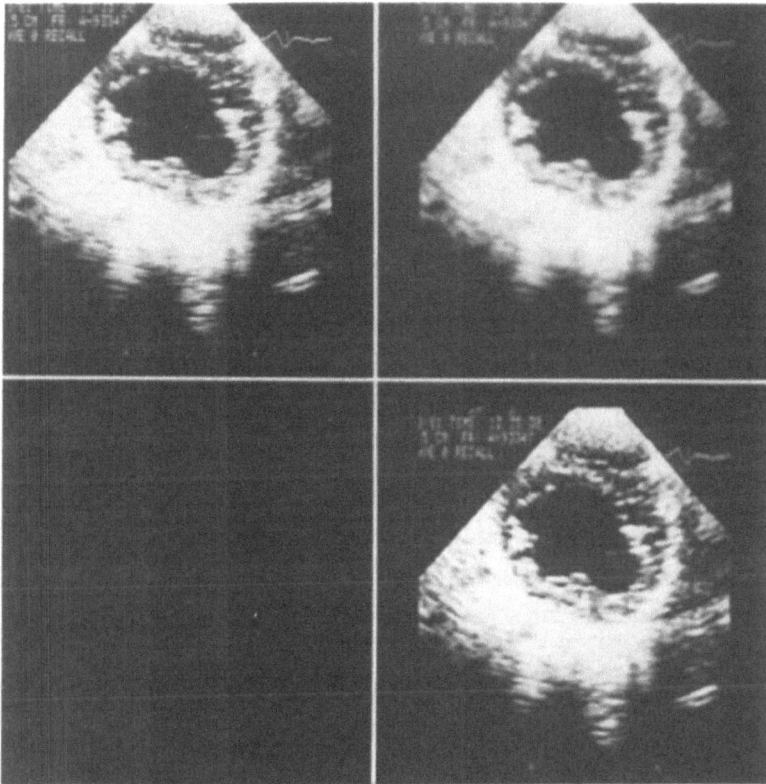

Figure 8. Window operations. The upper left image is an echocardiographic image. The upper right image is the result of using a 3 × 3 smoothing operation on the original image. Notice that the speckle texture appears to be reduced but at the same time the wall locations are blurred. The lower right image is the result of using a 3 × 3 edge enhancement operation known as the Laplacian operator [1]. The edges appear to be enhanced but the speckle texture has also been increased.

In the discussion above, all of the window operations were described on 3 × 3 windows. The current research in window operations is directed at using large window sizes, e.g. 9 × 9, 13 × 13, or 21 × 21. The philosophy in this work is that small window sizes only use local information and what one really needs to use is information that is more global in nature [10].

Edge detection

The ability to find gray level edge structures in images is an important image processing operation. We shall define an *edge* to be regions in the image where there is a large change in gray level over a relatively small spatial region. The process of finding edge locations in digital images is known as edge detection.

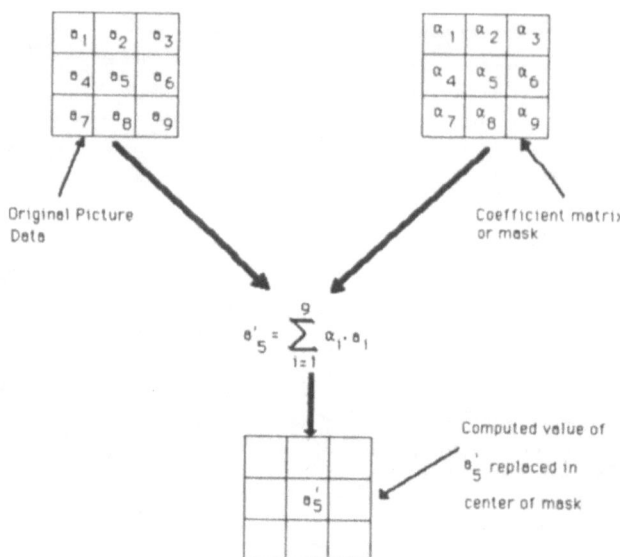

Figure 9. A typical 3×3 linear window operation.

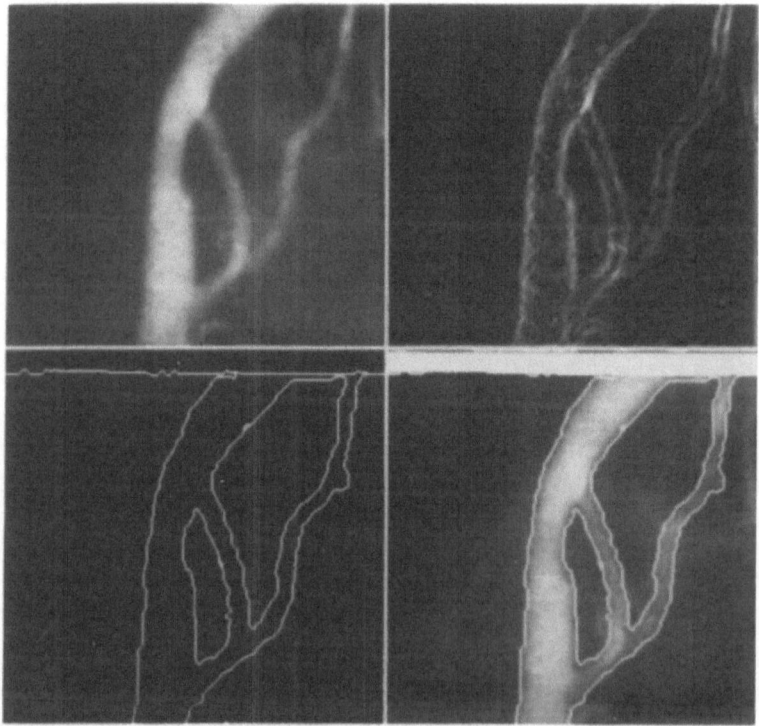

Figure 10. Edge detection. The upper left image is an original X-ray picture of a coronary artery. The upper right is the result after edge enhancement using the Sobel operator (see Figure 11). The lower left is the detected edge locations after thresholding and edge linking. The lower right is the edge image overlaid on the original image.

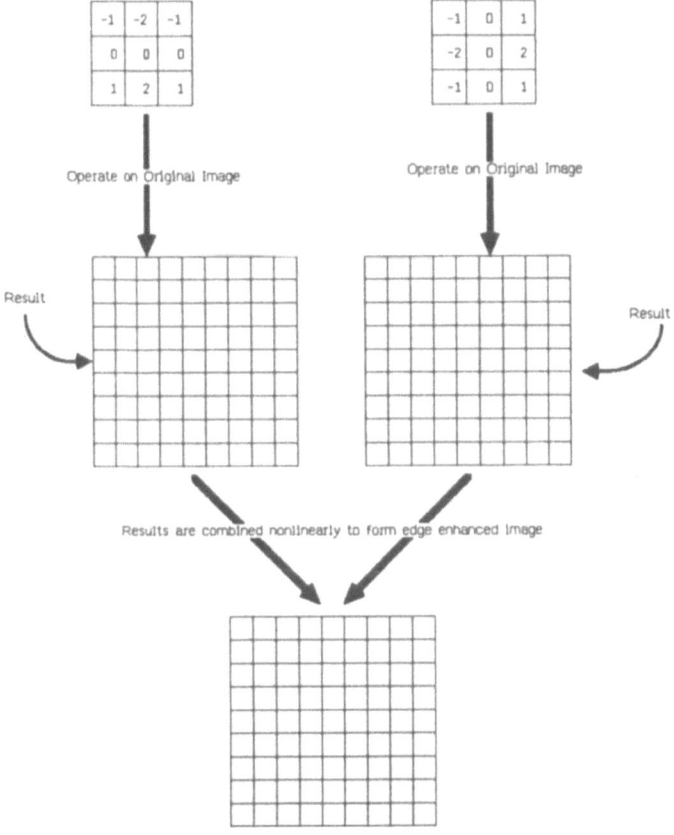

Figure 11. The Sobel operator used for edge enhancement and edge detection.

Most edge detection operators, also known as edge operators, are defined by the use of window operators to first enhance the edges in the image, followed by thresholding the enhanced image. In Figure 10, the edge enhanced image was obtained using a Sobel operator which was thresholded to obtain the edge locations or boundaries of the coronary artery.

There is a great deal of research being performed in the area of edge detection [1, 3, 10, 12, 47]. Some of the research issues include robust threshold selection, window size selection, noise response, edge linking, and the detection of edges in moving objects (e.g. the heart). While it is beyond the scope of this book to discuss these issues in detail, it is obvious that such things as threshold selection will greatly affect the performance of the edge detection algorithm. If the threshold is set too high then many edge points will be missed; if set too low then many 'false' edge points will be obtained due to the inherent noise in the image. The investigation of the 'optimal' choice of the threshold is an important research area [2]. Selection of the particular window operation to enhance the edges of an image, as an initial step in edge detection, has recently been based on using models of the performance of the human visual system in detecting edges [47, 48]. The use of classical edge operators, such as Sobel and Laplacian, has poor performance with respect to noise and false edge detection particularly in echocardiography [55]. The *Primal Sketch Operator* described by Marr & Poggio [47], which models the human visual system, has excellent performance and is being used more and more in medical imaging.

Feature extraction and scene analysis

Most applications of digital image processing techniques in cardiac imaging involve quantification or automatic analysis. The process of extracting useful measurements from an image or sequence of images is known as *scene analysis*. Before scene analysis can be performed one must first determine pertinent features or attributes of the heart, e.g. wall thickness, and extract information about these features [10, 18, 19, 27, 28, 34, 39, 40, 49]. The selection of which features in the image to measure must be chosen a priori based on empirical results. Most features used in cardiac imaging consist of shape properties or of shape change properties. These include wall thickness, ejection fraction, regional wall motion, blood flow, and area change. New features such as tissue characterization, local radius of curvature, change in myocardial wall shape, and coronary artery shape measures are becoming popular. The features are usually measured using the output of an edge detector which has determined boundary locations. After the features are extracted, one must then use the feature measurements to assess cardiac status. In the past simple pattern recognition algorithms, e.g. nearest neighbor classification [27], have been used to compare the feature measurements of an image to a set of feature measurements that correspond to a known type of cardiac status. A decision is then made whether or not the features of the image match those of the known type of cardiac status [7, 9, 18, 28].

Recently, there has been work in the application of *artificial intelligence* techniques to medical imaging [50, 51]. This approach, known as an *expert system*, is very much different from classical statistical pattern recognition in that the feature measurements are used in a different manner as part of a larger system that attempts to model every possible indication of cardiac status and in many ways tries to analyze the image the way an expert (i.e. cardiologist) performs the analysis. The initial results of this work look promising.

The fundamental goal of automatic analysis is that of minimizing intra- and inter-observer variability in the assessment of cardiac status, the measurement of regional function, and the ability to measure change in cardiac status over long time periods. The attainment of this goal requires more research in the area of scene analysis. Recent advances in dynamic scene analysis used in other areas, such as the robot vision, indicate that the dynamic cardiac imaging poses some interesting research problems for the future [6, 19].

Related subjects

There are other branches of digital image processing that are relevant to cardiac imaging, particularly in recent years two areas have become very important. The first area is three-dimensional real-time graphical display of the beating heart as a diagnostic tool to assess cardiac status, e.g. wall motion irregularities. This type of processing usually involves CT images or images obtained from two-dimensional echocardiograms of multiple views [8]. Real-time three-dimensional imaging requires very fast data acquisition and computer processing systems. Most of the current research is not performed in real-time but the images are reconstructed 'off-line'.

One of the problems in digital cardiac imaging is the large amount of data generated when acquiring heart images. With the advent of digital subtraction angiography, it is not unusual that 50 million bytes of image data per day need to be stored for future diagnostic use in a typical laboratory. This data must be stored cost effectively and be relatively easy to retrieve. A new branch of image processing, known as pictorial-data base systems, has been developed in the past few years to address these types of problems. These systems are also known as picture archiving systems or PACS [38, 53, 54]. PACS use techniques from database management analysis and image coding [54] so that one can easily store and retrieve large amounts of image data. The area of database management analysis addresses the larger issue of how one manages a large database of information with regard to query techniques, data structures, user friendliness, and efficiency. Image coding is the study of efficient data representation since in many cases it is possible to represent an image *exactly* with fewer bytes by exploiting some of the statistical properties of the gray values in the image [1]. PACS combine both of these areas to form systems that will make digital imaging more attractive in the clinical area.

In the future, other areas in image processing and computer vision, particularly artificial intelligence, will impact cardiac imaging. The future looks bright although many research issues need to be addressed.

Acknowledgements

The authors would like to thank Paul Eichel and Henry Chu for help in preparing this chapter. Support for the preparation of this manuscript under funding from the National Institutes of Health Grant 1-R01-HL29716-01A1 is gratefully acknowledged.

References

This is a list of various image processing books and journal articles. The list is by no means exhaustive.

1. Rosenfeld A, Kak AC: Digital picture processing. Vols 1 and 2. Academic Press, 1982.
2. Pratt WK: Digital image processing. John Wiley, 1978.
3. Gonzalez RC, Wintz P: Digital image processing. Addison-Wesley, 1977.
4. Macovski A: Medical imaging systems. Prentice-Hall, 1983.
5. Onoe M *et al.*: Real-time medical image processing. Plenum Press, 1980.
6. Meyer J *et al.*: Advances in noninvasive cardiology. Martinus Nijhoff, 1983.
7. Lieberman DE, Mosby CV: Computer methods: the fundamentals of digital nuclear medicine. 1977.
8. Shani U: Understanding three-dimensional images. UMI Research Press, 1984.
9. Hall EL: Computer image processing and recognition. Academic Press, 1979.
10. Ballard DH, Brown CM: Computer vision. Prentice-Hall, 1982.
11. Baxes GA: Digital image processing: a practical primer. Prentice-Hall, 1984.
12. Castleman KR: Digital image processing. Prentice-Hall, 1979.
13. Andrews HC *et al.*: Tutorial and selected papers in digital image processing. IEEE Computer Society, 1978.
14. Andrews HC: Computer techniques in image processing. Academic Press, 1970.
15. Huang TS: Picture processing and digital filtering. Springer-Verlag, 1975.
16. Andrews HC, Hunt BR: Digital image restoration. Prentice-Hall, 1977.
17. Herman GT: Image reconstruction from projections. Springer-Verlag, 1979.
18. Aggarwal JK *et al.*: Computer methods in image analysis. IEEE Press, 1977.
19. Huang TS: Image sequence analysis. Springer-Verlag, 1981.
20. Ahuja N, Schachter BJ: Pattern models. John Wiley, 1983.
21. Rosenfeld A: Image Modelling. Academic Press, 1981.
22. Pratt W: Image transmission techniques. Academic Press, 1979.
23. Ahmed N, Rao KR: Orthogonal transforms for digital signal processing. Springer-Verlag, 1975.
24. Oppenheim AV, Schafer RW: Digital signal processing. Prentice-Hall, 1975.
25. Rabiner LR, Gold B: Theory and application of digital signal processing. Prentice-Hall, 1975.
26. Brigham EO: The fast fourier transform. Prentice-Hall, 1974.
27. Fukunaga K: Introduction to statistical pattern recognition. Academic Press, 1972.
28. Duda RO, Hart PE: Pattern classification and scene analysis. John Wiley, 1973.
29. Papoulis A: The fourier integral and its applications. McGraw-Hill, 1962.
30. Bracewell R: The fourier transform and its applications. McGraw-Hill, 1965.
31. Papoulis A: Systems and transforms with applications in optics. McGraw-Hill, 1968.
32. Rabiner LR, Rader CM: Selected papers in digital signal processing. IEEE Press, 1972.
33. IEEE DSP Committee (ed.): Selected papers in digital signal processing II. IEEE Press, 1976.
34. Agrawala AK: Machine recognition of patterns. IEEE Press, 1977.
35. Bernstein R: Digital image processing for remote sensing. IEEE Press, 1978.
36. McClellan JH, Rader CM: Number theory in digital signal processing. Prentice-Hall, 1979.
37. Jayant NS: Waveform quantization and coding. IEEE Press, 1976.
38. Chang SK, Fu KS: Pictorial information systems. Springer-Verlag, 1980.
39. Fu KS: Digital pattern recognition. Springer-Verlag, 1980.
40. Pavlidis T: Structural pattern recognition. Springer-Verlag, 1977.
41. Fu KS: Syntactic pattern recognition and applications. Prentice-Hall, 1982.
42. Oppenheim AV: Applications of digital signal processing. Prentice-Hall, 1978.
43. Schachter BJ: Computer image generation. Wiley, 1983.
44. Mandelbrot BB: The fractal geometry of nature. Freeman, 1983.
45. Serra J: Image analysis and mathematical morphology. Academic Press, 1982.

46. McFarlane MD: Digital pictures fifty Years Ago. Proc of the IEEE, July 1972, pp 768–770.

47. Marr D, Poggio T: A theory of human stereo vision. Proc of the Royal Society of London 204: 301, 1979.

48. Granrath D: The role of human visual models in image processing. Proc of the IEEE 69: 552–561, May 1981.

49. Barrow H, Tenenbaum J: Computational vision. Proc of the IEEE 69: 572–595, May 1981.

50. Shortliffe E, Buchanan B, Feigenbaum E: Knowledge engineering for medical decision making: a review of computer-based clinical decision aids. Proc of the IEEE 67: 1207–1224, Sept. 1979.

51. Szolovits P, Pauker S: Computers and clinical decision making: whether, how, and for whom? Proc of the IEEE 67: 1224–1237, Sept 1979.

52. Marr D: Vision. WH Freeman & Co, 1982.

53. Chang SK (ed.): Special issue of IEEE Computer Magazine devoted to pictorial information systems. Nov 1981.

54. Duerinckx AJ, Duyer SJ, Prewit JMS: Special issue of IEEE Computer Magazine devoted to digital image archives system for medicine. Aug 1983.

55. McGuffin LJ, Delp EJ, Buda AJ: A stochastic model for two-dimensional echocardiography, Presented at the IEEE Frontiers of Engineering and Computers in Health Care, Los Angeles, Sept 1984.

3. Basic physical principles of cardiac imaging systems

CHARLES R. MEYER

The intent of this chapter is to provide an overview of the basic physics in cardiac imaging systems, excluding magnetic resonance imaging. A later chapter describes both the physics of magnetic resonance imaging as well as preliminary clinical results. Most current imaging systems can be classified into one of two categories, those generating images of projections and those generating tomograms.

Projection imaging

Since the early days of Roentgen's discovery, projection images of organ systems have been made using ionizing radiation from either X-ray tubes or radioactive isotope sources. By definition a projection is the integration of a multi-dimensional property along one dimension in order to yield a new property having one less dimension [1]. In conventional radiography the three-dimensional linear attenuation coefficient of the imaged object is modeled as having an integrated effect along a set of one-dimensional rays to yield a two-dimensional shadowgram, or projection image. In nuclear medicine the three-dimensional source activity is integrated along a set of rays to yield the source projection image. For X-ray photon energies in the range of ten to several hundred keV the linear attenuation coefficient at any one location in a three-dimensional object can be thought of as the sum of two terms, one due to the photoelectric effect and the other due to Compton scattering. The photoelectric term is proportional to the tissue density and the third power of the average atomic number, and inversely proportional to the third power of the photon's energy. The Compton scattering term is also proportional to the tissue density and nearly independent of all other effects [2]. It is easily seen (and demonstrated in Figure 1) that imaging with high keV photons creates images whose effects are primarily due to Compton scattering and demonstrate only density changes in the tissue. Imaging with low keV photons emphasizes the photoelectric effect and creates images effected by both atomic

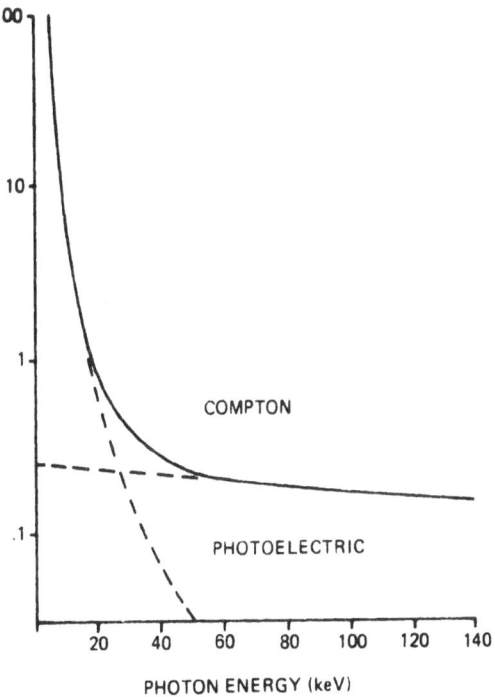

Figure 1. Compton and photoelectric attenuation as a function of photon energy (from Technicare Maintenance Manual, No. 961055, Rev. B, 1981).

number changes as well as density. Differentiation in soft tissues is best performed at lower keV where the more sensitive photoelectric effect predominates.

Angiography

Conventional and digital angiography share much of the same physical imaging principles. The system signal flow diagram shown in Figure 2 accounts for the significant stages in image generation for either system. X-rays are produced by the X-ray tube in either a continuous or pulsed mode. The continuous mode of X-ray production is called the fluorographic mode and allows continuous visualization. The pulsed mode is referred to as the cine or digital mode in which short pulses at higher tube current and X-ray fluence are used to produce images of the same quality as continuous exposures made at lower tube current and X-ray fluence in the fluoro mode. The shortened exposure time is needed to reduce motion blurring in each cinegraphic frame.

All systems suffer from non-zero focal spot size. The unsharpness created by the width of the focal spot can be increased or decreased by geometric factors as shown in Figure 3. Note that the unsharpness due to the focal spot size is multiplied by the ratio of distance between image receptor and object to distance

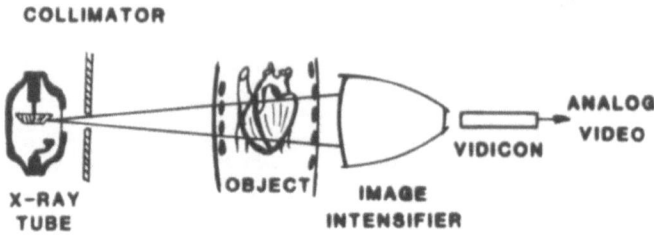

Figure 2. Signal processing chain for conventional and digital angiography systems.

between the focal spot and object. Vendors of X-ray tubes have attempted to resolve the conflict between reducing the focal spot size and the intense local heating incurred in a small focal spot by rotating the anode target and placing the region of electron bombardment at an oblique angle as demonstrated in Figure 4. This technique allows the use of a larger area to generate the focal spot and uses only the projection of the focal spot area at 90° to the tube axis as the effective focal spot size.

Unfortunately this approach to reducing focal spot size creates a non-uniform X-ray illumination over the receptor field referred to as the 'heel' effect. Most effective focal sport sizes are on the order of $1.0 \, mm^2$. In high resolution systems focal spot sizes are smaller, typically $0.25 \, mm^2$. It is important to point out that for a C-arm digital angiography unit with a $1 \times 1 \, mm^2$ focal spot in which the patient is located midway between the tube and receptor, overall system spatial resolution is limited to one line pair per millimeter (lp/mm) simply due to focal spot size and improper patient positioning.

The image intensifier plays an important role in the signal processing chain in both conventional and digital angiographic systems. The role of the image intensifier is to amplify and optimize the visible light output from the X-ray system for the characteristics of the vidicon (TV camera). Intensification can be

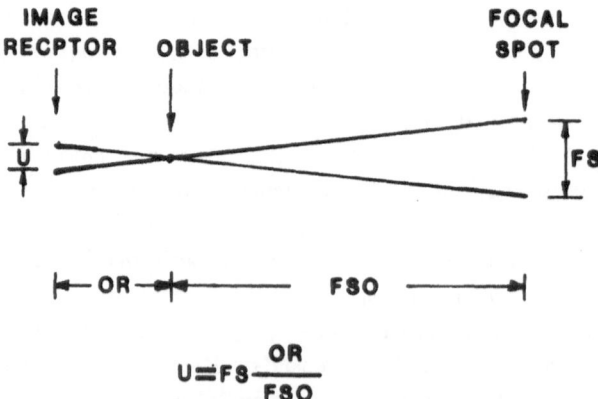

Figure 3. Unsharpness due to focal spot size and geometric factors.

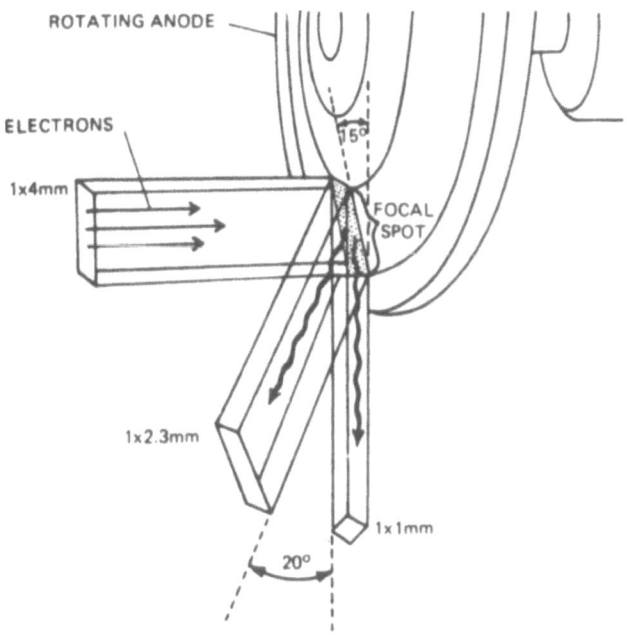

Figure 4. Design of anode in X-ray source tube (from Technicare Maintenance Manual, No. 961055, Rev. B, 1981).

thought of as occurring by two separate processes. The first process involves a simple area reduction in which the larger area of the incident X-ray beam is reduced to a much smaller area appropriate for the visualization by the vidicon. A second amplification process is effected by accelerating the free electrons ejected from the rare earth screen at the front of the image intensifier by the incident X-ray photons. The free electrons are accelerated by a high voltage gradient as they travel toward the smaller rear screen and possess more energy when they strike the rear screen. Spatial resolution for image intensifiers lies typically between 2 to 4 lp/mm referred to the front screen of the image intensifier [3].

In the fluorographic mode X-rays are produced continuously, amplified by the image intensifier, and viewed by the vidicon in the typical interlaced television mode, i.e. two frames each produced in a 60th of a second with each frame displayed sequentially but with scan lines from each frame interlaced. In the pulsed digital angiographic mode the vidicon acquires the integrated image from the image intensifier after the short X-ray pulse in a single frame with sequentially scanned lines (no interlacing).

In digital angiography the need to subtract two separate images to detect small contrast changes requires significant performance in signal-to-noise ratio from the vidicon compared to the signal-to-noise ratio needed for fluoro. Indeed, the signal-to-noise ratio and the bit depth of the digitizer following the vidicon in digital radiographic systems are intimately related. One bit is required for each 6

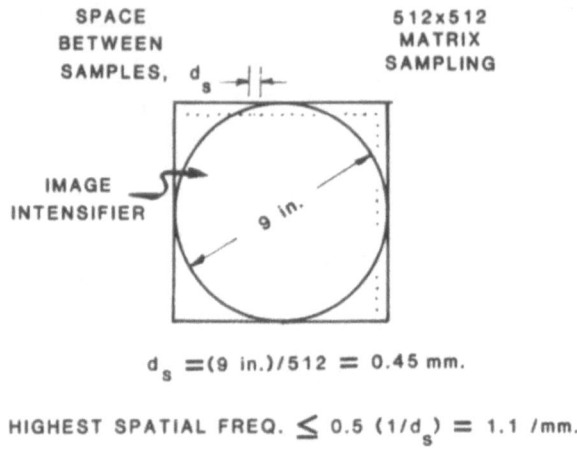

$$d_s = (9 \text{ in.})/512 = 0.45 \text{ mm.}$$

HIGHEST SPATIAL FREQ. $\leq$ 0.5 $(1/d_s) = 1.1$ /mm.

Figure 5. 512 × 512 sampling matrix on face of 9 inch image intensifier receptor face.

dB of dynamic range and the maximum dynamic range available is equal to the signal-to-noise ratio at the output of the vidicon. Thus, an 8 bit digitized word from a single pixel supports a 48 dB dynamic range in the video signal before digitization. Likewise, 10 bits support 60 dB, etc. There is no need for a 13 bit digitizer if the signal-to-noise ratio of the vidicon is only 50 dB. In the current state of the art 60 dB signal-to-noise ratios are commonly achievable and lead to the use of 10 bit digitizers in many systems.

The image sampling matrix, i.e. the number of pixels per frame, is another important parameter in digital angiography. The Nyquist sampling theorem indicates that we can uniquely reconstruct only those spatial frequencies that have been sampled at rates greater than twice their frequency [4]. All other spatial frequencies in the image which exceed half the sampling rate will be ambiguously aliased to lower spatial frequencies in the reconstructed image. The sampling theorem when applied to the equivalent sampling rate at the front face of the image intensifier tube allows us to estimate the highest spatial frequency that can be reconstructed uniquely. This places another upper limit on spatial resolution obtainable by the digital system. As seen in Figure 5 the equivalent digital sampling interval for a 512 × 512 pixel matrix referred to the front of a 9″ intensifier tube face defines a sampling interval of approximately 0.45 mm, or a sampling frequency of 2.2 mm^{-1}. Thus the highest spatial frequency capable of being reconstructed is 1.1 mm^{-1}, or approximately 1 lp/mm. Thus it is possible to see that a major upper limit in spatial resolution for digital angiography systems is due to the size of the image intensifier and pixel matrix. From this consideration it should be clear that the current goal of digital radiography is to increase low contrast resolution for larger objects with a resultant trade-off in spatial resolution.

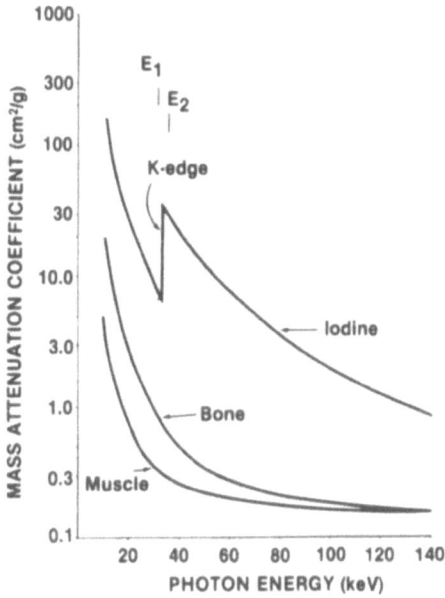

Figure 6. Plot of tissue and iodinated contrast material attenuation coefficients as a function of photon energy showing k-absorption edge for contrast material (from Digital radiology: an assessment of its potential impact on radiological practice, General Electric, 1980).

Another major problem in digital radiography is motion. Only with a cooperative patient capable of exercising good control of inspiration does the process meet its full goals of increased contrast resolution. Large structures with low spatial frequencies or non-uniformities such as the 'heel' effect are effectively removed by subtraction of two frames, but misregistration due to motion of high spatial frequency structures such as edges cause severe edge artifacts in the subtracted result. Edge artifacts can seriously degrade patency estimates of small vessels. In addition edge artifacts can significantly effect the estimates of flow for both simple and complex flow algorithms. Thus mask alignment over a local region of interest as well as perhaps warping of the mask before subtraction is critical. In the near future the use of dual energy techniques allowing the use of one pulse at a lower keV followed within milliseconds by another pulse at a higher keV will produce two images with no relative motion differences [5]. The two keV levels are chosen to be just below and above the k-absorption edge of the contrast material being used during an injection. At the higher keV the contrast material has a significantly increased attenuation coefficient as shown in Figure 6 and thus the major non-zero differences in the subtracted image are due to those regions containing only contrast material.

Conventional nuclear medicine

Conventional nuclear medicine is physically characterized as an imaging modality with poor spatial resolution. The imaging modality is clinically successful because isotopes have been found that mimic the physiological behavior including uptake or washout rates of ions such as iodine and calcium. Since the physiological uptake or washout is very ion specific, the low contrast resolution of the total imaging system including the source delivery mechanism is very good. Isotopes undergoing beta decay generate photons that are identical to X-rays. Thus the processes of photoelectric absorption and Compton scattering play major roles in conventional nuclear medicine imaging as well. The goal in nuclear medicine is to map the concentrations of the isotope after it has been injected into the patient and selective uptake or washout has begun. It is interesting to note that tissue attenuations which are the subject of mapping in angiography and conventional computed tomography are sources of error in nuclear medicine because they adversely affect estimates of source concentration within the patient.

A single pinhole collimator may be used to create a focused image of the photon source distribution on the detector, but this technique suffers from poor collection efficiency. Multihole collimators or coded apertures used to create projection images of the source have much higher collection efficiencies. The typical detector material in scintillation cameras is sodium iodide. The crystal's large, 3/8″ width and its high atomic number increase the probability of a photoelectric interaction between the incoming photon and the detector material. In the photoelectric interaction the incoming photon is totally absorbed and produces a free, energetic electron. The energetic electron loses energy by inelastic collisions with other loosely bound valence electrons which are kicked into the higher energy conduction band. Eventually electron-hole pairs recombine with the simultaneous production of optical or ultraviolet photons in a decay process called fluorescence [6]. A matrix of photomultiplier tubes behind the sodium iodide crystal record the intensity and position of the fluorescence. As demonstrated in Figure 7 a weighted network of capacitors or resistors forms pulses whose amplitudes are proportional to the X and Y coordinates of the event from the photomultiplier tube pulses. In addition, by summing these position pulses it is possible to obtain the intensity of the fluorescent flash which is directly proportional to the energy of the incident photon. This energy information channel is called the Z-axis. Nuclear medicine imagers which operate in the manner described here are called scintillation cameras, or Anger cameras in honor of Hal Anger, the first designer of such a camera [7].

Clearly it is desirable to make an image only from direct, primary photons as opposed to lower energy, scattered photons incident from random directions. Compton scattering occurs not only in the body of the patient but also in the detector crystal. In order to prevent photons other than primaries from participating in image formation, an energy window is used to exclude those events

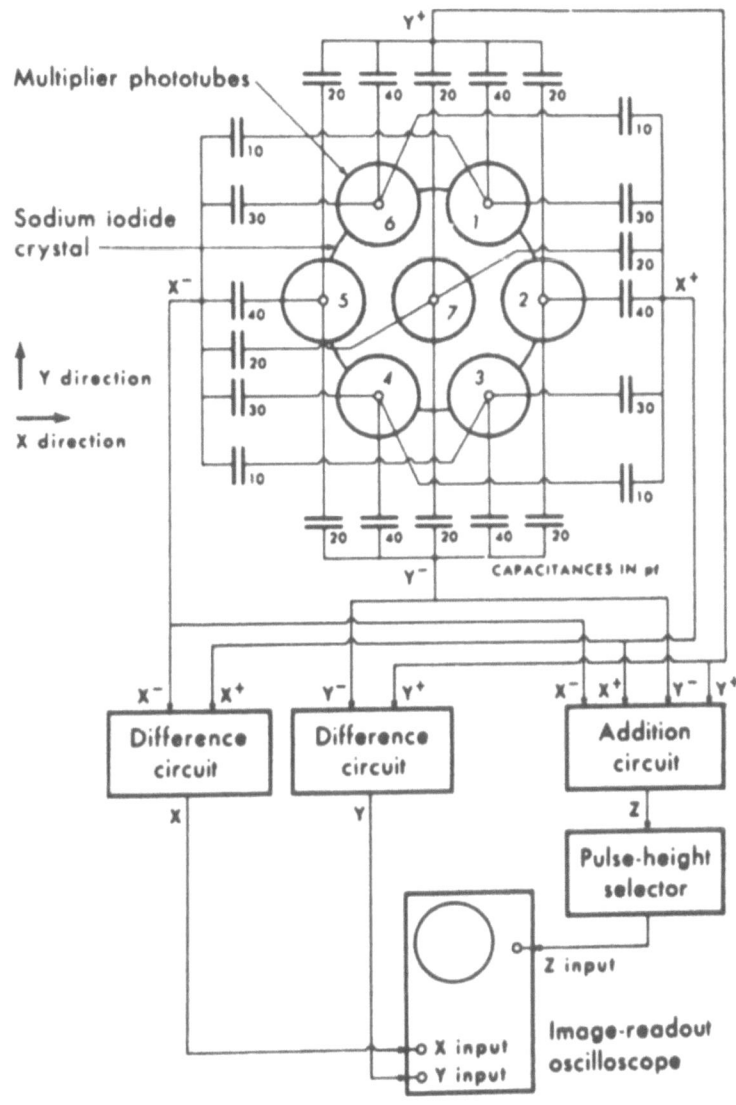

Figure 7. Basics of weighted capacitor network to convert fluorescent flash into amplitude modulated pulses corresponding to X and Y coordinates of flash (from H. Barret & W. Swindell, Radiological Imaging, Vol 1, Academic Press, 1981).

whose energies are above or below that produced by the isotope. The energy windowing is performed by an electronic pulse height analyzer and associated logic circuit operating on the Z-axis signal. The upper and lower thresholds of the window can be set by the operator to correspond to the isotope used. Thus the final image is sum of all detected fluorescent events that pass the energy window criterion. Accumulation of the image occurs in a digital computer memory by direct memory access where the contents of memory address corresponding to the X and Y coordinate of the fluorescent event are incremented by one for each event accepted by the energy window.

Most Anger cameras suffer from an upper detection rate limit. If the dose of the injected isotope is too large, the occurrence rate of events in the detector crystal will cause the weighted pulses from the photomultiplier tubes to coalesce. The summated Z-axis signal will be too large in general to pass the energy window criterion. In this mode detection efficiency is effectively reduced to zero.

Cardiac images are obtained by forming an image of the beating heart in the usual continuous manner, or by using temporal gating. The continuous imaging mode further reduces the spatial resolution in the moving object's image due to blurring. Even so, such techniques are still successful in detecting large cardiac wall abnormalities. Cardiac gating achieves stop-action imaging by forming images from event data acqured during specific phases of the cardiac cycle. Efficient gating is achieved with a newer technique referred to as a list mode acquisition. In list mode acquisition all events that satisify the energy window criterion are recorded along with the elapsed time since the last QRS complex of the electrocardiogram. After acquisition has ceased, the image for a particular phase of the cardiac cycle is formed by using only those events stored in the list that have the appropriate elapsed, post-QRS time for the desired cardiac phase. Images formed in this manner for a short phase of the cardiac cycle are more useful in detecting smaller lesions since motion blurring is effectively eliminated.

Tomographic imaging

Computed tomography

For the past ten years we have known that tomograms can be reconstructed from projection images if the images are gathered from enough viewing angles at a sufficiently high spatial sampling rate [8]. Indeed in the idealized world where we can imagine gathering continuous projections of the imaged object using infinitesimally thin, straight ray paths passing through the object, the commonly used, filtered back projection algorithm will yield the exact reconstruction of the object. When we step from this idealized setting back into the real world, problems as well as multiplicities of partial solutions result.

Several reconstruction algorithms have been proposed and used. The algebraic reconstruction technique (ART) is an iterative technique that systematically modifies an assumed reconstruction (guess) to yield projections through the assumed reconstruction that more closely approximate the actual projections gathered during data acquisition. In each iteration the remaining errors or differences between an actual projection and the projection from the assumed reconstruction are redistributed equally across the reconstructed field to correct the estimate for that projection. The redistribution process for one view obviously corrects that view, but causes errors for other views. The iterative process corrects sequential projections until the errors between the actual and estimated projections are sufficiently small.

The rationale supporting the filtered backprojection and Fourier techniques relies on the slice-projection theorem which states that the Fourier transform of the projection of an object is equal to the appropriately oriented, central slice of the two-dimensional Fourier transform of the object [9]. The orientation of the central slice is parallel to the projection. In the filtered backprojection technique the acquired projection is filtered via convolution with the 'rho' filter and then redistributed or backprojected through the reconstruction matrix.

Filtering can alternatively be accomplished in the frequency domain by multiplying the Fourier transform of the acquired projection by the Fourier transform of the 'rho' filter, i.e. w, where w is spatial frequency in radians per unit distance. The inverse Fourier transform of the product yields the filtered projection which can then be backprojected. In general the filtered backprojection technique is favored since the algorithm may begin after the collection of the first projection, as opposed to waiting for all views to be collected. In addition the technique is not iterative and the reconstruction process is complete with the backprojection of the last filtered projection. The combination of these two properties for the backprojection technique leads to a fast, high quality reconstruction algorithm.

The Fourier reconstruction technique places the Fourier transform of all projections in the reconstruction matrix with their appropriate angular orientations as guided by the slice-projection theorem. Unfilled matrix elements remaining must be interpolated and then a single two-dimensional, inverse Fourier transform is performed. This technique is infrequently used due to the undesirable results of interpolation in the frequency domain [10].

X-ray computed tomography

Since the beginnings of practical computed tomography four types, or generations, of geometry have been used for data acquisition. These are pictured in Figure 8. The first generation geometry was referred to as the translate-rotate geometry. In this scheme the single source and single detector were moved or translated together across the object to acquire one projection. The the gantry was rotated an angular increment and the translation was repeated. This translate-rotate process was repeated until views over at least 180° were acquired. In the second generation geometry several detectors were used such that several angular increments could be collected in one translation. Then the angular rotation increments of the gantry were made larger which led to a faster collection time. In the third generation systems no translation was needed since the number of detectors had grown to totally encompass all projections through the subject.

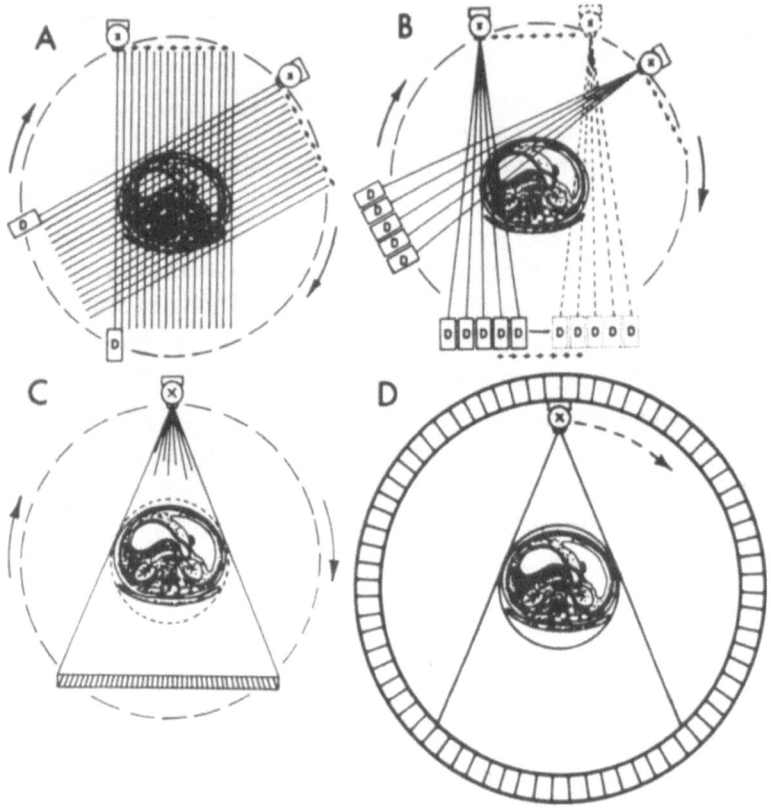

Figure 8. Generations of geometries for data acquisition in computed tomographies (from W. Hendee, Medical Radiation Physics, Year Book Medical Publishers, Inc., 1979).

Only concurrent rotation of the source and detector array was needed. In current fourth generation systems the detector array totally surrounds the subject and only the source must be rotated. Both third and fourth generation systems use fan beam sources to illuminate all ray projection paths through the subject.

In practice X-ray computed tomography units have many problems to overcome. The litany is long and an incomplete list follows: detector uniformity, calibration and drifting, data sampling rates and dynamic range, beam hardening, Compton scatter rejection, and most important of all for cardiac imaging, motion. New third and fourth generation scanners acquire data over angles greater than 180° in 1–3 s. Obviously such times are much too long for high resolution cardiac imaging. Low dose cardiac gated acquisition, e.g. list mode or otherwise, leads to a sparse data set with missing views corresponding to X-ray source positions at times other than the desired cardiac phase. To overcome this problem many limited angle reconstruction algorithms are under examination. Obviously all have met with limited success due to the lack of such products in the X-ray CT market place.

Cardiac X-ray computed tomography

A new device known as the cardiovascular computed tomography (CVCT) scanner is currently under development [11]. In this new scanner the interval between sequential scan acquisitions, each of which is a dual slice scan, is only 70 m. Such shortened scan times are achieved by the use of controlled magnetic fields to rotate the electron beam in the evacuated cone surrounding the patient. As seen in Figure 9 the large cone is the X-ray tube which allows the subject to be placed in the aperture at the base of the cone. The tube has multiple, adjacent anode rings which are placed in the base of the cone surrounding the subject. Also placed adjacent to the anode rings are the X-ray photon detectors. Fan beam geometry is assumed in the reconstruction algorithm.

SPECT and PET: computed tomography in nuclear medicine

Clinically available systems allow tomographic reconstruction of isotope source distributions using single photons emitted during isotope decay. The generic name of the system is descriptive of the process, i.e. single photon emission computed tomography (SPECT). A typical data gathering apparatus for SPECT includes one or two rotating Anger camera heads, each weighing several hundred pounds. With parallel hole collimation the camera(s) gather multiple, parallel-slice projections.

SPECT differs from X-ray computed tomography in several fundamental ways. In SPECT the goal is to reconstruct the source distribution within the body of the subject. Unfortunately estimates of source activity in the acquired projections are diminished by tissue attenuation, primarily from Compton scattering. In addition projections are collected along diverging rays which are narrowest in the holes of the collimator and diverge as the distance from the collimator increases. Rotation of the Anger camera heads can create uniformity problems in the fine tuning of the photomultiplier tubes (PMTs) since the PMTs are very sensitive to local magnetic fields including the earth's. Shielding of PMTs is necessary to ameliorate non-uniformities due to Anger camera rotations. While diverging rays are responsible for resolution loss, the most significant problem in SPECT is tissue attenuation. Several correction algorithms have been proposed. One approach uses a preinjection scan with an external source in order to reconstruct an attenuation map of the subject much like conventional X-ray CT. An advantage to using the external isotope source is that the reconstructed attenuation map is appropriate for the monoenergetic isotope source and does not contain beam hardening artifacts present in conventional CT. The computed reconstruction of attenuation is used to correct projections for the patient scan following isotope injection. Another more popular approach estimates body contours using Compton scattered photons accepted through a second, lower energy window. This approach implicitly assumes that all tissues have the same attenuation coefficient.

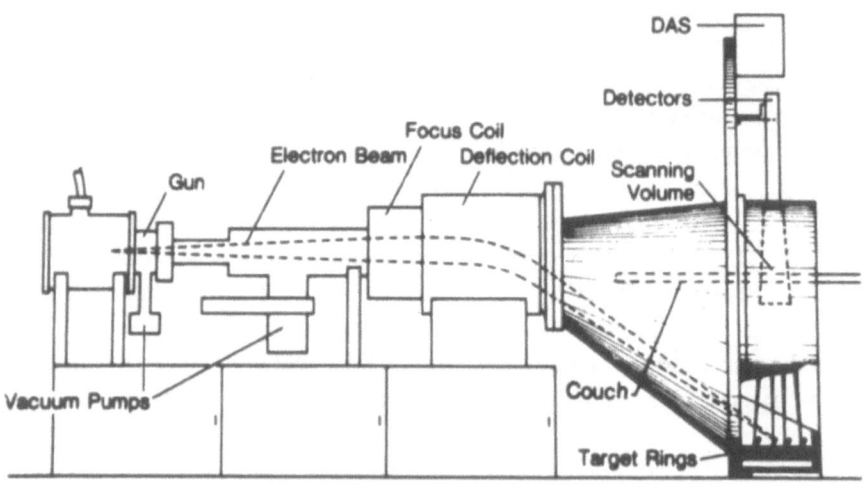

Figure 9. Schematic of cardiovascular CT scanner construction (from D. Boyd, Theorectical possibilities for CT scanner development, Diagnostic Imaging, Dec., 1982).

Recall from earlier discussions that Compton scattering at higher energies such as 140 keV is the dominant attenuation process and depends primarily on tissue density. Thus the knowledge of contours allows reasonably accurate estimates of attenuation projections for correcting source activity estimates.

Slice thickness and in-plane resolutions in SPECT are determined primarily by collimation and both resolution measures lie in the 10–25 mm range [12]. The duration of data collections is roughly proportional to the number of independent slices to be reconstructed. Cardiac gating is tyically implemented by list mode acquisition and increases even further the duration of the acquisiton period.

Positron emission tomography (PET) in nuclear medicine is available only at larger research institutions or at sites located conveniently near synchrotrons. Isotopes used in PET scanning typically have half lives on the order of 15 to 120 min and thus must be generated near the sites of usage in order to reduce delivery times. The isotope decay process results in the production of a positron which is soon annihilated by a neighboring electron. The annihilation results in two photons traveling nearly colinearly in opposite directions. Data acquisition systems surround the subject with parallel rings of detectors for gathering parallel slice projections. Coincidence circuits determine appropriate pairs of photons striking the detector rings. The locus of the decaying isotope source is assumed to lie on the straight line between the two detector pairs. Cardiac gating is typically implemented using the list mode acquisition. Recent advances in PET involve the measurement of the time of flight (TOF) differential in the detection of the two photons by the two opposite detectors. Time resolution in such a measurement is on the order of 500 ps. While this time resolution is insufficient to provide high resolution images using only TOF, its combined usage with the knowledge that the event took place along the straight line between the two detectors increases the signal-to-noise ratio in the resultant images on the order of 2 to 4 times [13].

Echocardiography

Tomograms are created by other imaging modalities directly without elaborate reconstruction algorithms. Backscattered ultrasound is employed daily in echo-cardiography to generate two dimensional maps of the heart at rates near 30 frames per second. In echocardiography outgoing pressure waves are generated by a piezoelectric transducer in which the application of a voltage transient causes a short, ringing mechanical deformation of the transducer. The ringing motion of the transducer generates a pressure wave that propagates into the adjacent tissues. Backscattering within the tissues due to variations in tissue density and bulk modulus cause echoes to return to the transducer. The echoes, or pressure waves returning to the transducer, cause the transducer to be deformed and generate a voltage which is detected by the sensitive receiver. The sources of the echoes are mapped to a position based on the assumption of an *a priori* propagation velocity in tissue of 1 540 m/s. In fact tissue velocities vary depending on tissue histology from the lower values for fat of 1 480 m/s to the upper values for scar tissue of 1 580 m/s [14]. Fortunately such variations are proportionately small, less than $\pm 5\%$. Low level backscattering is responsible for the general texture seen in structures such as the myocardium where the average radius of the scattering structures is much, much smaller than the wavelength (note that the wavelength for 3.0 MHz is 0.51 mm). Specular reflections, which are much stronger echoes, are produced by boundaries between structures of differing acoustic impedance whose sizes are much larger than a wavelength. Specular reflections follow the ray optics principle of angle of incidence equals angle of reflection and Snell's law for refraction [15]. Thus specular echoes are seen for objects only where they are perpendicular to the direction of ultrasound propagation.

The variations in echo signal strength from the largest signal returning from a close, specular reflector down to the smallest signal just above the noise floor of the transducer typically cover a 120 dB dynamic range, or a factor of 1 000 000. Since the dynamic range of the observer's eye is only 35–40 dB, it is necessary to compress the range of the input signal. This compression is achieved by both time-varying gain compensation and the use of grayscale preprocessing. For time-varying gain schemes the operator is responsible for adaptively creating a signal used to offset the attenuation the propagating wave suffers during its round trip. Grayscale preprocessing is typically implemented via look-up tables and allows operator selection from multiple logarithm-like functions to preferentially boost low level signals.

The direction of the outgoing pressure wave and the direction of sensitivity during reception is controlled either mechanically or electronically. In mechanical systems (often called wobblers) fixed disk transducers are mechanically angulated at rates up to 30 cycles per second. In other mechanical systems the transducer is stationary but an acoustic mirror is rapidly angulated. In still another configuration three transducer heads separated by angles of 120° are rotated continuously on a rotating drum (Figure 10). Nearly all mechanical transducers are mounted in a fluid bath that couples the moving transducer to the stationary face of the transducer. Classically mechanical scanners have been thought to be superior because of the low off-axis clutter and sidelobes. However, reverberations between face of the transducer and the transducer disk mounted in the fluid bath are a source of unwanted artifact. In addition fixed-focused transducers in mechanical systems have good lateral resolution only in the focal zone of the transducer.

Two-dimensional echo systems using annular arrays rely on both mechanical steering of the beam and electronic focusing. In these systems an oscillating acoustic mirror is typically used to steer the beam (Figure 11). Focusing of the transmitted wavefront and dynamic focusing during reception are identical to the phased array systems described below.

Electronically steered arrays, often referred to as phased arrays, are capable of both electronically varying the direction and focal length of the transmitted wave within the imaging plane as well as performing dynamic focusing along the desired look direction during reception. The out-of-plane focus is determined by the curvature ground on the face of the array or, if a lens is used, by its speed of sound and shape. While it is true that rectangular aperture, phased arrays may have poorer off-axis sidelobe performance than circular disk transducers, aperture apodization, i.e. shaping of the array elements vertical height or the equivalent electronic weighting of each element's contribution, can remove the theoretical difference (Figure 12). Careful attention must be paid to electronic and acoustic isolation between each piezoelectric element in the transducer head and amplifiers to eliminate unwanted off-axis clutter. Beam steering and focusing is accomplished by a combination of phase shifting and tapped delay lines. In current systems the received signal is viewed as the product of a high frequency carrier and a baseband modulator. During reception beam steering and focusing are accomplished by demodulating the received signal with the appropriately phase shifted carrier and then delaying the low frequency, baseband result by

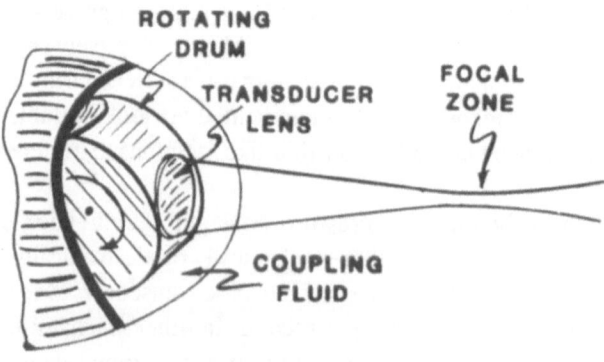

Figure 10. Disk transducer with fixed focal region.

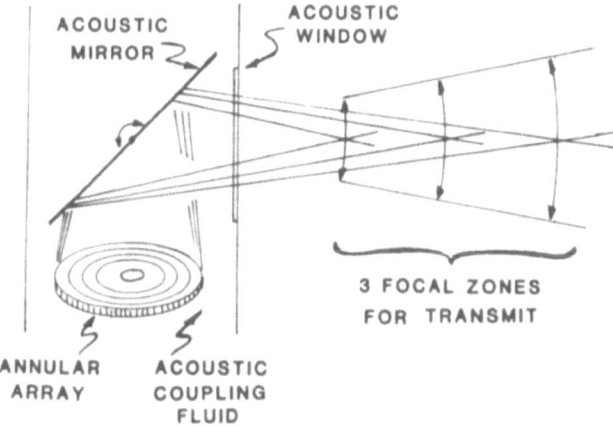

Figure 11. Annular array transducer with acoustic mirror and dynamic focusing.

selecting the appropriate taps on the delay lines using analog multiplexors (Figure 13) [16]. This approach allows use of lower cost delay lines since the cost of delay lines is directly related to the delay-bandwidth product. First generation systems used 32 array channels for both transmission and reception. Current generation systems use 64 channels and a new entry in the phased array market place uses 128 channels for both transmission and reception. In cardiac imaging the number of channels, or array elements, is important. The length of the physical aperture available for ultrasonic examination of the heart in short axis view is approximately 2 cm between the sternum and the flap of the left lung. Since resolution is improved by increasing aperture, it is desirable to fill the natural acoustic window. However the maximum width of each element in the array is limited by the same Nyquist sampling theorem to sizes less than or equal to 1/2 wavelength, or 0.15 mm for 5.0 MHz arrays. Thus it would take a minimum of 130 elements to fill the 2 cm wide aperture between sternum and lung and satisfy the sampling theorem. Violating the sampling theorem leads to the presence of off-axis grating lobes, or directions of major sensitivity in addition to the desired main lobe, and

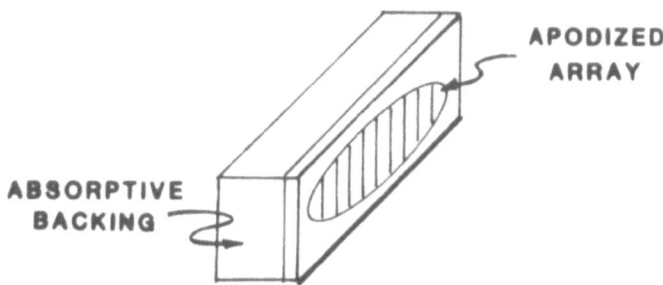

Figure 12. Face of phased array with apodized aperture.

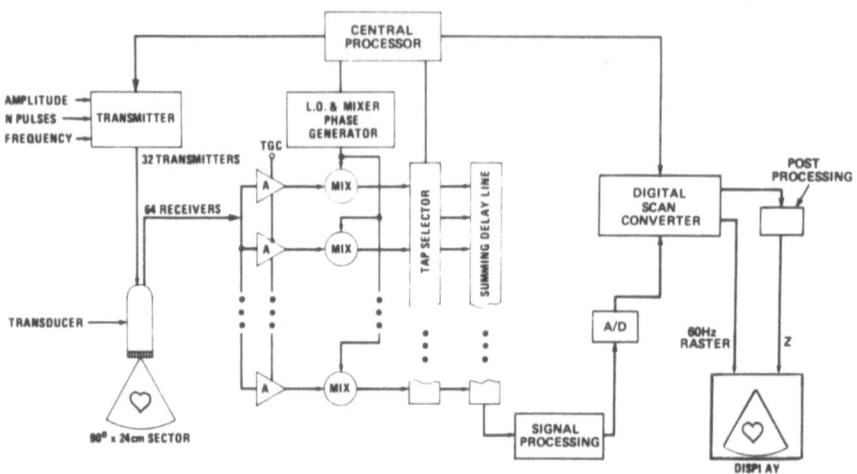

Figure 13. Schematic of signal processor for phased array imaging system (from H. Karrer *et al.*, A phased array imaging system for medical use, in Acoustical Imaging, Vol 10, P. Alais (ed.), Plenum Press, 1982).

should be avoided. The presence of grating lobes can lead to aliased, or duplicated structures as well as reduced, overall contrast sensitivity.

Two-dimensional echo also offers the possibility of tissue characterization. Initial efforts using texture measures have not been successful. Texture variations have been shown to be dependent on range even in uniform tissues [17]. However, other parameters of ultrasonic backscattering show significant promise in detection of older infarct scars as well as ischemia. Integrated backscattered power doubles within seconds of the onset of ischemia [18]. In fact cyclic periodicities in integrated backscattering during the normal cardiac cycle associated with wall thickening have been reported [19]. In addition assessment of the extent of older infarct scarring may be computed in the future from quantitative estimates of the regional ultrasonic attenuation coefficient. Scars contain significant concentrations of collagen, and the ultrasonic attenuation coefficient is highly correlated with collagen concentration [20]. While all of these possibilities exist, accurate quantitative mappings of ultrasonic backscattering and attenuation are difficult to compute. Quantitative estimates of backscattering require good estimates of attenuation in the intervening tissues between the transducer and the backscattering site. Estimates of attenuation based on spectral estimates from low level backscattering require many independent estimates, i.e. significant tissue volumes, due to the random nature of backscattering to arrive at estimates whose variances are sufficiently low to be meaningful [21]. Estimates of attenuation based on more local specular echoes are more deterministic and can be made for smaller tissue volumes, but suffer from variations in angle of incidence with off-normal structures [21]. As of now tissue characterization in echocardiology is a topic for research only.

Acknowledgements

Support in part for the preparation of this manuscript under funding from DHHS PHS grant 1 RO1 HL29716 is gratefully acknowledged.

References

1. Barrett HH, Swindel W: Radiological imaging, Vol 2. Academic Press, New York, 1981, p 534.
2. *ibid*, Vol 1, pp 317–323.
3. Mistretta CA: X-ray image intensifiers. In: Haus A (ed.), The physics of medical imaging: recording system measurements and techniques. Am. Institute of Physics, New York, 1979, p 188.
4. Papoulis A: The fourier integral and its applications. McGraw-Hill, New York, 1962, pp 50–52.
5. Kruger RA, Mistretta CA, Crummy AB *et al.*: Digital k-edge subtraction radiography. Radiology 125: 243–245, 1977.
6. Barrett HH, Swindel W: Radiological imaging, Vol 1. Academic Press, New York, 1981, pp 220–229.
7. Anger HO: Scintillation camera. Rev Sci Instrum 29: 27, 1958.
8. Hounsfield GN: Computerized transverse axial scanning tomography. Part I, description of the system. Brit J Radiol 46: 1016–1022, 1973.
9. Bracewell RN: Strip integration in radio astronomy. Aust J Phys 9: 198–217, 1956.
10. Mersereau RM, Oppenheim AV: Digital reconstruction of multi-dimensional signals from their projections. IEEE Proc 62: 1319–1338, 1974.
11. Boyd DP: Theoretical possibilities for CT scanner development. Diagn Imaging, Dec 1982, pp 32–60.
12. Knoll GF: Single-photon emission computed tomography. IEEE Proc 71: 320–329, 1983.
13. Ter Pogossian MM, Ficke DC, Yamamoto M, Hood JT Sr: Super PETT I: a positron emission tomograph utilizing photon time-of-flight information. IEEE Trans Med Imaging 1: 179–187, 1982.
14. Gross SA, Johnston RL, Dunn F: Comprehensive compilation of empirical ultrasonic properties of mammalian tissues. J. Acoust Soc Am 64(2): 423–457, 1978.
15. Wells PNT: Biomedical ultrasonics. Academic Press, New York, 1977, p 16.
16. Karrer HE, Dias JF, Larson JD, Pering RD, Maslak SH, Wilson DA: A phased array accoustic imaging system for medical use. In: Alais P (ed.), Acoustical imaging, Vol 10. Plenum Press, New York, 1982, pp 47–63.
17. Skorton DJ, Collins SM, Woskoff S, Melton HE Jr: Range- and azimuth-dependent variability of quantitative texture measures in two-dimensional echocardiographic images. Ultrasonic Imaging (abstr) 4(2): 183, 1982.
18. Mimbs JW, Bouwens D, Cohen RD, O'Donnell M, Miller JG, Sobel BE: Effects of myocardial ischemia on quantitative ultrasonic backscatter and identification of responsible determinants. Circ Res 49: 89–96, 1981.
19. Madaras EI, Barzilai B, Perez JE, Sobel BE, Miller JG: Systematic variations of myocardial backscatter during the cardiac cycle in dogs. Ultrasonic Imaging (abstr) 4(2): 185, 1982.
20. O'Donnell M, Mimbs JW, Miller JG: The relationship between collagen and ultrasonic attenuation in myocardial tissue. J Acoust Soc Am 64(2): 512–517, 1979.
21. Kuc R: Estimating acoustic attenuation from reflected ultrasound signals: comparison of spectral-shift and spectral-difference approaches. IEEE Trans Acoust, Speech and Signal Processing 32(1): 1–6, 1984.
22. Meyer CR: Preliminary results on a system for wideband reflection-mode ultrasonic attenuation imaging. IEEE Trans Sonics and Ultrasonics 29(1): 16, 1982.

4. Computer hardware considerations in digital imaging

EDWARD J. DELP

Introduction

In this chapter we describe some of the issues involving computer hardware used in cardiac imaging. Cardiac imaging, with respect to computer hardware, is not greatly different than image processing used in any other application except that more recently there has been great interest in real-time acquisition systems for use in digital subtraction angiography, echocardiography, and other forms of cardiac imaging.

In this chapter we shall discuss three areas relative to digital cardiac imaging hardware. These areas are acquisition systems, computers, and storage technology. We shall overview some of the recent research issues in image processing systems with particular reference to the use of parallel processing techniques. Finally, we will conclude with some issues in image processing software.

We shall not discuss the image creation hardware such as X-ray tubes, ultrasound transducers, etc. We are assuming that these systems are in place and that they have converted the imgaging energy to an electrical signal that will be digitized (see Chapter 2). While it is true that so-called *integrated* cardiac imaging systems have image formation and digitizers together in one total system, for discussion purposes, we will concentrate on the *digital* part of the system.

Acquisition

The first step in any image processing application is that of image digitization or data acquisition. This process, as described in Chapter 2, consists of spatial sampling and gray-level quantization.

In the past, acquisition systems were very slow and did not allow the true motion of the heart to be captured. It is still common for cardiac processing to be performed on images that are obtained at end-systole and end-diastole. However, the motion of the heart is rich in information and cardiac motion must be captured digitally before this information can be extracted. This requires a real-time acquisition system capable of digitizing images at a rate of 20–30 images/s for several cardiac cycles. It should be emphasized that real-time acquisition does not necessarily mean that the images must be *processed* or *analyzed* in real-time. However, the acquisition system must be capable of digitizing the images at this rate and then storing them somewhere, usually in a computer memory system or a storage disk. The acquisition/storage system must be capable of handling a large amount of data at a high rate to capture cardiac motion. At 30 images/s with a spatial sampling grid of 512×512 pixels and 8 bits of gray scale resolution, the acquisition system must be capable of handling data a 7 864 320 bytes/s. In fact, the typical minicomputer used in most cardiac imaging systems cannot handle data at this rate. Thus, special hardware must be used to accomplish real-time cardiac image acquisition.

Special integrated circuits have been developed to allow image data to be acquired at these high rates. At the center of every real-time system is a special integrated circuit known as a *flash converter* that performs the A/D conversion process [1]. The development of the flash converter has greatly lowered the cost of high-speed acquisition systems. Most of the current hardware issues, as far as real-time acquisition is concerned, are relative to storage (or processing) of the image data after it has been acquired at these high rates.

The real-time system described above is necessary when the cardiac images are acquired on a rectangular grid, such as in digital subtraction angiography or nuclear cardiology. In echocardiography the data should be acquired using a polar-type grid. This type of real-time acquisition, known as *line mode* acquisition, is very useful when acquiring either envelope detected echo data or the RF data used in tissue characterization [2]. It is very important to acquire the data, in whatever format it exists, as close to the imaging sensor as possible to minimize noise and capture all the detail (e.g. motion) that exists in it.

Computers and related processing hardware

The computer system and its related peripherals are the parts of the cardiac imaging system that perform the actual image processing operations. Computer systems are usually characterized by the speed with which they can perform operations, usually arithmetic operations, and the accuracy or resolution of the resultant operations. The speed of operations is usually measured in millions of operations per second (sometimes called mega flops) and the accuracy of the resultant operation is usually measured in the number of bits used to represent a number in the computer memory. More typically this is indicated by the fundamental number of bits used to represent any computer instruction which is commonly known as the *word length* of the computer. Most typical cardiac imaging systems use minicomputers that have word lengths of 16 bits. These systems are capable of running at speeds of 0.5 megaflops.[1] Small microprocessor systems, such as those based on the Intel 8008, are only 8 bit systems. Whereas, large mainframe computers have word lengths of 64 bits and larger. In the future, more and more image processing systems will be based on 16 bit and 32 bit microprocessors. As a result of future research, cardiac imaging systems will include larger word lengths and faster speeds.

These types of computers are classified as *serial* computers in that only one instruction is performed at a time in a step-by-step fashion. The serial nature of these computer systems limits the processing speed, which can be augmented by using various special purpose peripheral devices attached to the main computer. These devices include array processors [3], pipeline processors [5], and video processors [6, 7].

Array processors are devices attached to a computer system that perform highly specialized operations, such as floating point multiplication, very quickly. These devices are relatively expensive and are usually needed in applications requiring very precise computational accuracy. They have been used extensively in digital subtraction angiography [4].

Pipeline processors are used in image processing to perform window operations (see Chapter 2) at real-time rates.[2] Various pipeline processors have been built for medical image processing. The initial application of pipeline processors has been in areas such as cytology, histology, and the analysis of coronary arteries [8].

Video processor is a term being used in this chapter for the latest generation of image display/processors [7]. These systems are capable of performing a large number of image processing operations including window operations, pseudo-coloring, look-up table modification, zooming, registration, and even real-time image acquisition. In fact, many of these video processors have pipeline processors and array processors imbedded in them. These systems are capable of performing many of the image processing operations with the computer, usually called the *host* computer, used for passing commands to the video processor and/ or image data. The host computer is used to perform operations that the video processor cannot perform.

Another approach in image processing to increase the speed of operations is the use of more than one serial computer to perform an image processing operation. This is known as *parallel processing*. The philosophy here is simple in that if it takes, for instance, 1 second to perform an operation on an image then if one splits the image in half and two processors are used, each operating on part of the image to perform the same operation, then that operation should only take

---

[1] The reader who is not familiar with typical computer systems should see [3].

[2] A pipeline processor is one of many types of *computer architectures*. It can be used for other image processing operations besides window operations. The reader should see [3, 5] for detailed description of pipeline processors and other computer architectures.

0.5 s. This reduction in processing time is known as the *speedup* of the parallel processor [3, 5]. If one uses N processors to perform the operation together then it may be possible to obtain the results in $1/N$ s. This, of course, depends on the particular type of operation being performed. In some cases, such as window operations, a particular processor may need the result obtained in another processor before it can obtain its results so that the speedup will not be a factor of N.[3]

Parallel processors are just now becoming available for use in cardiac imaging. A new system, known as PASM,[4] is being developed at Purdue University for various image processing applications including echocardiography and digital subtraction angiography [8]. This system will have 64 serial processors and has been designed for use in image processing and pattern recognition.

As the current cardiac image processing work moves from the research laboratory to the clinic there will be more demand for higher speed computer systems to allow adequate patient throughput. Therefore, parallel processing techniques will be necessary to meet these needs.

Storage systems

After the image is acquired or processed it is necessary to store the image data somewhere. Typical storage mediums include magnetic tape, magnetic disks, and computer memory. Magnetic tape is the oldest storage technology and is used mainly for archival storage of image data. Large magnetic tape libraries are often used with picture archiving systems (see Chapter 2).

Magnetic disks are also a relatively old technology. For small intermediate storage, floppy disk systems are used in many imaging systems. Floppy disks are not very efficient for storage of a large number of images. The small Winchester type of 'hard' disk is becoming more popular with storage capabilities up to 500 megabytes. Disk speeds are increasing and hard disks that can handle image data in real-time are being incorporated in digital subtraction angiography systems now in use at larger research centers. At present, magnetic tapes and disks are mainly used for intermediate or long-term storage.

With the reduction in the cost of computer memory systems, these systems are becoming attractive for short-term and intermediate storage particularly in real-time acquisition systems. Other storage technologies such as bubble memories and digital microfilm will also soon impact cardiac imaging relative to archival storage.

[3] The nature of the largest speedup one can obtain is discussed in [3, 7].
[4] PASM is an acronym for Partitionable SIMD/MIMD Machine [9].

Image processing software

It is important to emphasize that the image processing hardware is useless without adequate supporting software. This software gives the computer hardware detailed instructions on how to perform the processing operations. Software is often the neglected part of a cardiac imaging system. This author feels strongly that presently available cardiac imaging systems have poor software and, in many cases, the software does not fully exploit the available hardware.

There are various issues in the design of cardiac imaging software. The most important are ease of use (i.e. user friendliness), the ability to be modified by the user so that new image processing operations can be developed, the issue of portability, i.e. how easily the software can be moved from one system to another, and finally the concern of how well the software uses all the capabilities of the hardware.

In a clinical environment where little, if any, research is performed the first and last issues, discussed above, are the overriding concerns of the user. *Turnkey* cardiac imaging systems are available from various sources that support typical image analysis algorithms. However, in a research environment all of the issues are equally important (in fact some would argue that user-friendliness is not an issue in a research environment). There has been a great deal of work in the area of portable image processing software, however, this author believes that as the hardware configurations of cardiac imaging systems get more complicated, the goal of portability will become more difficult to meet. At present, there are software systems being developed that have as a goal *hardware transparency*, i.e. the user could run this software on 'any' hardware and the software would exploit all the properties of the given hardware system. The use of hardware transparent software systems in cardiac imaging systems will not appear for about five years but there is a potential of some very powerful software being available to address some of the difficult issues in cardiac imaging.

Conclusions

New advances in image processing hardware (and software) are in the very near future. The demands of cardiac imaging will drive the development of real-time systems that will allow the true motion (of the heart and blood flow) to be captured.

Acknowledgements

Support for the preparation of this manuscript under funding from the National Institutes of Health grant No. 1-RO1-HL29716-01A1 is gratefully acknowledged.

References

1. Baxes GA: Digital image processing: a practical primer. Prentice-Hill, 1984.
2. Buda AJ, Delp EJ *et al.*: Digital two-dimensional echocardiography: linemode data acquisition, image processing, and approaches to quantitation. In: Meyer J *et al.* (eds), Advances in noninvasive cardiology. Martinus Nijhoff, 1983.
3. Hayes JP: Computer architecture and organization. McGraw-Hill, 1978.
4. Alexander P: Array processors in medical imaging. IEEE Computer 16: 17–30, June 1983.
5. Hwang K, Briggs FA: Computer architecture and parallel processing. McGraw-Hill, 1984.
6. DeAnaza IP8500 product description. Gould/DeAnaza Corp.
7. Reader C, Hubble L: Trends in image display systems. Proc of the IEEE 69: 606–614, May 1981.
8. Special issue of IEEE Computer devoted to computer architectures for image processing, Jan 1983.
9. Siegel HJ *et al.*: PASM: a partitionable SIMD/MIMD system for image processing and pattern recognition. IEEE Trans on Computers C-30: 934–947, Dec. 1981.
10. Siegel HJ: The PASM system and parallel image processing. In: Freeman H, Pieroni GG (eds), Computer architecture for spatially distributed data. Springer-Verlag, 1984.

5. Physiologic concepts in cardiac imaging: Flow-function relations in acutely ischemic myocardium

KIM P. GALLAGHER

Several concepts from basic cardiovascular physiology have and are being applied to clinical imaging. The purpose of this chapter is to review recent studies which addressed the relationship between regional myocardial blood flow and regional contractile function. The abbreviated term we have used to describe this subject is myocardial 'flow-function relations'.

In the last few years, we have examined regional function by using systolic wall thickening (measured with sonomicrometry) as a parameter of regional contractile performance. Wall thickening provides an integrated measure of mechanical function across all 'layers' of the myocardium and it avoids a potential limitation of myocardial segment length measurements which may be affected by improper alignment relative to local fiber orientation [1, 2]. It also has the advantage of having direct counterparts in clinical use. This is particularly appropriate in the context of cardiac imaging because dynamic assessment of regional myocardial function as systolic wall thickening is possible with several different clinical modalities, such as echocardiography, digital ventriculography, CT scanning, and magnetic resonance imaging. As detailed in this chapter, systolic wall thickening provides a reliable index of the adequacy of myocardial perfusion during acute ischemia. The sensitivity of transmural function (measured as wall thickening) to changes in deep myocardial blood flow and relative insensitivity to alterations in outer myocardial perfusion are the salient features that have emerged from recent studies.

Effects of ischemia on wall thickening

Experimental studies on wall thickening dynamics have been performed with a variety of techniques (see references in [3]) and the utility of this parameter as a descriptor of normal cardiac function is well established [4, 5]. Until recently, ischemic effects on wall thickening were examined primarily in studies focusing on the influence of changes in total coronary inflow, usually in anesthetized, open-chest preparations [6–9]. For example, Kerber *et al.* [7] measured mean transmural blood flow with microspheres and wall thickening with M-mode echocardiography. Alterations in the extent of systolic excursion and thickening velocity correlated well with relative reductions in mean blood flow during various levels of circumflex coronary artery narrowing. Stowe *et al.* [9], using a flowmeter to measure coronary blood flow in anesthetized pigs, produced stepwise reductions in blood flow through the left anterior descending artery. Systolic wall thickening (measured with sonomicrometers) was reduced by 55% when coronary inflow decreased approximately 25% from the control level. When inflow was less than 25% of control, systolic thinning replaced thickening in the affected area. A significant linear relationship was documented between total coronary inflow and wall thickening.

More recent studies have addressed the functional consequences of changes in myocardial blood flow distribution produced by coronary stenosis or occlusion. Most of these studies have examined the response of subendocardial segment shortening to acute restriction of coronary flow. Vatner [10], for example, created different levels of partial stenosis in conscious dogs in order to correlate alterations in subendocardial blood flow and segmental shortening measured in the same area. The flow-function relation determined in this study was best described by an exponential expression. Weintraub *et al.* [11], in anesthetized dogs, also documented a non-linear relationship between subendocardial blood flow and segment shortening. In other studies using subendocardial segment shortening, however, linear relationships were observed in anesthetized dogs [12], conscious dogs during gradual ameroid occlusion [13], or in collateral dependent zones of exercising dogs [14]. Thus, conflicting results have been reported concerning the shape of the relationship between regional myocardial blood flow and function (measured as segment shortening) during ischemia.

Myocardial flow-function relations

Resolving conflicting results such as these are important because we think the shape of the flow-function relationship and its position have significant implications for understanding wall motion disorders during acute myocardial ischemia. To illustrate this point three different hypothetical flow-function relations are shown in Figure 1 to briefly discuss the implications of different types of flow-function relations.

Blood flow is plotted on the x-axis and contractile function (measured either as segment shortening, wall thickening, or another parameter of mechanical performance), expressed as a decimal fraction of the control value, is plotted on the y-axis. The relation labeled with A (dashed lines) is strongly non-linear. Reductions in blood flow less than 50% are associated with minimal change in function. As shown with the arrows, at 50% reduced flow, systolic function is only mar-

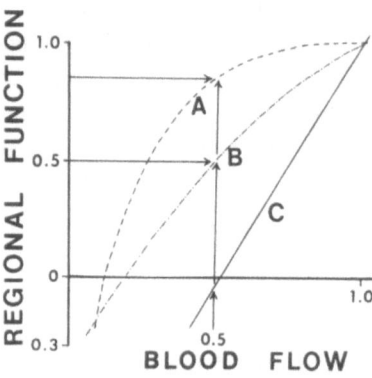

Figure 1. Three different hypothetical flow-function relations. Blood flow is plotted on the x-axis and regional function on the y-axis. Both parameters are plotted as decimal fractions of control (equal to 1.0) values.

ginally affected. Thereafter, the relation steepens and additional decreases in flow are associated with large decrements on the y-axis. If this type of relationship existed, which is suggested by Vatner's subendocardial flow-function data [10], for example, it could be interpreted to indicate that coronary flow exceeds requirements during control conditions. Moderate reduction of flow would produce minimal dysfunction because there is a 'reserve' of flow available (within limits). Alternatively, oxygen delivery (rather than blood flow) is maintained by increased extraction, thereby sustaining relatively normal contractile performance. If this relationship was observed for transumral wall thickening, rather than segment shortening, versus subendocardial flow it might suggest that outer wall function was compensating for subendocardial ischemia, thereby maintaining or buffering the change in overall function and minimizing the degree of transmural dysfunction.

The linear or nearly linear relation depicted in B shows a closer correspondence between blood flow and function at all levels of perfusion. As shown with the arrows, 50% reduction in blood flow is in this case associated with roughly 50% decrease in wall thickening, a major change. The implication in B, different from that in A, is close dependence of function on myocardial blood flow and is similar to the results on the subendocardial flow-segment shortening relationship reported by Tomoike *et al.* [13], Hill *et al.* [14], and Gross *et al.* [12]. This type of relationship for wall thickening (or transmural function) versus subendocardial blood flow would suggest that deep myocardial perfusion plays a major role in total wall thickening.

The line shown as C, suggests poor coupling between flow and function, in that large changes in wall motion occur with relatively small changes in blood flow. A 50% reduction in flow is associated with severe dysfunction. This type of relation might imply that wall motion is affected by factors other than flow reduction alone. These factors could include tethering between ischemic and non-ischemic muscle which somehow constrains motion in the near normally perfused myocardium [7, 15].

Using the shape and position of flow-function relationships to aid in analysis of acute wall motion disorders is made difficult by the complex geometry of the ventricle. Consequently careful experimental correlations must be established between blood flow (and its transmural distribution) and different parameters of myocardial function. Previous studies on subendocardial shortening have established a strong dependence of this parameter on changes in blood flow (although the shape of the relation remains controversial). Extrapolating subendocardial shortening to conventional clinical parameters of regional myocardial function, however, requires the assumption that segment shortening is a precise indicator of function across the entire wall. This has not been fully verified. Systolic wall thickening, on the other hand, clearly provides an integrated measure of transmural contractile function which is used clinically thereby facilitating extrapolation of experimental findings to clinically relevant situations (with the usual precautions).

Flow-function relations at rest in conscious dogs

The flow-function analysis of how wall thickening is affected by acute ischemia is complicated by the non-uniform distribution of blood flow produced by coronary narrowing. Consequently it was our view that we should explore the relationships between blood flow in different 'layers' of the myocardial wall and transmural function measured as wall thickening. Accordingly, several studies were conducted at the Seaweed Canyon Laboratory (under the direction of Dr John Ross, Jr) in conscious, chronically instrumented dogs. The instrumentation we used is diagrammatically depicted in Figure 2. At sterile surgery a high fidelity micromanometer (Konigsberg, P7) was inserted through the apex to measure left ventricular pressure. Catheters were placed in the left ventricle (to calibrate the pressure gauge), left atrium (to inject tracer labeled microspheres) and aorta (to withdraw a reference arterial sample for calculation of myocardial blood flows). A hydraulic occluder was placed around the circumflex artery to produce variable degrees of coronary narrowing. In some dogs a pulsed Doppler flowprobe was positioned proximal to the occluder to simultaneously measure coronary blood flow velocity.

Regional myocardial wall thickness was measured with ultrasonic dimension gauges in the posterior wall of the left ventricle. One crystal of the pair was inserted tangentially through the myocardium to the subendocardium, as shown in the lower right inste (Figure 2). The second crystal, attached to a dacron patch, was sewn to the epicardial surface over the position of the subendocardial crystal. This point was determined by locating the spot corresponding to the smallest

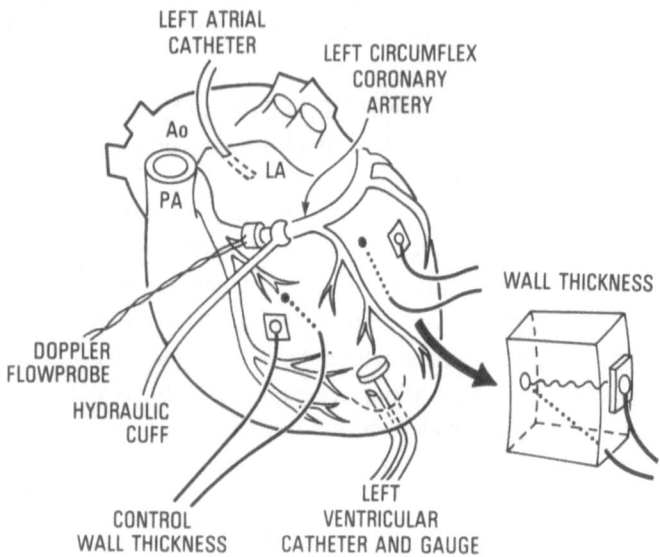

Figure 2. Schematic representation of instrumentation used in conscious dogs to study the relationship between myocardial blood flow and regional function during acute coronary inflow restriction. Regional function was measured as systolic wall thickening with ultrasonic dimension gauges (lower right inset).

distance between the crystals while monitoring the signals with an oscilloscope [5]. The position of the crystals was routinely examined carefully at the time of necropsy to verify correct alignment. When imprecise alignment was detected, data from such gauges were not used.

The transmural pattern of myocardial perfusion was determined during control conditions and during varying levels of flow restricting coronary stenosis. The reference withdrawal method was used to calculate blood flows using tracer labeled microspheres injected into the left atrium [16]. Full wall thickness sections of the left ventricle containing the dimension gauges were obtained. Each block of tissue was divided into three pieces of approximately equal thickness, to enable measurements of flow in the subepicardial, midmyocardial, and subendocardial thirds. Additional samples were obtained around the samples containing pairs of ultrasonic crystals to insure that the wall thickness measurements had been made in the ischemic zone and not in tissue at its edge, where intermediate levels of blood flow were observed (probably representing perfusion of mixed ischemic and non-schemic origin).

During resting conditions, while the dogs laid on their sides on a table in the laboratory, control recordings and a first microsphere injection were made. Then coronary stenosis was produced with the hydraulic occluder while monitoring wall thickness in the ischemic area. When stable conditions were achieved, characterized by a steady level of reduced wall thickening, another set of microspheres was injected. After completing the reference withdrawal, the coronary stenosis was released. When regional function had recovered, a second stenosis was created and the procedure was repeated. As many as five different degrees of stenosis were produced in some of the dogs.

An example of recorded tracings and blood flow data from one of these experiments is shown in Figure 3. In this example two different degrees of dysfunction are presented, a mild (middle panel, labeled 'stenosis') and a severe wall thickening abnormality (right panel, labeled 'occlusion'). In the upper rows are shown tracings from two-dimension gauges measuring wall thickness in the ischemic zone. End-diastole and end-systole are indicated with the solid vertical lines. In the left panels are control tracings with the normal pattern of thickening evident from end-diastole to end-systole. The succeeding panels show the effects of ischemia, the most evident change being reduction in the extent of systolic thickening compared with control.

In the lower row of Figure 3 are shown the transmural patterns of myocardial blood flow in the tissue surrounding these pairs of crystals. In the far left panel is the control distribution of blood flow from subendocardium to subepicardium. The usual pattern of blood flow is evident, with subendocardial flow exceeding subepicardial flow. In the second panel the major change in blood flow is limited to the subendocardial third and was associated with aproximately 50% reduction in systolic thickening. This example suggests that transmural function is very sensitive to changes in deep myocardial perfusion. In the third panel, blood flow was reduced transmurally and net systolic thinning (or paradoxical motion) occurred.

Flow-function plots from experiments in which several levels of coronary stenosis were produced during resting conditions are shown in Figure 4, which illustrates changes in wall thickening as a function of subendocardial and sub-epicardial blood flows. Blood flow data are presented on the x-axis as normalized values. The data were normalized by expressing blood flow as decimal fractions of simultaneously measured blood flow in control regions of the left ventricle, remote from the ischemic area. On the y-axis are plotted normalized systolic wall thickening data, expressed as decimal fractions of systolic thickening during control conditions.

It is quite clear that systolic wall thickening varies closely with changes in subendocardial blood flow, indicating consistently strong dependence of trans-mural function on deep myocardial perfusion. Regression lines for subendocar-dial data are shown with the heavy dashed lines and they were characterized by excellent fits (r^2 varying from 0.87 to 0.99). Subepicardial blood flow, however, related relatively poorly to changes in transmural function in that large reductions in thickening occured before subepicardial blood flow was reduced by coronary narrowing. Only two of the subepicardial flow-transmural function relations (shown with light dashed lines in plots 1 and 3 of Figure 4) were statistically significant and they were shifted substantially rightward from the subendocardial flow-function relations.

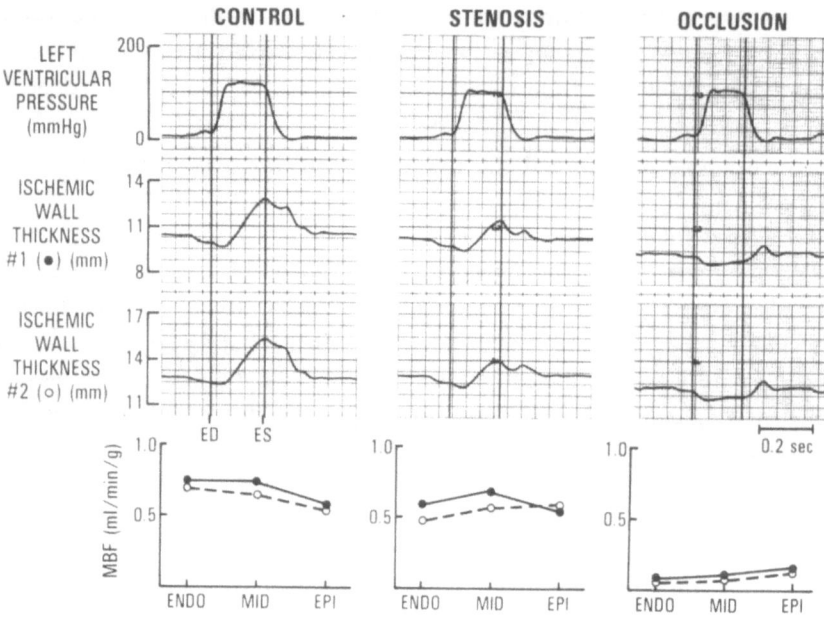

Figure 3. Example of analog tracings and blood flow data from one of the experiments with coronary stenosis and occlusion at rest, in a conscious dog. Myocardial blood flow (MBF) distribution in the dimension gauges is shown in the lower row. Blood flow is shown in three layers across the wall, from subendocardium (ENDO) to subepicardium (EPI).

To facilitate analysis of data from all of the dogs, the data were categorized into six groups by the effect on systolic wall thickening. The average data from 15 dogs on normalized subendocardial and subepicardial flow versus changes in wall thickening by category (defined by progressive reductions in thickening in multiples of 20%) are shown in the left panel of Figure 5. Normalized mean transmural blood flow (average of flows in the three layers across the wall) versus wall thickening is presented in the right panel (Figure 5). Statistically significant changes in blood flow from control are indicated with asterisks. Consistent with the individual examples (Figures 3, 4) presented above, reductions in subendocardial blood flow exert a substantial influence on transmural thickening. Transmural function was reduced by approximately 13% in the first category of dysfunction and from a practical standpoint this could be considered the detectable limit of wall thickening impairment due to ischemia using the methodology we have described. Frankly, when the data were subdivided by decrements in wall thickening less than 20%, we were unable to show significant reductions. This degree of dysfunction (category 1), was associated with a relatively small decrease in subendocardial blood flow (approximately 20%) which stresses the sensitivity of transmural function to changes in deep myocardial perfusion. Additional reductions in subendocardial flow were closely associated with further decreases in systolic wall thickening [17].

The mildly non-linear trend of the average subendocardial data are similar to

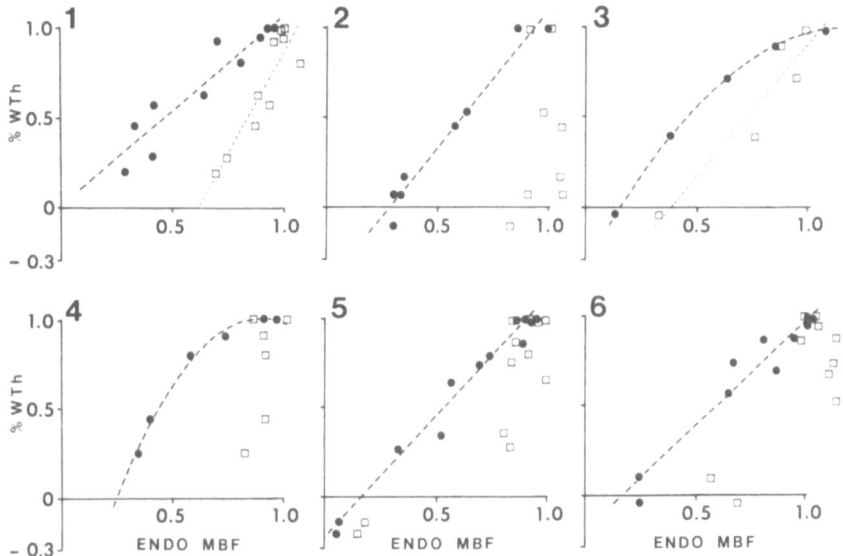

Figure 4. Flow function plots from six individual experiments in which several levels of coronary flow restriction were produced. Blood flow is on the x-axis as decimal fractions of simultaneously measured flow in control areas. Both subendocardial and subepicardial blood flow data are presented versus normalized systolic wall thickening. The heavy dashed line in each plot is the most appropriate regression line for the subendocardial flow-wall thickening relationship. Excellent fits are evident. Subepicardial data, on the hand, were characterized by a varible and poorly correlated relationship.

the B relation shown in Figure 1. Although a linear regression equation described the data well, there was small but significant improvement by using a quadratic expression to describe the overall relationship between normalized subendocardial blood flow and wall thickening.

Nonetheless, we think the shape of the subendocardial flow-transmural function relationship can be considered linear, with little loss of accuracy. Had the relationship been markedly curvilinear (like that shown as A in Figure 1) with large reductions in subendocardial flow accompanied by relatively minor changes in wall thickening it would have implied the existence of compensatory function in well-perfused outer layers of the myocardium. This was not the case, however, suggesting that the outer wall contributes minimally to sustaining overall transmural function when the deeper myocardium is underperfused. The data presented here, obtained in conscious dogs, confirm our previous conclusion (based on studies in anesthetized dogs [3]) and that of Roan *et al.* [18] that transmural thickening is largely dependent on deep myocardial blood flow.

Changes in systolic wall thickening also correlated well and in linear fashion with reductions in mean transmural blood flow (Figure 5, right). The close correspondence between mean blood flow and thickening is similar to the report by Savage *et al.* [19] which was based on studies in conscious pigs with acute coronary occlusion, rather than progressive degrees of coronary narrowing. Although our data were obtained in conscious dogs, this relationship is also

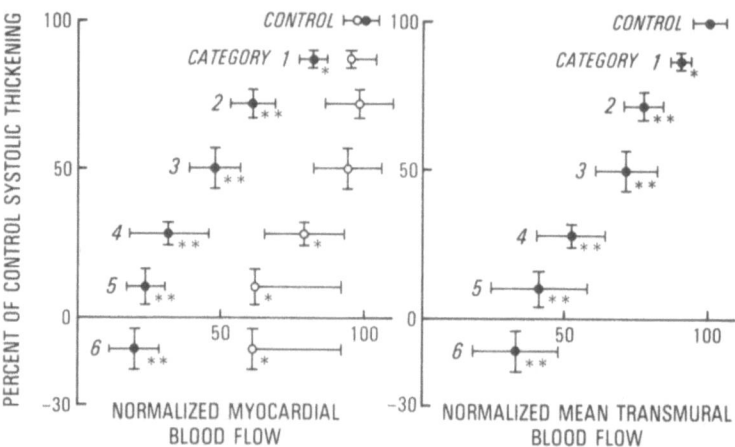

Figure 5. Average data in six categories of dysfunction due to coronary stenosis. On the left, normalized subendocardial (closed circles ●) and subepicardial (open circles ○) blood flow data are plotted versus changes in systolic wall thickening, by category. Wall thickening data are presented as percentages of wall thickening during control conditions. Normalized mean transmural versus wall thickening data, in the same categories, are presented on the right. Significant differences in blood flow data from control are indicated with asterisks and data are presented as mean ±SD. (Used with permission of the American Heart Association.)

similar to the data obtained in earlier studies using anesthetized animals [7–9].

The correlation between wall thickening and subepicardial blood flow is relatively poor. Wall thickening was significantly reduced in the first three categories, but there was no significant change in subepicardial blood flow. Even a 50% reduction in wall thickening (category 3) was characterized by normal perfusion in the outer third of the wall (Figure 5, left). In categories 4, 5, and 6, when coronary stenosis was severe enough to restrict subepicardial blood flow, more substantial transmural dysfunction was evident and decrements in thickening and outer wall perfusion appeared to change in parallel. The scatter in the subepicardial blood flow data is substantial, however (especially in categories 5 and 6), emphasizing the high degree of variability in this relationship. As depicted here (Figure 5) and in Figure 4, subepicardial blood flow seems to play a relatively small role in determining what happens to transmural function during acute ischemia. The distribution of the subepicardial flow-transmural function data are similar to the relationship shown as C, in Figure 1, which was characterized by large functional deficits associated with relatively small decrements in blood flow.

Flow-function relations during exercise

Additional experiments were performed in dogs instrumented in the same manner and trained to run on a treadmill. The objective of these studies was to examine the relationship between myocardial perfusion and transmural function (measured as wall thickening) during exercise [20]. In addition to defining regional flow-function relations when conditions were greatly altered compared with the resting state, it also allowed us to test the contention that relative changes in systolic wall thickening constitute a reliable index of the adequacy of myocardial blood flow under widely different conditions.

The effects of exercise on regional flow-function relations have received relatively small attention [20, 21, 14] and no prior comparison of this relationship at rest with that during exercise has been made. Previous studies showed that partial coronary stenosis leads to maldistribution of myocardial blood flow [22, 23] and in other studies, regional mechanical dysfunction during exercise with coronary flow restriction was demonstrated [24–26]. Because of the difficulties associated with correlation of data between different studies and by different investigators, we combined flow and function studies in order to relate particular patterns of transmural blood flow to specific degrees of wall thickening dysfunction during exercise [20].

After training dogs for 2–4 weeks to run on a treadmill, the animals were instrumented as described previously. The dogs were allowed to recover and when they exhibited normal activity (including the ability to run 10–13 km/h at 5% grade on the treadmill), the studies were performed. The experimental treadmill runs were preceded by control recordings at rest and an initial injection of microspheres was made while the dogs stood quietly on the treadmill. Then the dogs were run on the treadmill at speed and grade sufficient to increase heart rate to approximately 200 beats/min or more and another injection of microspheres was made. At least 30 min were allowed for recovery. Thereafter, coronary stenosis was produced by adjustment of the hydraulic occluder and the treadmill run was repeated at the same speed and grade, at which time another injection of microspheres was made. It was sometimes necessary to further adjust the occluder during the exercise period to attain sufficient myocardial dysfunction and additional time was allowed for establishment of steady state conditions before injecting microspheres in these circumstances. One to three treadmill runs with coronary stenosis were performed in each dog.

An example of slow paper speed tracings from one of the experiments is shown in Figure 6. This exercise run was performed with a relatively mild restriction of coronary blood flow. Phasic and mean coronary blood flow velocity recordings are shown in the two lower rows; flow velocity was 35% lower than the control exercise level although the treadmill was set at the same rate and inclination as control exercise. This degree of flow restriction led to mild regional dysfunction (29% reduction compared with control exercise) in the myocardium supplied by the stenosed circumflex artery. The ischemic zone wall thickness (ischemic WTh) rapidly achieved a steady level of reduced thickening after minor adjustments were made in the occluder setting (during the first 30 s of the run).

A reference withdrawal sample was obtained after stable conditions were

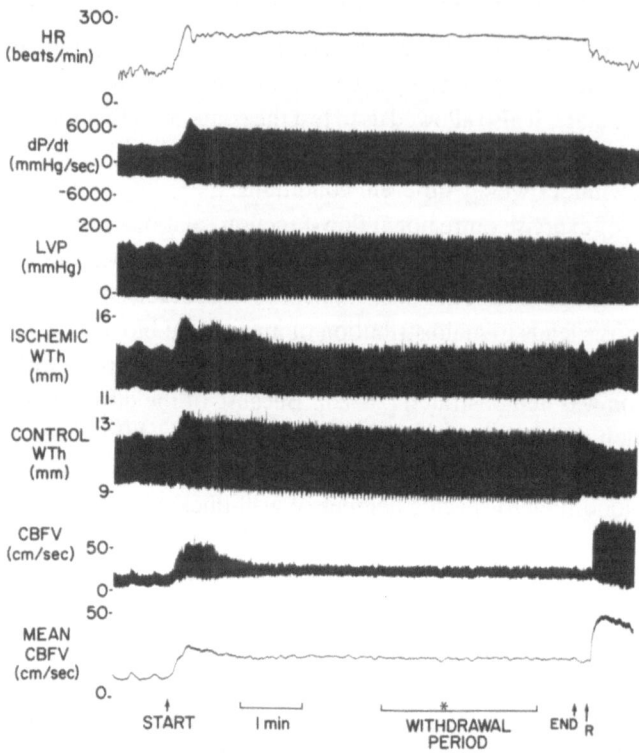

Figure 6. Example of recordings at slow paper speed from one experiment to illustrate hemodynamic and dimensional changes during treadmill exercise with coronary stenosis. Abbreviations: HR = heart rate; LVP = left ventricular pressure; WTh = wall thickness; CBFV = coronary blood flow velocity.

established ('withdrawal period') and microspheres were injected to document myocardial blood flow (indicated with the asterisk). After stopping the treadmill (END), the stenosis was released (R) and a reactive hyperemic response was evident which confirmed that ischemic conditions existed during the exercise period with coronary narrowing.

To more clearly illustrate the changes in wall thickening associated with exercise plus coronary stenosis, examples of tracings obtained at fast paper speed (from a different experiment) are presented in Figure 7. Control zone wall thickness (Ctl WT) and ischemic zone (Is WT, in the area supplied by the circumflex artery) are shown in the upper two rows. Phasic coronary blood flow velocity is in the lower row. Normal patterns of systolic thickening from end-diastole (ED) to end-systole (ES) are evident in both dimensions during control conditions, at rest, while the animal stood on the treadmill (panel A). The pattern of coronary blood flow velocity is normal, with a low systolic component and high diastolic component.

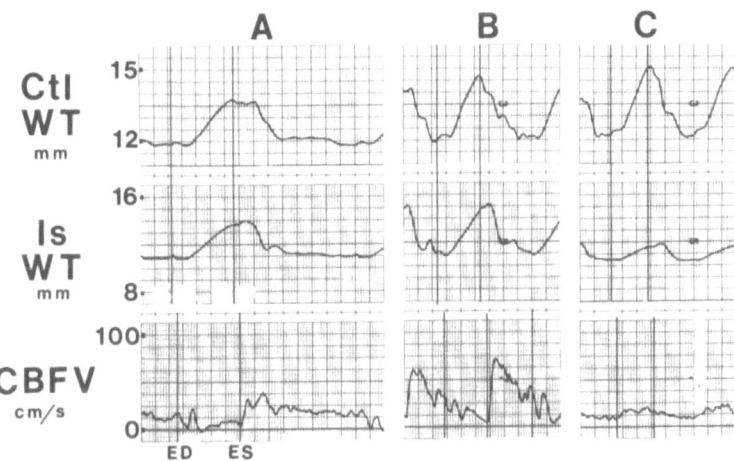

Figure 7. Example of analog tracings at fast paper speed from an exercise experiment. In panel A are control recordings, at rest; in panel B, recordings from control exercise; in panel C, recordings during exercise with restriction of left circumflex coronary inflow. Abbreviations: Ctl WT = control wall thickness; Is WT = ischemic wall thickness; CBFV = coronary blood flow velocity.

In panel B are shown recordings during exercise without coronary stenosis. Heart rate was greatly elevated and the extent of systolic wall thickening was augmented similarly in the two dimensions. Coronary blood flow velocity was increased substantially, as well, with maintenance of the usual diastolic dominant flow pattern. In panel C, exercise in the presence of coronary stenosis is shown. Wall thickening in the control area was maintained but in the ischemic area, it was reduced by 70% compared with control exercise. Associated with the severe degree of regional hypokinesia was elevated left ventricular end-diastolic pressure, reduced systolic left ventricular pressure, and diminished positive dP/dt. Coronary flow velocity through the narrowed circumflex artery is clearly restricted, as shown in the figure. Mean flow velocity was restricted to the resting level and the phasic pattern was altered greatly, with primarily systolic rather than diastolic flow.

The transmural pattern of myocardial blood flow in this experiment is presented in Figure 8. On the left is blood flow in the anterior wall (or control area) and on the right is blood flow in the posterior wall (or ischemic area) containing the pairs of dimension gauges measuring wall thickness. Blood flow is shown in three layers across the wall, from subendocardium (#1) to subepicardium (#3). Mean transmural blood flow (M) is indicated with the isolated symbols. Blood flow at rest was comparable in both zones with slightly higher subendocardial than subepicardial flow, the usual pattern. During control exercise blood flow was similarly elevated in both regions and subendocardial flow remained higher than subepicardial flow. In the control area, during exercise with coronary stenosis, the blood flow data were similar to the control exercise. In the ischemic

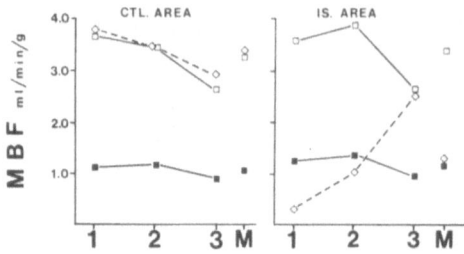

Figure 8. Myocardial blood flow (MBF) data from the experiment shown in Figure 7. On the left is blood flow in the tissue sample containing the control wall thickness dimension gauges (CTL. AREA); on the right, blood flow in the ischemic area (IS. AREA). Blood flow is shown in three layers across the wall (1 = subendocardium; 2 = midmyocardium, 3 = subepicardium). Mean transmural (M) blood flow is presented as the isolated symbols. Data from three conditions are depicted: at rest (■—■), during control exercise (□—□), and during exercise with coronary stenosis (◇---◇).

area, which exhibited greatly reduced systolic wall thickening, there was a large reduction in mean transmural blood flow compared to control exercise. Although the mean level of blood flow was the same as control flow at rest (consistent with the coronary flow velocity recordings shown in Figure 7), there was a marked alteration in the transmural distribution of myocardial perfusion. Subendocardial blood flow was greatly reduced and midmyocardial flow (#2) was not changed compared with resting conditions, but subepicardial blood flow was augmented to a level similar to the control exercise.

Like the findings in conscious dogs at rest with coronary stenosis discussed earlier, substantial transmural dysfunction was evident despite minimal change in subepicardial blood flow. The degree of dysfunction appeared more closely related to changes in deep myocardial perfusion. Although the absolute levels of blood flow differ between resting and exercise conditions, the close correspondence between subendocardial flow alterations and wall thickening during coronary stenosis appear similar. Individual data points from 13 dogs are plotted in Figure 9 to illustrate the relationships determined in the experiments with exercise during coronary stenosis. As suggested by the example in Figures 7 and 8, subendocardial blood flow (normalized in the same fashion as in Figure 4) correlates well and closely with changes in systolic wall thickening. A linear expression described the data best but it is interesting that to fill the gap between the available data during exercise with coronary stenosis and control exercise, a non-linear component seems to be required (suggested by the light dashed line in Figure 9). The subepicardial flow-transmural function data were also comparable to the resting data shown in Figures 4 and 5. Minimal change in subepicardial blood flow was associated with decrements in wall thickening of approximately 50%. Thereafter coronary stenosis was severe enough to also reduce outer perfusion. The regression equation describing these data had a significantly lower slope than the subendocardial data. A non-linear component appears necessary

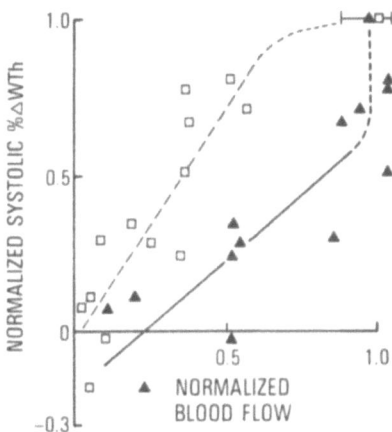

Figure 9. Relationship between normalized subendocardial and subepicardial blood flow and normalized systolic wall thickening during exercise with acute coronary stenosis. Blood flow data are presented as decimal fractions of flow in control areas; thickening data are presented as decimal fractions of control exercise values. Like the relationships at rest, changes in systolic wall thickening appear to correspond closely with alterations in deep (subendocardial □–––) myocardial perfusion but relatively poorly with changes in outer (subepicardial ▲—) blood flow.

with this relationship, as well, and is suggested by the dashed line connecting the subepicardial regression line to the control data (at 1.0) which also emphasizes the difference between the subendocardial and the subepicardial flow-transmural function relations. Thus, there is considerable similarity between the resting (Figures 4, 5) and exercise flow-function (Figure 9) relations when expressed in relative terms, supporting our contension that wall thickening provides an accurate index of myocardial perfusion during acute ischemia over a wide range of hemodynamic conditions.

Factors contributing to the importance of subendocardial blood flow

The most prominent finding of the studies reviewed here is the dependence of systolic wall thickening on changes in subendocardial blood flow. We believe that two factors may contribute importantly to this observation: (1) the non-uniform manner in which the wall thickens during systole, and (2) transmural tethering between ischemic (subendocardial) and non-ischemic (subepicardial) muscle. Based on simple theoretical considerations, the fractional contribution of the inner portion of the wall to total thickening should exceed that of the outer muscle. This is also predictable from a more complex model of left ventricular mechanics, which takes into account differences in fiber orientation across the wall, proposed by Arts *et al.* [27] and has recently been confirmed experimentally. When ischemia affects only the inner third of the myocardial wall, a large reduction in transmural thickening will be evident simply because this layer does most of the thickening during systole. Even if wall thickening in the outer third remains completely normal when the deeper muscle is ischemic, its fractional contribution to transmural thickening is relatively small thereby limiting its apparent importance in terms of total systolic wall thickening.

A tethering effect may be defined as constraint of motion in normally (or near normally) perfused muscle adjacent to an ischemic area. Previous studies have examined the response of subepicardial segment length shortening to ischema limited to the subendocardium in open-chest, anesthetized dogs. We studied this phenomenon and observed that the subepicardial segmental response was strongly dependent on the alignment of the dimension gauges relative to local fiber orientation [2]. Gauges aligned parallel with surface fiber orientation were not affected by subendocardial or midmyocardial ischemia while gauges aligned parallel with the minor axis (approximately 50 degrees off the surface fiber orientation) were severely affected. We concluded that tethering-related effects occur in the subepicardium but our data suggested the effect was more limited than previous investigators had suggested. Moreover, we concluded that persistent epicardial contraction had little effect on overall wall motion. Thus, the relative contribution tethering may make to overall wall motion abnormalities is not certain. However, we speculate that the non-uniform nature of wall thickening may be the predominant factor with tethering contributing in a less substantial, variable manner. The relative roles of these two factors in acute wall motion abnormalities are far from conclusively established and we think that additional studies will be required to specifically address this issue. Although flow-function analysis constitutes an incompletely developed investigative approach, it may prove useful in examining this and other aspects of wall motion changes due to ischemia.

Acknowledgements

Supported in part by American Heart Association grant-in-aid 81-1161, NIH Ischemic Heart Disease SCOR grant (HL-17682), NIH New Investigator Award HL-30067, and NIH grant HL-29716.

References

1. Bugge-Asperheim, Leraand S, Kiil F: Local dimensional changes of the myocardium measured by ultrasonic technique. Scand J Clin Lab Invest 24: 361–371, 1969.
2. Gallagher KP, Osakada G, Hess OM, Koziol JA, Kemper WS, Ross J Jr: Subepicardial segmental function during coronary stenosis and the role of myocardial fiber orientation. Circ Res 50: 352–359, 1982.
3. Gallagher KP, Kumada T, Koziol JA, McKown MD, Kemper WS, Ross J Jr: Significance of

regional wall thickening abnormalities relative to transmural myocardial perfusion in anesthetized dogs. Circulation 62: 1266–1274, 1980.

4. Gould KL, Kennedy JW, Frimer M, Pollack GH, Dodge HT: Analysis of wall dynamics and directional components of left ventricular contraction in man. Am J Cardiol 38: 322–331, 1976.

5. Sasayama S, Franklin D, Ross J Jr, Kemper WS, McKown D: Dynamic changes in left ventricular wall thickness and their use in analyzing cardiac function in the conscious dog. Am J Cardiol 38: 870–879, 1976.

6. Goldstein S, de Jong JW: Changes in left ventricular wall dimensions during regional myocardial ischemia. Am J Cardiol 34: 56–62, 1974.

7. Kerber RE, Marcus ML, Ehrhardt J, Wilson R, Abboud FM: Correlation between echocardiographically demonstrated segmental dyskinesis and regional myocardial perfusion. Circulation 52: 1097–1104, 1975.

8. Kerber RE, Marcus ML, Wilson R, Ehrhardt J, Abboud FM: Effects of acute coronary occlusion on the motion and perfusion of the normal and ischemic interventricular septum. An experimental echocardiographic study. Circulation 54: 928–935, 1976.

9. Stowe DF, Mathey DG, Moores WY, Glantz SA, Townsend RM, Kabra P, Chatterjee K, Parmley WW, Tyberg JV: Segment stroke work and metabolism depend on coronary blood flow in the pig. Am J Physiol 234 (Heart Circ Physiol 3): H597–H607, 1978.

10. Vatner SF: Correlation between acute reductions in myocardial blood flow and function in conscious dogs. Circ Res 47: 201–207, 1980.

11. Weintraub WS, Hattori S, Agarwal JB, Bodenheimer MM, Banka VS, Helfant RH: Relationship between myocardial blood flow and contraction by myocardial layer in the canine left ventricle. Circ Res 48: 430–438, 1981.

12. Gross GJ, Lamping KG, Warltier DC, Hardman HF: Effects of three bradycardic drugs on regional myocardial blood flow and function in areas distal to a total or partial coronary occlusion in dogs. Circulation 69: 391–399, 1984.

13. Tomoike H, Inou T, Watanabe K, Mizukami M, Kikuchi Y, Nakamura M: Functional significance of collaterals during ameroid-induced coronary stenosis in conscious dogs. Interrelationships among regional shortening, regional flow and grade of coronary stenosis. Circulation 67: 1001–1008, 1983.

14. Hill RC, Kleinman LH, Tiller WH Jr, Chitwood WR Jr, Rembert JC, Greenfield JC Jr, Wechsler AS: Myocardial blood flow and function during gradual coronary occlusion in awake dog. Am J Physiol 244 (Heart Circ Physiol 13): H60–H67, 1983.

15. Guth BD, White FC, Gallagher KP, Bloor CM: Abnormal wall thickening in myocardium adjacent to ischemic zones in conscious swine during brief coronary artery occlusion. Am Heart J 107: 458–464, 1984.

16. Heymann MA, Payne BD, Hoffman JIE, Rudolph AN: Blood flow measurements with radionuclide labeled particles. Prog Cardiovasc Dis 10: 55–79, 1977.

17. Gallagher KP, Matsuzaki M, Koziol JA, Kemper WS, Ross J Jr: Regional myocardial perfusion and wall thickening during ischemia in conscious dogs. Am J Physiol (in press).

18. Roan PG, Buja LM, Izquidedo C, Hashimi H, Saffer S, Willerson JT: Interrelationships between regional left ventricular function, coronary blood flow, and myocellular necrosis during the initial 24 hours and 1 week after experimental coronary occlusion in awake, unsedated dogs. Circ Res 49: 31–40, 1981.

19. Savage RM, Guth B, White FC, Hagan AD, Bloor CM: Correlation of regional myocardial blood flow and function with myocardial infarct size during myocardial ischemia in the conscious pig. Circulation 64: 699–707, 1981.

20. Gallagher KP, Matsuzaki M, Osakada G, Kemper WS, Ross J Jr: Effect of exercise on the relationship between myocardial blood flow and systolic wall thickening in dogs with acute coronary stenosis. Circ Res 52: 716–729, 1983.

21. Matsuzaki M, Gallagher KP, Patritti J, Tajimi T, Kemper WS, Ross J Jr: Effects of a calcium

entry blocker (diltiazem) on regional myocardial flow and function during exercise in conscious dogs. Circulation 69: 801–814, 1984.

22. Ball RM, Bache RJ: Distribution of myocardial blood flow in the exercising dog with restricted coronary artery inflow. Circ Res 38: 60–66, 1976.

23. Sanders TM, White FC, Peterson TM, Bloor CM: Characteristics of coronary blood flow and transmural distribution in miniature pigs. Am J Physiol 235: H601–H609, 1978.

24. Tomoike H, Franklin D, McKown D, Kemper WS, Guberek M, Ross J Jr: Regional myocardial dysfunction and hemodynamic abnormalities during strenuous exercise in dogs with limited coronary inflow. Circ Res 42: 487–496, 1978.

25. Kumada T, Gallagher KP, Shirato K, McKown D, Miller M, Kemper WS, White F, Ross J Jr: Reduction of exercise induced regional myocardial dysfunction by propranolol: studies in a canine model of chronic coronary artery stenosis. Circ Res 46: 190–200, 1980.

26. Tomoike H, Franklin D, Kemper WS, McKown D, Ross J Jr: Functional evaluation of coronary collateral development in conscious dogs. Am J Physiol 241: H519–H524, 1981.

27. Arts T, Reneman RS, Veenstra PC: A model of the mechanics of the left ventricle. Ann Biomed Eng 7: 299–318, 1979.

6. A geometric foundation for the study of left ventricular motion: Some tensor considerations

FRED L. BOOKSTEIN

The tensor description of deformation

Information about the heartbeat is of most value when it is geometrically distributed: the *regional* description. This descriptive task begins with the Cartesian motion of little bits of wall that we can't help perceiving upon the imaging screen. Because the heart is moving in the chest as it beats, much of the observed motion of edge elements is passive translation and rotation, irrelevant to the assessment of contractile function. To analyze the function of one bit of myocardium, one must somehow cancel out the motion imputed to it by contraction elsewhere.

The essence of this biometric problem is the presence of information from two distinct sources: geometrical location and biological homology. Each point of the outline has a particular identity as a bit of tissue, and many of these, the *landmarks,* are quickly recognizable upon the image of the shape at different moments in time. The nature of a landmark varies with the biometric context: the abutment of two bones, the origin of a valve, a reliable 'corner', a metallic implant or marker, and so on. Change of form is a matter of change in configuration of the set of landmarks and the edge-arcs connecting them. Automatic recognition of the landmark configuration is a difficult problem specific to the details of each type of scene. But it is straightforward to analyze changes in these configurations once they are recognized.

The basic unit for the study of biological shape change is a homologous pair of *triangles* of landmarks, Figure 1a. In the absence of other information we may take the transformation sampled by these limited data to be uniform between each homologous pair of edges and throughout the interiors of the triangles. The homogeneity of the transformation is indicated clearly in the *transformation grid* after the style of D'Arcy Thompson, Figure 1b.

The visual impression this leaves is a function of orientation of the square grid on the starting form, an orientation irrelevant to our goal of describing change. We may draw the transformation much more generally in terms of the collection of lines in all directions, Figure 1c. The deformation we are observing, driven by

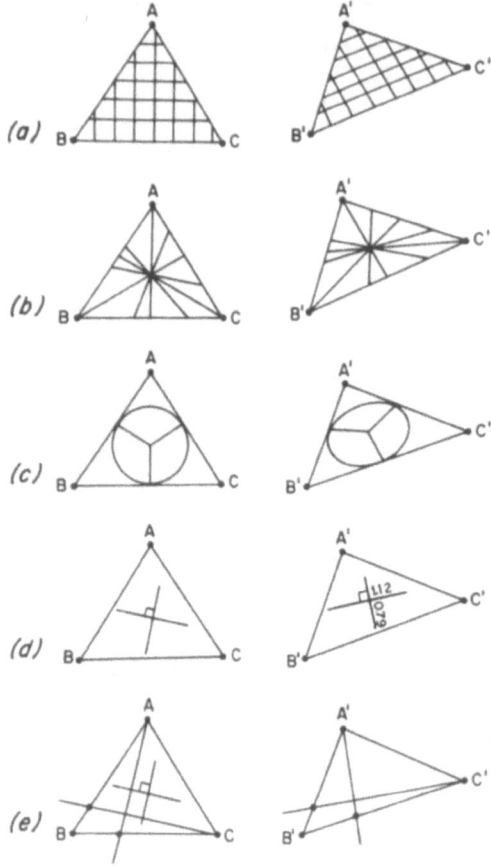

Figure 1. Discrete analysis of change in landmark configurations. (a) We abstract the form into a collection of deforming triangles; (b) The change of any triangle is modeled as a uniform deformation of the interior, an abstract space; (c) This deformation alters distances between homologous pairs of points in all directions; (d) We can observe these rates directly by observing the shape into which a circle is deformed under the transformation – it is an ellipse; (e) The ellipse may be wholly described by the lengths and orientation of its principal axes.

the displacements of those landmarks at the corners, will deform these lines into others which divide the edges in the same fractions. That is, the deformation takes edges to edges, median lines (dividing the opposite sides in the ratio 50:50) to medians, and so on.

Principal axes computed from triangles of landmarks. To fully describe a change of form, it is sufficient to know ratios of lengths of corresponding lines in the two triangles. These ratios are called *strains* or *extensions;* they are dimensionless. They determine the deformation completely, up to the rigid motions we are attempting to nullify. We could compute the strains explicitly by taking quotients of corresponding lengths, direction by direction; but it is easier to perform the division implicitly, by reference to lines of a length constant before deformation: that is, diameters of a circle. We can actually *draw* the circle, Figure 1d, whose deformation we wish to observe, and the oval into which the uniform shear takes it.

Under the assumption of homogeneous (linear) transformation, this oval is an ellipse, precisely. Being an ellipse, the image of the circle has two axes of symmetry, which lie at 90°. One is the largest diameter of the ellipse, one the smallest. The diameters of the circle which transform into them are likewise at 90°.

Recall that the lengths of the radii embody the strain ratios as a function of direction. One of the axes of the ellipse is therefore the direction of *greatest* strain, the greatest rate of change of length, and one is the direction of *least* strain. The diameters that were mapped into them are determined by corresponding fractions of intersection along edges of the triangles. In Figure 1e we have drawn them alone; the remaining information about strains in intermediate directions may be readily reconstructed. These axes are called the *principal axes* of the deformation, and the rates of change of length along them are the *principal strains*. Together they completely describe the change in form of this triangle of landmarks. The area of the triangle changes by the product of the strains – $1.12 \times 0.79 = 0.885$ – while the most sensitive descriptor of shape change is the proportion between lengths measured in these two directions, which changes by the factor $1.12/0.79 = 1.42$. Note that we are not 'measuring' the triangles separately at all. The shapes themselves have merely been archived; no preconceptions of specific variables have interfered with the technique's construction of optimal descriptions of change.

The analysis of shape change in this wise is not new. Engineering mechanics has long known this formalism as the strain tensor for simple finite elements [1–3]. Its application to problems of description in non-mechanical or abstract systems, however, is recent. In this version, the 'interior' of a morphometric triangle is not a homogeneous biological substance but an arbitrary mosaic of tissues, fluid, or air. The shape change of this interior is a useful descriptive device for reporting changes in the configuration of its vertices, whose locations are the real biometric data of these exercises. A more lengthy exposition of these matters, including a statistical praxis for systematic group differences in shape or shape change, is presented in Bookstein [4].

Two analyses of one cardiac cycle

I now apply this analysis to images from a single human heartbeat. The data (Figure 2), taken from a published figure ([5], Figure 3), are the positions of nine small tantalum screws implanted in a human heart during coronary bypass

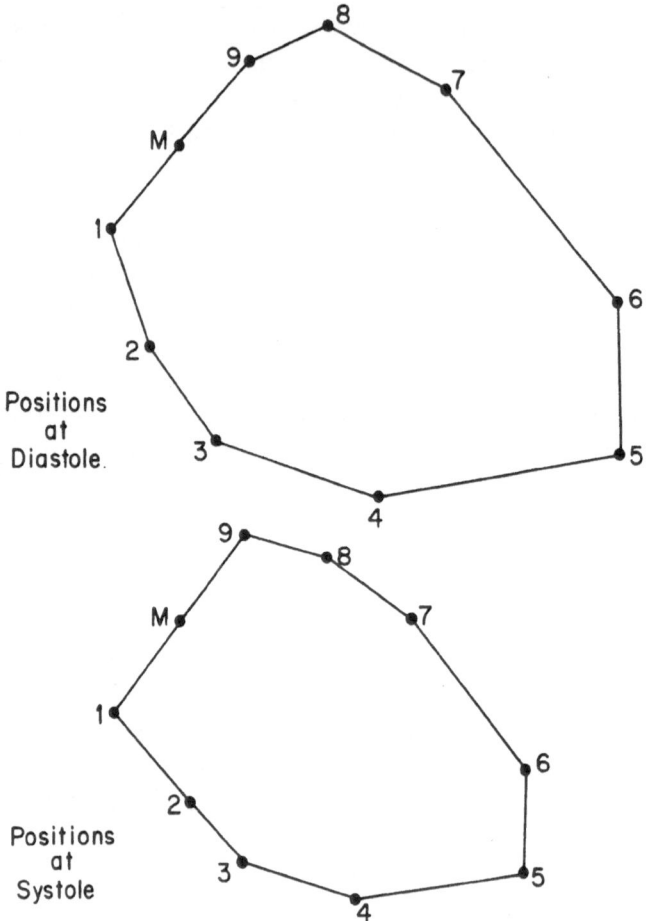

Figure 2. Nine tantalum implants approximating the silhouette of a healthy human left ventricle at systole and diastole, after Ingels *et al.* (see text).

surgery. The view is 30° right anterior oblique; the apex is at marker 5; the base spans markers 1 and 9.

The method of Figure 1 was used to describe the deformations from diastole to systole of the triangles formed from all sets of three implants out of the nine. From the computed tensors derives the report of Figures 3 and 4. In these diagrams, the principal strains for each triangle are drawn at the center of its inscribed circle. The coordinate systems of the configurations separately are irrelevant to the conclusions we draw.

From Figure 3 there immediately emerges a remarkable fact. Triangles 3–7–6 and 3–6–5 are each contracting nearly uniformly, and at the same rate: some 31% ± 2% in every direction. Fully half the area (at diastole) of the ventricle in this projection is accounted for by these triangles. Furthermore, although marker 4 is not moving according to this same homogeneous contraction, its displacement from marker 7, which is nearly on the normal to the ventricular contour at marker

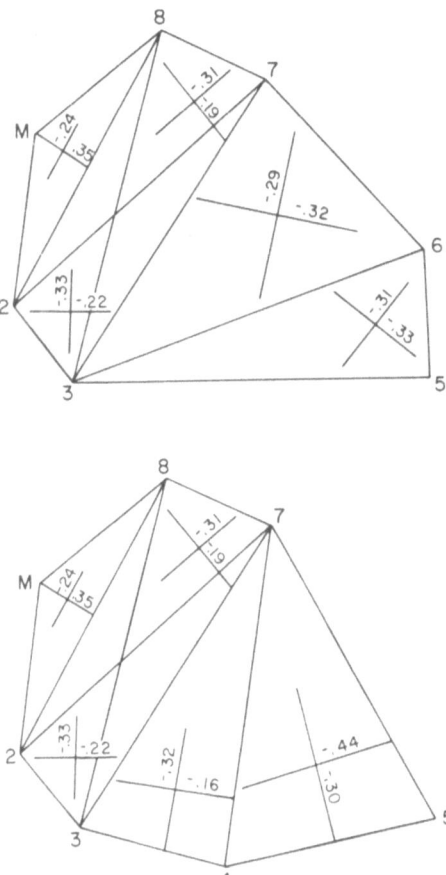

Figure 3. Principal strains (ratios of contraction) and directions of the shape change over the cardiac cycle for two carefully selected mosaics of triangles using the landmarks in Figure 2.

4, contracts at the same 30% rate. Relative to the uniform contraction, marker 4 is displaced only tangentially, away from 3 and toward 5. (Some of this heterogeneity is surely due to twisting of the heart with respect to the projection plane.)

This same contraction of about 31% persists quite far from the apex. In triangles 2–3–7 and 8–3–7, which overlap in Figure 6, the maximum contraction is at this same rate. The minimum contraction in these triangles, 19% or 22%, can be thought of as a weakening of the 32% by a superimposed extension of markers 2 and 8 outward by about 11% of their separation from the 3–7 baseline.

We join markers 2 and 8 to the midpoint of the aortic valve, M in the figures, to form an uppermost triangle for this analysis. As the bottom of the ventricle contracts, the top expands under hydrodynamic pressure. This top triangle contracts across its base by 24% (the same 30%, perhaps, corrected for the apparent divergence of the translations at 2 and 8 just noted); but its height (that is, its projection along the axis of the heart) increases by 35% from end-diastole to

70

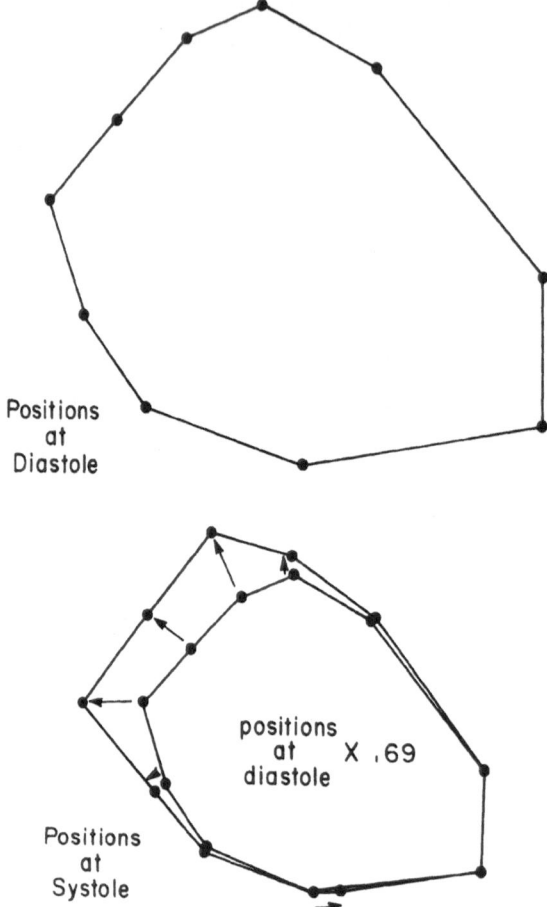

Figure 4. The analyses of Figure 3 suggest a vector summary of the deformation using a scale change of 0.69 and superimposing over the lower two-thirds of the ventricle.

end-systole. Relative to the general change of scale by 0.68, this height has doubled.

These aspects of the description may be abstracted into the simple, nearly symmetric scheme of Figure 4. Superimposed on a uniform contraction of 31% are outward displacements at markers 2, 1, 9, and 8 as shown, together with a lateral adjustment (presumably unrelated) at marker 4. Note the rotation of the axis of the heart relative to the aortic valve ring.

Biorthogonal grids for the same data. There is an alternate analysis of these data in which the role of marker 4 is not exceptional. The method of triangles computes one tensor per three landmarks, a tensor supposed to apply homogeneously to every point inside the triangle. But the data are not a set of triangles – they are one set of points, a polygon. The method of *biorthogonal grids* [6], a generalization of D'Arcy Thompson's *Cartesian grids* [7], is appropriate for such extended configurations. At the outset it computes a single smooth deformation (Figure 5a) relating the interiors of two polygons by extending the boundary correspondence inward according to a suitable interpolation formula. In the top (diastolic) form, the set of mesh points constitutes a conventional square (Cartesian) grid; the positions imputed to these points after the 'deformation' which is the heartbeat make up the distorted mesh inside the bottom form. These two meshes correspond point for point, as can be seen by comparing their relationship to the implants, points whose correspondence from diastole to systole we know quite reliably. The position and orientation of that starting square grid, although arbitrary, do not affect any of the subsequent stages in the description of this change. Like the deformations of triangles, this is an abstract transformation. It does not describe what is 'really there' but instead expresses the change of boundary form in a geometrically convenient metaphor.

From the derivative of this map a principal strain tensor can be computed at every point (Figure 5b). These are the infinitesimal directions corresponding to those in Figure 1e as applied to 'very small' triangles. The principal directions are orthogonal both before and after deformation; of the rates of change of length in all directions through this point and its computed homologue, the rate along one of the principal directions is greatest, and is least along the other. Curves can be constructed (Figure 6) which run parallel to one arm or the other of the crosses at every point through which they pass. These curves constitute a grid orthogonal in both forms, before and after deformation: a coordinate system not beholden to features of the forms separately but customized for this particular shape change. The locations at which similarly placed curves intersect, top and bottom, correspond exactly under the interpolated deformation of Figure 5a. The gross deformation is described, like that for the triangles, by the lay of these curves upon the forms, by the principal strains (rates of change of length) and their gradients along the curves, and by the differences of the pair of principal strains at every point (every intersection of curves). In Figure 6, these strains, indicated within the diagram of diastolic form, are the actual contraction ratios, length in systole divided by length in diastole, for the abstract segments upon which they are drawn.

With marker 4 treated as equivalent to all the others (that is, with no freedom to select particularly helpful triangles on subsets of the markers), the transformation no longer presents the aspect of uniform contraction anywhere. Rather, there is clearly indicated a long axis of least contraction, from M at the base to a point between markers 4 and 5. The strain in this direction is graded from a compression of some 30% near the apex (as we saw in the triangles) to expansion near the base. This long axis is one of a system of parallels filling the interior, all showing this same gradient. They are all slightly curved. Perpendicular to these lines are the short-axis curves of greatest contraction, likewise graded from 15%–25% near (but not at) the base to better than 40% near the apex, representing the movement of 4 toward 5 by 44% that we saw in the discrete analysis. Everywhere the little grid rectangles become narrower faster than they become shorter.

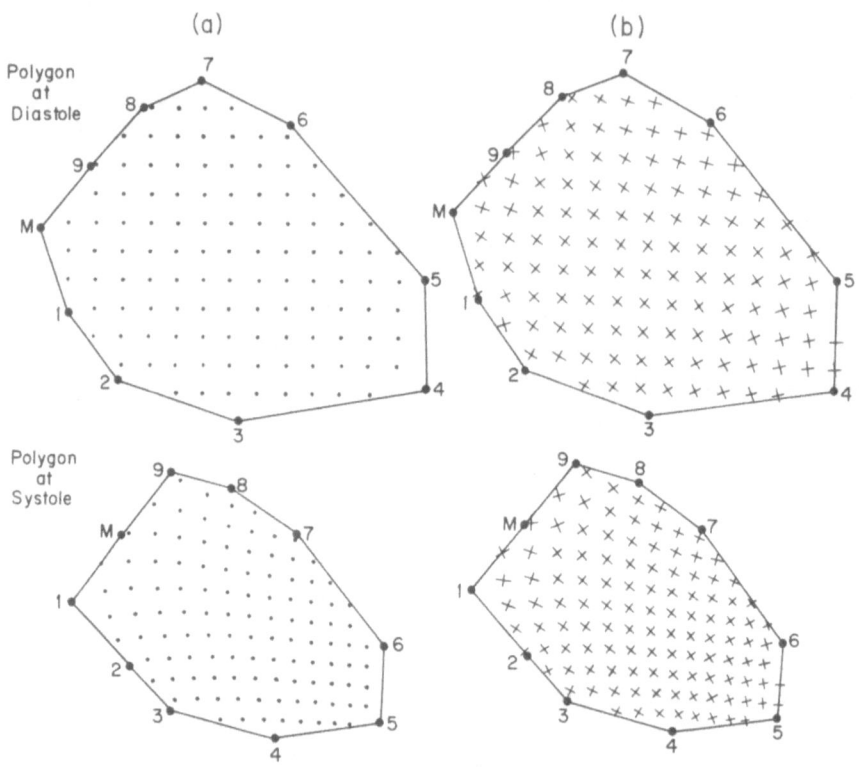

Figure 5. Continuous analysis of change in landmark configurations. (a) The interiors of two polygons may be related by a smooth interpolated non-linear transformation; (b) This transformation has principal strains at every point, computed from the derivative of the mapping in (a).

This smooth biorthogonal description, Figure 6, is as simple as the discrete analysis of Figure 4. Although it uses a quite different geometric language, it is expressing the same observed change of configuration. For instance, marker 4 now appears to participate homogeneously in a shortening of the septal wall 2–4, a shortening less marked than the long-axis shortening along the free wall 7–5; this asymmetry is equivalent to the rotation of the valve ring with respect to the heart axis noted in Figure 4.

Using tensors to characterize cardiac dysfunction

The preceding section invoked two styles of tensor analysis to describe one single cardiac contraction: to show its intrinsic magnitudes and directionality and to suggest measurement schemes and parameters. The tensor fields shown in Figures 3 and 6 are two representations of this single shape change. In the study of cardiac function, however, our interest is concentrated upon *effects upon* these

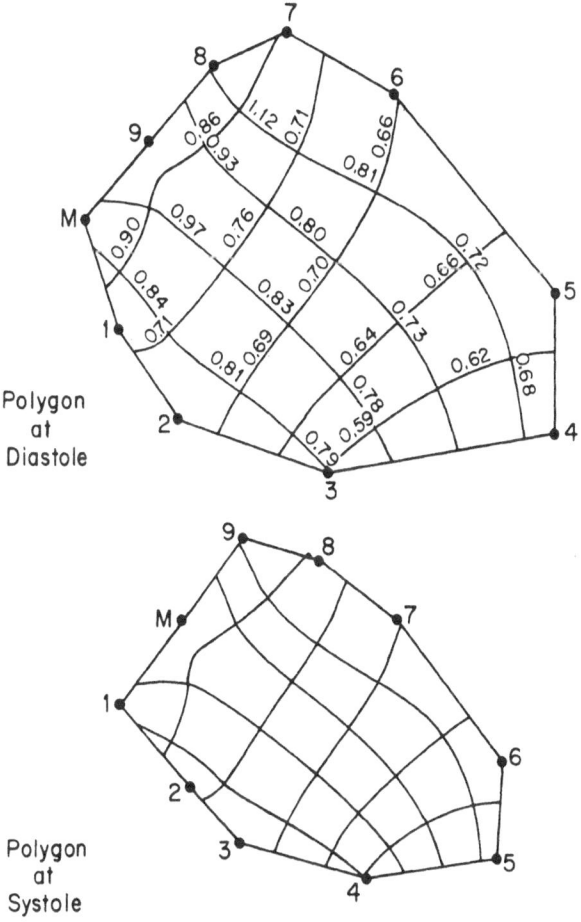

Figure 6. Biorthogonal grids for the transformation implied by the data of Figure 2 (interpolated as in Figure 5), with selected strain ratios.

changes, that is, systematic differences in them across diverse conditions of the heart muscle. The tensor method may be used to study these as well. Just as a single contraction can be represented by a pair of directions at 90° – one along the direction of least relative decrease of length, the other along the direction of the greatest relative decrease – so does a pair of typical contractions, condition A versus condition B, determine a pair of directions nearly at 90°. One is the direction of greatest *excess* of contraction in condition A as compared with condition B, the other the direction of greatest relative *shortfall* of contraction in condition A [4, 8].

I exemplify the comparative tensor method using data from a study-in-progress [12] dealing with experimentally produced occlusions in a canine model. For this example, Dr. Gallagher implanted seven 2-mm lead shot in the left ventricle of a 24-kg adult male dog, along with a balloon occluder about his left circumflex artery. The implants, which we believe were positioned nearly mid-wall, lay

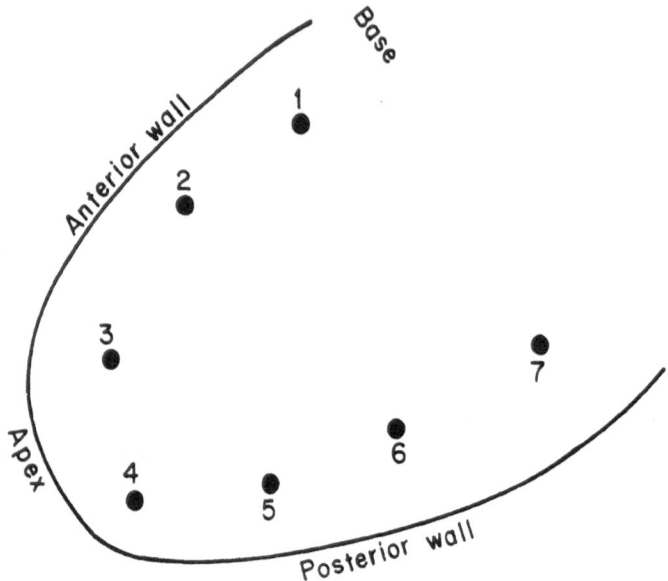

Figure 7. Sketch of the left ventricle of an experimental dog, showing estimated positions of the seven midwall implants used in this study.

approximately in a plane normal to the central beam of the LAO projection direction. They delineated the lower two-thirds of the left ventricle as sketched in Figure 7. With the animal under phenobarbitol sedation, cineroentgenograms were recorded for a few cardiac cycles before, during, and after the inflation of the left circumflex occluder and during and after its release. The complete findings of this study will be reported in detail elsewhere. In the present exposition, the geometry of contraction sixty seconds after the onset of occlusion will be compared with the basal geometry observed prior to occlusion. The data as represented here are averages of three consecutive contractions, from diastole to systole as determined by a consideration of area inside the ventricular contour.

Just as we analyzed the geometry of the normal contraction by two different tensor diagrams – uniform deformation of triangles or continuous deformation of polygons – so we may analyze the effect of occlusion on the geometry of contraction in two separate styles. For the biorthogonal grids of Figures 8 and 10, analysis is of a single composite contraction relating the mean positions of the implants at systole to their mean positions at diastole [9]. The analysis of the single triangle in Figure 12 instead averages the three individual contractions, each diastole to the corresponding systole [4], a calculation that cannot yet be performed for polygons other than triangles.

The contraction of the whole lower two-thirds of this left ventricle is modeled here as a smooth deformation of the polygon bounded by the implants, as in Figure 8. (The artificial straightness of the boundary edge at upper left does not alter the inferences to follow about the effect of occlusion.) In using data from only a single plane cine series, we ignore the rotation and twisting of the implants'

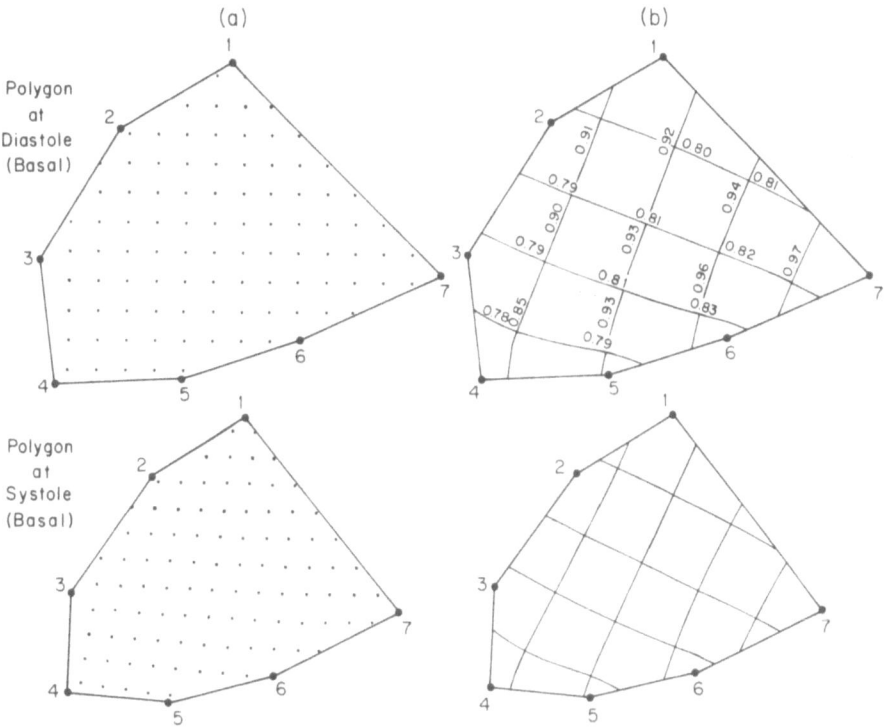

Figure 8. The basal heartbeat, displayed as a deformation of a polygon through the mean positions of the implants at diastole and at systole. (a) The Cartesian grid; (b) The biorthogonal grid pair showing major and minor principal strains.

'plane' during the cardiac contraction, and also the differences between normal and infarcted conditions in the amount of rotation or twist that we are ignoring. This geometrical imprecision should soon be corrected by biplane recording [3]. In this pilot study it is the analytic mode, not anatomical realism, which most interests us.

The basal heartbeat. Figure 8a shows the conventional Cartesian grid (cf. Figure 5a) representing the dog's basal heartbeat as a deformation. In the biorthogonal grid of Figure 8b, this same deformation is expressed by its directions of maximum and minimum contraction. This grid, itself nearly Cartesian, is oriented at some 45° to the direction conventionally taken as the 'axis' of the heart. The principal direction of greater contraction runs approximately northwest-southeast in this figure, with the strain ratios gently graded from 0.78 to 0.83. That is, the lengths at systole of the little elements of mathematical myocardium aligned in this direction have contracted by some 17% to 22% from the lengths they bore at diastole. Perpendicular to this set of curves is a family of directions of least contraction (strain nearer 1.0); this direction runs steadily northeast-southwest and bears a rate of contraction from 5% to 10%, except for the area nearest the apex.

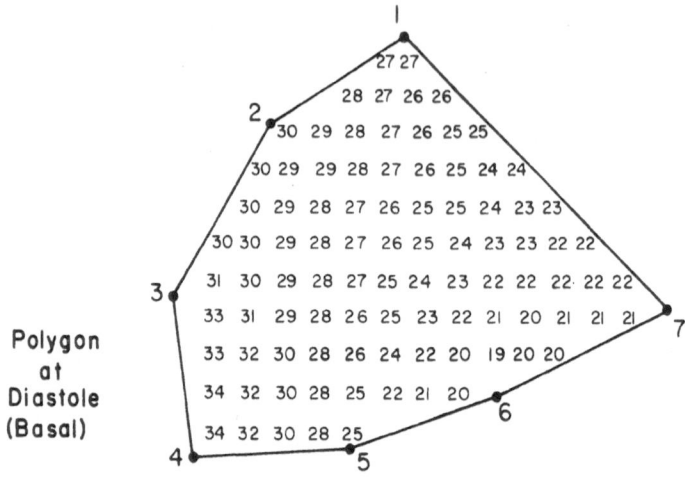

Figure 9. Regional ejection fraction for the basal heartbeat. The quantities of this scalar field are products, point by point, of the two principal strain ratios shown in Figure 8b. Each represents the ratio of an area-element at systole to the corresponding area-element at diastole in this mathematically deforming plane.

The deformation drawn here is, of course, a mathematical abstraction of the real myocardial shape change sampled by those projected implant locations. The (approximate) plane of the polygon represents a section right through the middle of the ventricle. It is filled not with muscle but with blood which flows, rather than deforming, during the cardiac cycle. Yet because the implant locations tell us most of what we need to know about this heartbeat, we gain considerable precision of analysis when we represent the geometry of contraction as a smooth transformation in this way.

For instance, everywhere within the region delimited by the landmarks we may compute a ratio of change in area for each little grid cell, area at systole divided by area at diastole.* There emerges a truly *regional* ejection fraction, a function of position throughout the interior. The field of these proportions is indicated in Figure 9 for the mesh points of Figure 8a. Although we presume uncommonly precise knowledge of the true correspondence of myocardium from diastole to systole – patients do not ordinarily present with a plane of implants – the analysis which results is wholly coordinate-free. It makes no reference to any arbitrary 'center' or 'axis' – it is a mathematical comparison determined solely by the reconfiguration of implants around the boundary of the ventricle, not by their motions in *any* coordinate system.

For the basal contraction geometry of this ventricle, the regional ejection fraction is graded smoothly along the same direction as the principal strain of

---

* Mathematically, this quantity is the determinant of the jacobian derivative of the mapping shown in Figure 8.

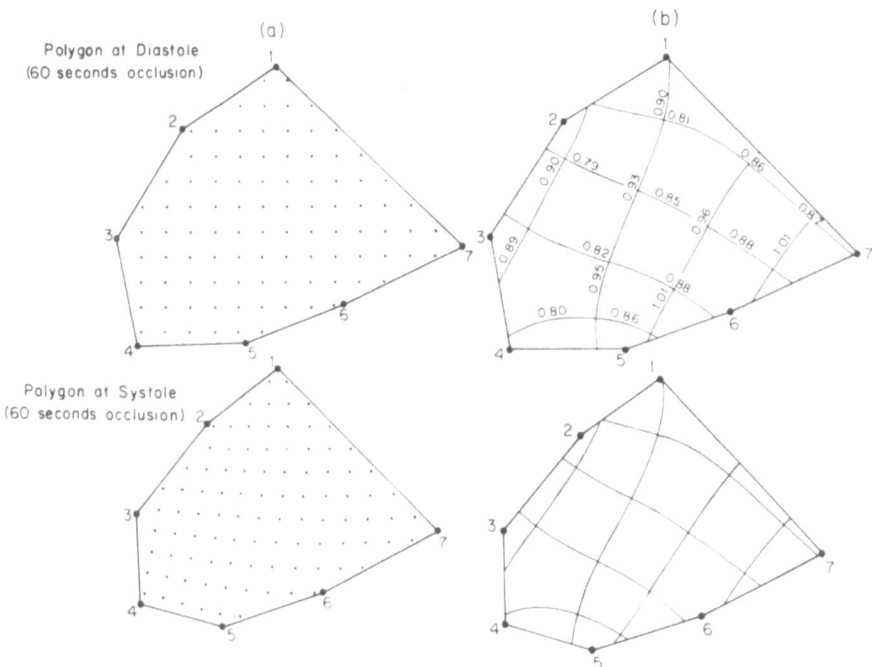

Figure 10. The cardiac contraction 60 s after onset of occlusion, represented as a deformation, diastole to systole, of the polygon through the mean positions of the same implants. (a) The Cartesian grid; (b) The biorthogonal grid pair.

greater contraction. The ratio of change in area is generally some 30% at the septal wall, 20% at the free wall, and peaks at about 34% at the apex. Note that the angle made at the apical implant by the segments joining it to its two nearest neighbors has closed slightly over this contraction.

The ischemic heart. We performed this same biorthogonal analysis for three consecutive cardiac cycles imaged about sixty seconds after the onset of occlusion. The configuration of mean positions of the implants at diastole may be related to that at systole by the smooth deformation shown in Figure 10. This deformation differs from the healthy contraction of Figure 8 in all aspects of the tensor description: both the directions and the magnitudes of the principal strains. We describe these differences in two stages.

The two magnitudes may best be summarized by the regional ejection fractions, which are computed without regard for direction. These, presented in frame (a) of Figure 11, show a rather steep gradient from some 30% at the septal wall of the ventricle to about 10% at the free wall. Because the shape of the ventricle at diastole is not much changed from its basal shape (compare the upper polygon of Figure 10 with that in Figure 8), we can subtract the two ejection fractions, basal from occluded, point by point upon the meshes of Figure 8a or

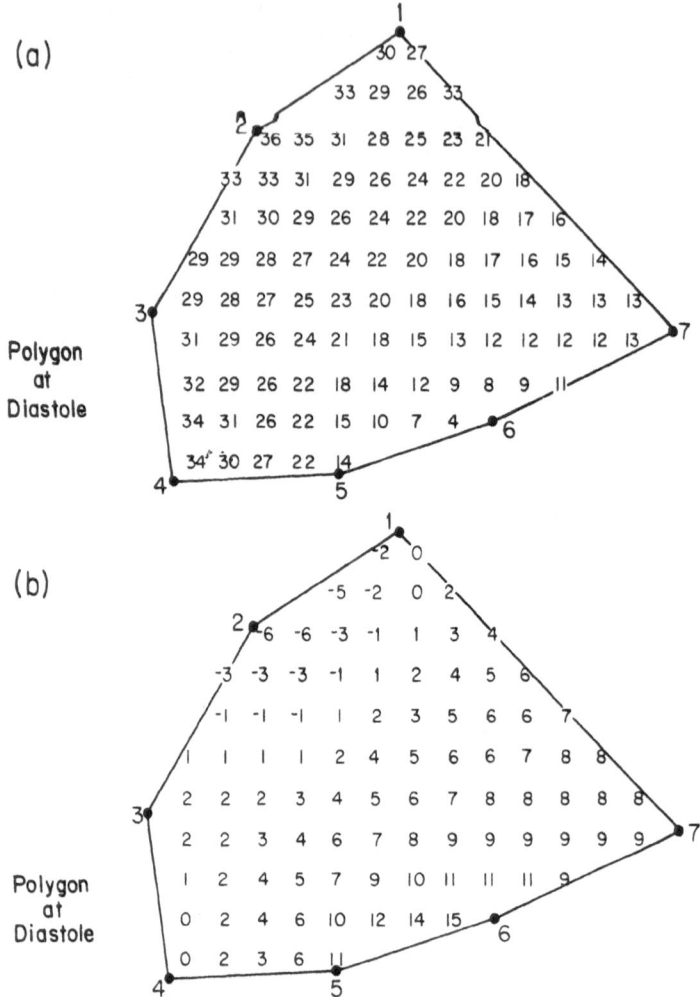

Figure 11. Effect of occlusion on the regional ejection fraction. (a) Regional ejection fraction for the heartbeat of the previous figure; (b) Difference between the fields of (a) and Figure 9: the explicit effect of occlusion upon this mathematical model of ejection.

10a. There results the *map of functional deficit* in Figure 11b, the explicit effect of occlusion on the computed regional ejection fraction.

The difference is clearly largest – that is, the shortfall from normal decrease of area is greatest – near the free wall, the portion of myocardium supplied by the left circumflex artery we occluded. The peak shortfall of 15% is located in the immediate vicinity of implant 6, the very center of the putative ischemic region. There is a hint of compensation by increased contraction along the opposite edge.

Notice that the vertex angle of the implant polygon at implant 4, an angle which closed over the course of the basal contraction, now becomes larger from diastole to systole. This reversal is associated with the unconformity of the grid in its vicinity that may be seen in Figure 10b. Sixty seconds after occlusion, near the apex there is a singularity [11] of the tensor field: a point at which contraction is directionally disorganized, proceeding at the same rate in every direction. Compare the systematic directional dominance of the contraction under the baseline condition as shown in Figure 6 or Figure 8b.

The functional deficit map summarizes changes in amount of contraction between the conditions. Changes in the directions of these contractions are most easily shown by an integrated display in which, as in Figure 3, we represent change as homogeneous over an extended region. The largest triangle we can form from this set of implants is the triangle 1–4–7; its deformations are the subject of Figure 12.

The change in shape of this triangle over the average contraction observed in the three basal beats is shown in panel (a) of the figure. The deformation manifests a major axis of greatest contraction (18%) and a minor axis of least contraction (11%); these vary hardly at all over the three consecutive beats studied. These numbers and directions are quite consistent with the grid of Figure 8b, but bear less information in that regional gradients are ignored.

Figure 12b presents the deformation tensor for the three beats observed after sixty seconds of occlusion. Notice that the principal cross has rotated some 45° upon the form. The least contraction, which used to be at 11% and along the septal wall, now is at 10% and lies along the free wall, at which the ischemia is concentrated. The direction of greatest contraction has also rotated by 45°, and bears a maximum rate of contraction that has dropped from 18% to 15%. Because of the steep regional gradient of change in area, this cross does *not* resemble the regional pattern, Figure 10b, of which it is a strict average.

The difference between these changes may be modelled [4, 8] as a tensor in its own right. It is displayed in Figure 12c by means of its own principal cross: the directions of algebraically greatest and least differences of contraction rate between the conditions. Along one of these directions, aligned loosely with the previous direction of greatest contraction, the net contraction of the myocardium across the ventricle is 7% less after occlusion than before. Another direction, perpendicular to this one and close to the direction bearing the least contraction during the baseline beats, contracts 3% *more* after occlusion than it did at baseline. This tensor thus presents the compensation of contractile failure during the 'adjustment to occlusion' very clearly.

An empirical origin for measurement protocols

The mathematics appropriate for the study of deformation is tensor analysis: coordinate-free consideration of rates of change in all directions, reported in terms of their maxima and minima. This chapter has shown how, when implant data are available, the analysis of the cardiac cycle as a deformation may proceed

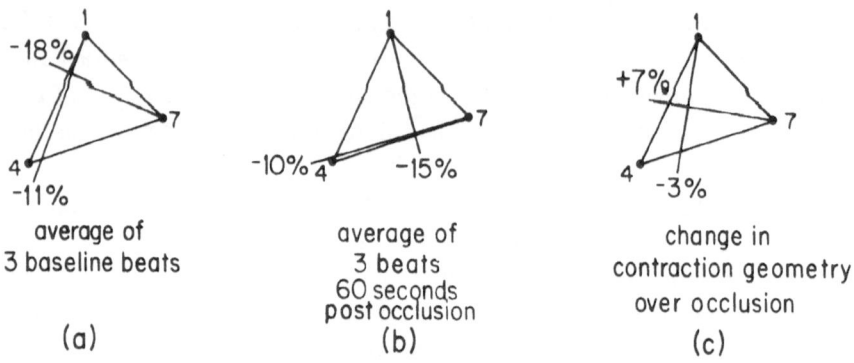

Figure 12. Large-scale analysis of directional differences in contraction geometry, occlusion versus baseline. (a) Baseline contraction of a large triangle of implants, drawn as a single tensor; (b) Observed contraction of the same triangle sixty seconds after occlusion; (c) Effect of occlusion upon the geometry of contraction: the relative tensor showing directional extrema of differences in rate of contraction between the mean deformations of (a) and (b). The principal directions of this relative tensor are not aligned with those of either of the contractions, baseline (a) or occluded (b), separately.

in this classical fashion. The major thrust of this mode of study is not its computation of rates of contraction – a straightforward strategy whatever one's methodological persuasion – but the specification of two particular directions in which those ratios *ought* to be measured. From the tensor analysis of implant data, indeed, we extract instructions for analyzing data taken from the ordinary clinical setting.

Nowhere in the literature of wall motion analysis have I been able to find an earlier assertion of this simple point: a pattern of distances used in studies of left ventricular wall motion ought to have been derived from prior data, data bearing the additional information required if one is to choose those directions rationally. As the primary purpose of this chapter is to sketch the tensor foundation for measurement of wall motion, I shall not review earlier articles dealing with the application of specific coordinate-based schemes in cardiology. Such articles tend to be fully competent in matters of experimental or natural sampling, geometric data collection, and careful statistical method – everything except the rationale for the selection of distances actually measured.

Tensor analyses report the geometry of the heartbeat by reference to particular empirical directions summarizing the motion as observed from implants. Statistical summaries of natural and experimental populations, not explicitly demonstrated in this chapter, likewise proceed in terms of these directions [4]. The conventional methods, however, report the motions of edge-elements by reference to some pre-assigned coordinate system, a center-of-contraction or an axis, toward which the edges are presumed to contract. In the tensor analysis there is no equivalent of such an interior terminus for length measures, but there is a computation of directions bearing the *principal* strains, those which are largest or smallest, and of gradients of these strains across the form.

In what way does the detection of the principal directions constitute a prescription for design of measures? Consider again the effect of occlusion on the shape change of one large triangle of implants, Figure 12c. The experimentally-produced occlusion has induced considerable shortfall of the contraction ratio in one direction (that bearing a relative strain of +7%), but also has induced an *increase* in the contraction ratio in another principal direction (relative strain −3%). These principal directions, of course, are at 90° to each other. There is no reason that the direction of greatest dyskinesis under LCx occlusion should be the same as that representing the pattern of contraction in the baseline condition, before the onset of occlusion. We see from a comparison of Figures 12a and 12c that there has been a rotation of some 20° between the direction of greatest normal contraction and the direction of greatest dyskinetic effect.

Distances measured in intermediate directions will show changes of contraction ratio intermediate between these extremes. For instance, lines at ± 45° to these principal directions will show changes of contraction ratio by the mean of the two principal relative strains, or +2%, from basal to occluded geometry; this difference is clinically negligible. In fact there are two directions near these 45° lines for which the effect of occlusion upon the contraction ratio is precisely zero. If this single canine ventricle is typical, these null directions are fairly close in orientation to the usual long axis of the left ventricle and its perpendicular; therefore, those are not very good directions for measuring the effect of LCx occlusion or detecting its presence.

Directions at ± 45° to the true principal axes begin at 90° but change their *angle* at nearly the fastest rate of any angle measureable upon the implant polygon [10]. Hence the measurement of changes in distances 'along' the null directions, instead of along the principal directions, conceals great tangential components of shear along the (inappropriate) reference axis. In the absence of implant data we cannot verify this shear, but we may surely heed the advice of the implant-based analyses and not make ourselves susceptible to it. The principal directions recommended here for measurement, defined as those of greatest or least rate of contraction, may be equivalently characterized as those directions for which the component of shear perpendicular to the direction measured, the component necessarily ignored in implant-free analysis, tends to be zero [10].

A research program for kinematics of the left ventricle

In this way the findings of a tensor analysis based on implant data may be reinterpreted as instructions for measurements to be made in the absence of implant data. I believe it very important that these instructions be extracted by reanalysis of existing data and clarified by new experiments in animal models, replicating and extending the single canine example reported here. Phrased in terms of such landmarks as can be located – for the long axis, apex and base; for the short axis view, the papillary muscles – these instructions would direct us to measure contraction ratios in particular directions for the optimal detection of particular anomalies. When implant data become available on extensive populations of experimentally modified contractions, the statistical analysis of populations of deformation tensors, which has matured in its other fields of application, can support all the usual biometric inquiries and inferences. For instance [9], the algebraic techniques exist for finding the pattern of distance-measures which best discriminates normal kinematics from wall motion under infarction of various extents in various regions. Distance-measures prescribed for detection of different abnormalities of motion will, in general, be different, as we saw in the example just considered.

Any analysis of a single triangular configuration will find that the distance whose contraction ratio announces the dyskinesis most clearly is measured all the way across the outline of the ventricle, from edge to edge. The restoration of 'sidedness' to this analysis – the measurement of distance 'from an axis' more or less along the midline – corresponds to the presence in the tensor analysis of gradients of relative strain along the curves of the biorthogonal grid. These gradients become visible, as in Figures 8 or 10, whenever the number of implants available for the delineation of areas is four or more [11].

There is little chance that the mode of analysis just demonstrated will be in routine clinical use any time soon. My collaborators A.J. Buda and K.P. Gallagher and I are concentrating our current research on several of the problems which must be resolved first. For instance, the map of functional deficit can be informative in general only if the variability of regional ejection fractions for the 'basal' human heartbeat excludes the sort of highly graded factor of deviation exemplified in Figure 11b. In addition to the distance-based discriminators suggested by straightforward reading of the relative strain tensors, as in the preceding exposition, we must explore the role in diagnosis of other coordinate-free morphometric variables, such as measures of the curvature of the endocardial boundary region by region. (Changes in such quantities are algebraic modifications of the same strain fields that underlie the tensor representation.) And, of course, we must extend the analysis to data in three dimensions. These advances will be driven as well by ongoing applications of the tensor morphometric techniques in other biomedical fields, notably plastic surgery, radiology, craniofacial growth, and embryology.

But these technical difficulties should not obscure the reader's sense of how far we have come. In analysis of the experimentally produced occlusion, the tensor method identified the locus of the perturbation with considerable apparent precision. With hindsight, one can supply amply justification of this success from morphometric theory [8]: the tensor technique is independent of all arbitrary centering rules and thereby is able to make full use of all the information borne by the implant locations. But it also must be the case that the parameters suggested by the tensor analysis – the directions and magnitudes of principal relative strain – are appropriate. descriptors of the heart's actual response to the perturbation which is occlusion. For instance, the clinically crucial components of the discriminatory information – that is, the spatial gradients in the functional deficit map exemplified in Figure 11b – will need to be estimated from whatever data is at hand: if not boundary landmarks then, perhaps, boundary curvature patterns.

If tensor analysis motivates an examination of the foundations of geometric cardiometry, it will have served its purpose. If, further, it engenders increased precision in diagnosis and treatment monitoring of patients with coronary artery disease, it will represent a considerable methodological advance indeed.

Acknowledgements

Preparation of this chapter was supported by NIH grants DE-05410 to Fred L. Bookstein, DE-03610 to R.E. Moyers, and HL-29716 to Andrew J. Buda. The canine experiment of which one fragment is described here was executed by Andrew J. Buda and Kim P. Gallagher at the University of Michigan.

References

1. Skalak R, Dasgupta G, Moss ML, Otten E, Dullemeijer P, Vilmann H: A conceptual framework for the analytical description of growth. J Theor Biol 94: 555–577, 1982.
2. Meier GD, Bove AA, Santamore WP, Lynch PR: Contractile function in canine right ventricle. Am J Physiol 239: H794–H804, 1980.
3. Meier GD, Ziskin MC, Santamore WP, Bove AA: Kinematics of the beating heart. IEEE Transact Biomed Engin 27: 319–329, 1980.
4. Bookstein FL: A statistical method for biological shape comparisons. J Theor Biol 107: 475–520, 1984.
5. Ingels NB Jr, Daughters GT II, Stinson EB, Alderman EL: Left ventricular midwall dynamics in the right anterior oblique projection in intact unanesthetized man. J Biomech 14: 221–233, 1981.
6. Bookstein FL: The measurement of biological shape and shape change. Lecture notes in biomathematics, Vol 24. Springer-Verlag, 1978.
7. Thompson DAW: On growth and form, abr. ed., J.T. Bonner (ed.) The University Press, Cambridge, 1961 (1917, 1942).
8. Bookstein FL: Foundations of morphometrics. Ann Rev Ecol Syst 13: 451–470, 1982.
9. Bookstein FL: Tensor biometrics for changes in cranial shape. Ann Hum Biol 11: 413–437, 1984.
10. Bookstein FL: The geometry of craniofacial growth invariants. Am J Orthod 83: 221–234, 1983.
11. Bookstein FL: Transformations of quadrilaterals, tensor fields, and morphogenesis. In: Antonelli PL (ed.), Mathematical essays on growth and the emergence of form. University of Alberta Press, 1985 (in press).
12. Bookstein L, Gallagher KP, Buda AJ: Mean tensor analysis of left ventricular wall motion. IEEE Computers in Cardiology, 1984 (in press).

7. The analysis of left ventricular function with digital subtraction angiography

G.B. JOHN MANCINI, ANDREW J. BUDA
and CHARLES B. HIGGINS

Imaging of the chambers of the heart, pulmonary circulation and great vessels by intravenous contrast injection was clinically implemented as early as 1939 [1], but it was not until the achievement of relatively recent advances in digital electronics, image intensification and television technology that a major resurgence of interest in this technique occurred. The technicological advances and the pioneering work from the Universities of Kiel, Arizona and Wisconsin provided the basis for the exciting preliminary application of digital subtraction angiography for the assessment of cardiovascular dynamics [2–9]. These results, in turn, initiated a widespread clinical evaluation of the use of this imaging modality in cardiac diagnosis. The purpose of this chapter is to summarize the recent applications of digital subtraction angiography in the quantitative assessment of global and regional left ventricular function.

Technical considerations

Digital fluoroscopy is a technique in which detected X-ray information is converted into digital form so that contrast enhancement and quantitative analysis of the images can be performed. Adequate images of the relatively large ventricular chamber have been obtained by first recording the video signal on videotape and later digitizing and processing the images with the computer. This technique of post-processing, while introducing some noise, has proved to be adequate for assessing left ventricular (LV) function because the LV is a relatively large structure with predictable non-random periodic motion enabling effective frequency filtering of random noise during processing [10, 11]. Ideally, however, the video signals are directly digitized and immediately processed so that the images are not degraded by the introduction of noise. Higher resolution of the LV chamber and of the much smaller and relatively stationary peripheral arteries can be best achieved by direct digitization of the amplified video signal. Currently, the direct video image from a Plumbican television with a 1000:1 signal-to-noise ratio is digitized through a 10-bit analog to digital converter into a digital disc with a 7 megabyte per second storage capacity. A commercial minicomputer which is LSI-23 controlled operating with a 2 megabyte visual memory and a floating point array processor is used for the image manipulation (subtraction, filtering, etc.). The digital data can then be converted by a digital-to-analog converter back into an analog (video) form for display on a video monitor or in a film format.

The capabilities of the image processing computer necessary for evaluating cardiac function are different from those considered optimal for evaluating vascular morphology. Compared to peripheral vessels, the left ventricle is a large structure so that spatial resolution is less critical. Moreover, after intravenous administration of contrast media the heart is a relatively contrast laden structure compared to peripheral arteries so that contrast resolution is also less critical. On the other hand, temporal resolution needs to be considerably greater for evaluation of cardiac function compared to that necessary for depicting vascular morphology. Accordingly, most systems designed for cardiac work provide a temporal resolution of at least 30 frames per second and the spatial resolution obtained with a 256×256 pixel matrix is generally adequate for evaluating the left ventricle.

Technique for clinical studies

For cardiac imaging, the radiation dose per frame can be considerably lower than that required for vascular imaging. Compared to vascular imaging, which mandates X-ray milliamperage (mA) greater than 300, cardiac studies can be performed using either continuous fluoroscopy (60–70 kvp; 7–10 mA) or standard, pulsed cineradiographic exposure levels. In both cases, the radiographic parameters must be constant throughout the entire sequence of image acquisition. Opacification is produced with 30 to 40 ml of iodinated contrast injected intravenously over 1.5–2 s through a catheter positioned in the superior vena cava. The same processes of subtraction and contrast enhancement can be used to advantage in obtaining diagnostic left ventriculograms with very small doses of contrast materials injected directly into the left ventricle. This approach has been successfully used in several centers and will be discussed subsequently.

Subtraction methods

Several different types of subtraction techniques have been used for cardiac studies. Subtraction methods can be divided into two broad categories: temporal (time difference) subtraction and energy (energy difference) subtraction [12]. Temporal techniques include: mask mode subtraction, time interval difference

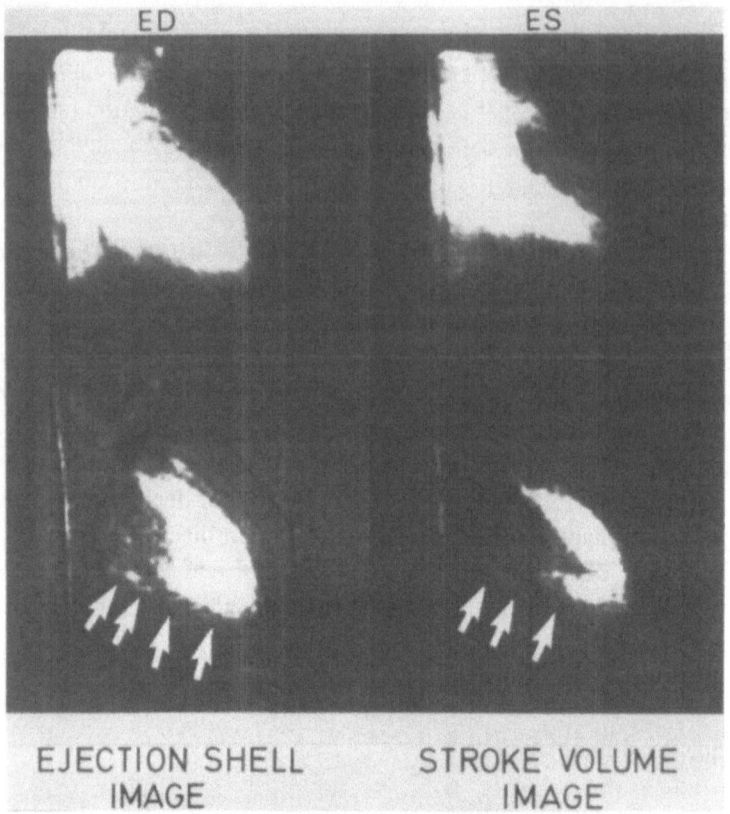

Figure 1. Mask mode images and functional images from a patient with inferior akinesis. The ejection shell and stroke volume images graphically display this abnormality (arrows). (Reproduced with permission from Mancini *et al.*, Cardiovasc Intervent Radiol 6: 252–262, 1983.)

(TID) subtraction, and functional subtraction. Temporal techniques are critically sensitive to motion (breathing, coughing, etc.). Since the time separation between image frames is greatest for mask mode subtraction, motion degradation occurs most frequently with this, but can be alleviated by remasking, pixel shifting and rotating programs now available with image processing computers.

In mask mode subtraction (Figure 1) the digitized data from peak opacified frames is subtracted from single or averaged frames of the same area before the arrival of the contrast media. Overlying non-vascular structures that do not contain contrast material at the instant when the cardiac structure is maximally opacified are erased from the image, thereby improving the visibility of faintly opacified vascular structures.

Another form of subtraction is time interval difference subtraction (TID). In TID subtraction the sets of frames subtracted from each other all contain contrast media but are separated only slightly in time. Consequently, the resultant subtracted image (TID image) is a display of the difference in contrast levels between the two sets of frames. In this way, all stationary elements in the field of view are still suppressed, and an image that provides an indication of instantaneous changes in contrast levels throughout the ventricle during the cardiac cycle is produced (Figure 2). An advantage of this method is that non-recurrent or non-cyclical motion due to slight patient motion is seen only briefly, and the brief motion artifact does not degrade the entire image sequence.

An important type of subtraction used to evaluate left ventricular contraction is functional subtraction [13]. Functional subtraction can be accomplished by taking the mask mode image at end-diastole and end-systole and subtracting one from the other. The end-diastolic and end-systolic images can be selected by reference to a computer generated transmission vs. time curve. An ejection shell image is created by subtracting the end-systolic (ES) from the end-diastolic (ED) image and a functional paradox image is created by subtracting the ED from the ES image (Figures 1, 3).

Assessment of left ventricular dimensions and ejection fraction

Experimental studies

The reliability and accuracy with which digital intravenous ventriculography can be used to quantify cardiac function has been investigated in several experimental canine studies. Carey *et al.* [14] examined the relationship between cardiac output measurements obtained by the thermodilution technique compared to heart rate and stroke volume measurements determined from digital intravenous ventriculograms in dogs. They found a high correlation (p = 0.89) between these two measurements of cardiac output. Slutsky *et al.* [15] compared LV volume measurements from mask mode images and non-subtracted ventricular images with thermodilution and sonomicrometer measurements. In this study the beat analyzed was identical for both the direct contrast and mask mode images, the only difference being the data manipulation used to obtain the final digital image. They found that the mask mode images correlated well with the direct contrast images, although the mask mode images consistently underestimated the direct contrast images by approximately 12% accounting for smaller stroke volume measurements. These results suggest that the image processing technique may slightly alter quantitative measurements. Several clinical studies [16, 17] noted similar results using different mask mode subtraction processes and different imaging systems. On the other hand, other clinical studies have not found this [18, 19]. However, except for the study of Vas *et al.* [16], most clinical studies have not analyzed the identical beat pre- and post-processing.

A further contribution of the study of Slutsky *et al.* [15] was the demonstration of a high correlation (r = 0.91) between LV end-diastolic and end-systolic volumes determined by area-length analyses of digital ventriculograms and vol-

88

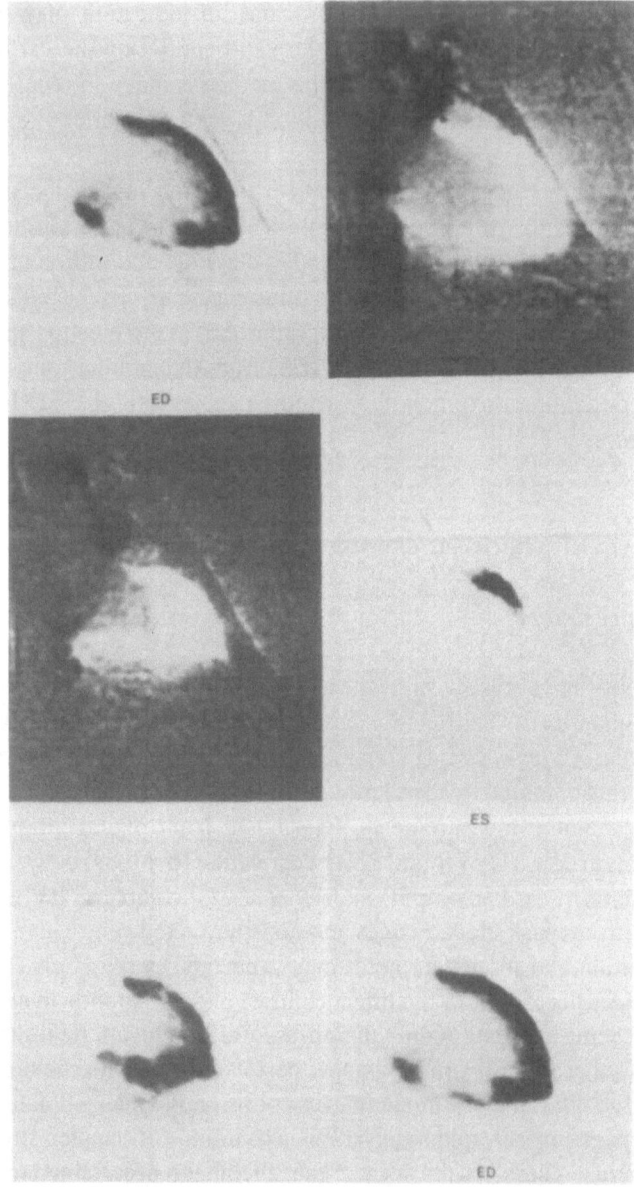

Figure 2. Selected frame from a digital intravenous ventriculogram processed by the time-interval-difference (TID) technique. This patient had a right coronary occlusion and hypokinesis of the inferobasal wall. In addition, early relaxation of the anterior wall (ES frame) is seen. These phase differences in systolic and diastolic wall motion are readily demonstrated by this technique. ED = end-diastole; ES = end-systole. (Reproduced with permission from Higgins *et al.*, Radiology 144: 461–469, 1982.)

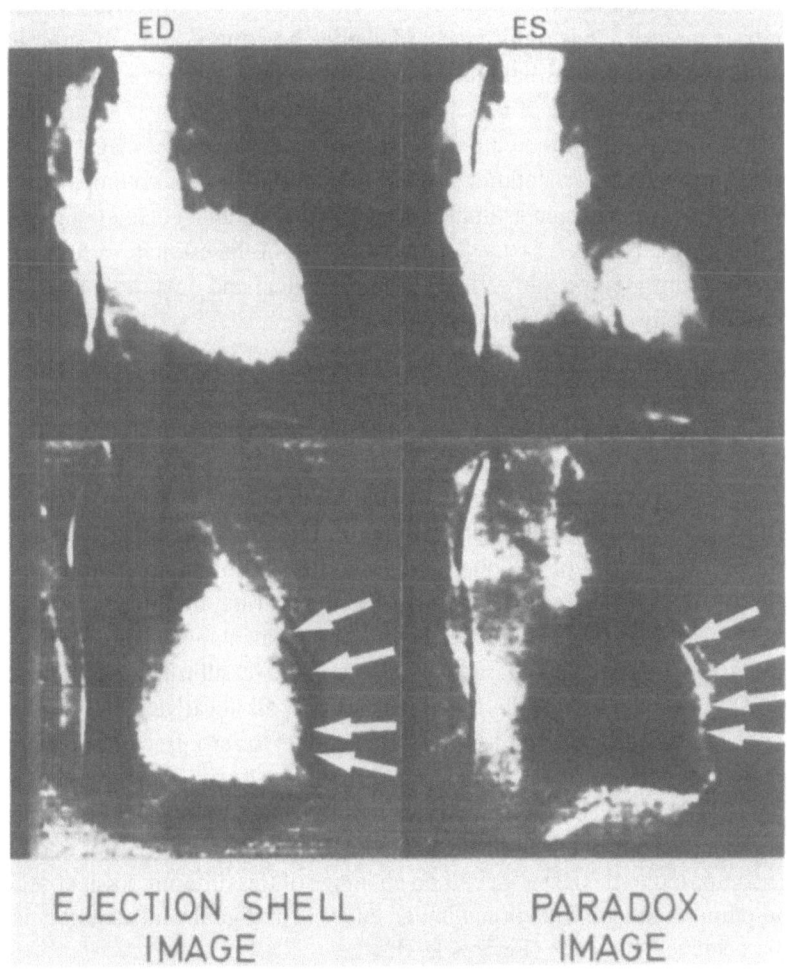

Figure 3. Mask mode and functional images in a patient with occlusion of the left anterior descending artery. The ejection shell image shows no excursion of the antero-apical segments, whereas the paradox image displays dyskinesis in this area. (Reproduced with permission from Mancini *et al.*, Cardiovasc Intervent Radiol 6: 252–262, 1983.)

umes determined by a non-imaging, independent method. The latter volumes were obtained by measuring the major and minor axes of the LV with ultrasonic dimension crystals. The sonomicrometer crystals provided a measurement of the long axis and only one minor axis of the LV, so that it might be anticipated that the correlation between volume measured in this fashion and volumes derived from the digital images might be decreased in the presence of regional contraction abnormalities.

Radkte *et al.* [20] used direct intraventricular injections of contrast material in pigs to determine the ability of biplane digital techniques to visualize not only the endocardial contour of the opacified ventricle but also the myocardial perfusion of contrast material. The outer myocardial edge was thus visible. By subtracting the volume of the endocardial outline from the volume of the epicardial outline, an estimate of the volume of muscle could be obtained. This was determined by videodensitometry from the end-diastolic and the end-systolic images and compared to post-mortem calculations of left ventricular muscle volume. The end-systolic angiocardiographic estimate of myocardial volume correlated best with the post-mortem results ($r = 0.938$, standard error of the estimate = 5.9 ml). An extension of this method allowed this group to detect and quantitate myocardial perfusion deficits caused by infarction.

Further animal experimentation has demonstrated that the measurement of free wall thickening from digital fluoroscopic images during the cardiac cycle in response to inotropic stimulation and ischemia closely approximates ultrasonic crystal measurements ($r = 0.98$) [21].

Alternative approaches to regional wall motion detection in response to ischemia have been used by several laboratories [6, 13]. Gerber *et al.* [13] were able to quantitate the severity of regional, ischemic dysfunction in a canine model by calculation of regional area displacement and the average amplitude of excursion of the anterior and postero-inferior walls. These calculations were made from functional ejection shell and paradox images created by subtracting end-diastolic and end-systolic images. In the functional images, all negative pixels (algebraic sign opposite that arbitrarily set as positive) were set to zero. Because all negative pixels in the functional image were set to zero, an image showing motion of a LV segment was observed on the ejection shell only when that segment was larger on the ED compared to the ES image. Likewise, if a segment was larger on the ES image compared to the ED image, then an image of this difference was contained on the paradox image. Functional image analysis of digital ventriculograms can also be achieved clinically (Figures 1, 3).

Clinical studies

Digital intravenous ventriculography. The clinical application of digital angiography has generally paralleled the animal studies outlined above in an effort to determine the potential clinical utility, accuracy and limitations of this technique in the evaluation of patients with coronary artery disease. In particular, several studies have now compared intravenous digital subtraction angiography and direct contrast left ventriculography for quantitative cardiac assessment.

The early report of Vas *et al.* [16] included four patients studied by both techniques. End-diastolic, end-systolic and ejection fraction measurements were very similar, but the venous-injected images showed a 2 to 7% systematic underestimation of volumes, probably related mainly to the subtraction and contrast enhancement process.

Tobis *et al.* [22] studied 27 patients by both techniques in which the two studies were separated by 24 hours. End-diastolic volumes and ejection fractions correlated well (r = 0.82 and r = 0.96, respectively) and without systematic errors. End-systolic volumes correlated very well (r = 0.93) with only a small systematic underestimation.

Kronenberg *et al.* [17] also showed high correlations between the techniques for volume and ejection fraction calculations (r = 0.91 and r = 0.89, respectively). Of interest in this study systematic underestimation of volumes was noted in the processed intravenous images, but not in similarly processed images produced by low-dose intraventricular injection of contrast. The authors suggest that these differences may have been due to the fainter borders seen on the intravenous studies and errors on estimating valve plane location, or both.

Goldberg *et al.* [18] showed very high correlations between the intravenous digital technique and direct contrast ventriculography in 31 patients (end-diastolic volume, r = 0.96; end-systolic volume, r = 0.97; ejection fraction, r = 0.98). No systematic errors were noted. This group was uniformly successful in obtaining diagnostic images of the left ventricle in the 30 degree right anterior oblique projection, even in patients with an ejection fraction less than 30%. This was not the experience of Tobis *et al.* [22] who were unable to adequately visualize the left ventricle by the intravenous injection method when the ejection fraction was very low. These latter authors suggest that imaging in the left anterior oblique projection may obviate this problem, whereas Goldberg's group points out that a more rapid (1.5 s) bolus injection into a central vein may still allow adequate left ventricular imaging, even in the right anterior oblique projection and despite a low ejection fraction.

Norris *et al.* [23] demonstrated comparable correlative results (end-diastolic volumes, r = 0.88; end-systolic volumes, r = 0.89; ejection fraction, r = 0.81), but volumes appeared to be systematically underestimated compared to direct left ventriculography (Figure 4). Although the cause of this disparity remains speculative for this study and those of other groups, it may partially represent a loss of sensitivity of edge detection caused by the lesser density differential between the diluted opacified blood nearest the endocardium in comparison with the soft tissue density of myocardial muscle.

Felix *et al.* [24] studied 46 patients with coronary artery disease who had direct ventriculography and digital subtraction angiography studies separated by a mean of approximately 3 months. Very high correlations were obtained for ejection fractions (r = 0.938), end-diastolic volumes (r = 0.979) and end-systolic volumes (r = 0.925). They reported a systematic overestimation of end-systolic volumes when the ejection fraction was less than 36%. This led to consistently lower ejection fraction results from the digital studies compared to the direct cineventriculograms when the ejection fraction was depressed to this extent. This study included a relatively large proportion of patients with a depressed ejection fraction but no specific difficulty in studying these patients was reported. In fact, they concluded that intravenous digital subtraction ventriculography was more

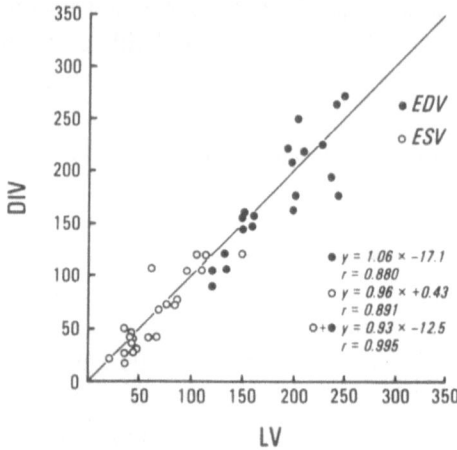

Figure 4. Left ventricular volumes in patients as determined by digital intravenous ventriculography (DIV) are plotted against the volumes determined by direct left ventriculography (LV). EDV = end-diastolic volumes; ESV = end-systolic volumes. (Reproduced with permission from Norris *et al.* [23].)

sensitive than cineventriculography because of more homogeneous and complete opacification of the apical areas with the intravenous technique and the ability to enhance the contrast of the images.

Nissen *et al.* [25] recently evaluated 40 patients, including 21 with prior mycardial infarctions. They showed very similar correlations compared to prior studies (end-diastolic volumes, $r = 0.88$; end-systolic volumes, $r = 0.92$; ejection fraction, $r = 0.93$). Technically adequate studies were obtained in all patients, including patients which had ejection fractions of 50% or less. However, they experienced some difficulty with edge definition in certain cases due to persistent right ventricular or left atrial opacification. This problem was most common in the setting of a low cardiac output or right ventricular failure, and it led to significant discrepancies in individual cases in volume measurements between the direct and digital intravenous ventriculograms. These findings are congruent with those of other groups, and they were encountered despite the fact that a rapid central venous injection of contrast (30 cc over 1 s) was used.

All of the previous investigations used mask mode imaging as the primary subtraction technique, whereas Engels *et al.* [26] reported ventricular assessments in 20 patients using time-interval-difference processing of digital intravenous ventriculograms. Absolute volumes were not reported, and their study included only patients with ejection fractions greater than 50%. Ejection fraction determined from the time-interval-difference images correlated with direct left ventriculography with an r value of 0.81.

The cited studies demonstrate that ventricular volumes and ejection fractions can be obtained from digital intravenous ventriculograms with a sufficiently high level of accuracy to make the technique diagnostically useful. Furthermore, the experience regarding the study of patients with depressed contractile function has not been uniformly unsuccessful. Although more investigation is needed, it appears that this subgroup can be adequately studied as long as there is optimization of the contrast injection, subtraction and enhancement techniques, and that alternate views are considered.

Low dose intraventricular digital angiography. Because the intraventricular and intravenous injection of ionic contrast materials can induce toxic effects and substantial hemodynamic derangements [27, 28], a practical use of digital subtraction angiography is in the study of left ventricular function through intraventricular injection of very small doses of contrast. Several groups have shown that through mask mode subtraction and contrast enhancement provided by digital subtraction angiography, diagnostic ventriculograms can be obtained that provide accurate quantitative assessments of left ventricular function.

Sasayama *et al.* [19] studied 16 patients with normal sized ventricles by obtaining ventriculograms in a conventional manner and also by digitally processing ventriculograms obtained with a 5 cc direct, intraventricular injection of contrast. Applying an automatic edge detection algorithm [29] and area-length techniques to both of the ventriculograms, they demonstrated excellent correlations between end-diastolic and end-systolic volumes measured by each technique (r = 0.95 and 0.98, respectively). The very small contrast injection provided adequate opacification only after subtraction and contrast enhancement. Furthermore, in order to ensure optimal mixing of contrast with blood, patients with large ventricles were excluded from the study, and the injection of contrast was initiated at the rapid filling phase of diastole by an electrocardiogram-triggered injector.

Kronenberg *et al.* [17] used 5 to 10 ml injections of contrast medium and compared ventricular volume measurements with conventional direct left ventriculography in 12 patients. They reported a technically inadequate image in one patient with a very large, poorly contracting ventricle studied with a direct injection of 5 ml of contrast. Otherwise, they showed a high correlation of volume measurements and ejection fractions from high dose and low dose ventriculograms (r = 0.96 and 0.91, respectively) but separate correlations for end-diastolic and end-systolic volumes were not given.

Nichols *et al.* [30] performed a similar study but used 7 ml of ionic contrast diluted in 43 cc of saline which was injected at 15 ml/s for three seconds. Despite an effective framing rate of only 10 frames per second for the digital studies, they showed high correlations between volumes from digital ventriculograms and conventional studies but not unexpectedly, the standard estimates of error were particularly high (23.4 cc for end-diastolic volume, 15.4 cc for end-systolic volume). Nevertheless, the dilution of small amounts of contrast allowed them to inject larger volumes over a longer period of time, thus providing better opacification than with small, rapidly injected doses of undiluted contrast. Furthermore, this group was able to obtain diagnostic studies even in patients with low ejection fractions and large ventricular volumes.

Tobis *et al.* [31] used 10 ml because of inconsistent visualization with 5 ml injections. Even with this higher, undiluted dose they were able to show only a modest correlation between conventional and low-dose ventriculograms in measuring end-diastolic volumes (r = 0.77), although end-systolic volumes showed a better correlation (r = 0.95). Inadequate opacification of the ventricle would be expected to cause indistinct visualization of the ventricular margins that are difficult to outline and that would predispose to random errors in volume measurements depending on the unpredictable effects of intraventricular streaming of contrast. These problems might have been compounded in this study since Tobis *et al.* [31] studied patients with generally larger ventricles than those included in the study of Sasayama *et al.* [19]. Nichols *et al.* [30] suggest that a more generally applicable technique for low contrast dose imaging of the left ventricle would be to use small doses of contrast media diluted in larger volumes. In the authors' experience adequate images can be obtained in almost all patients with 10 cc of contrast diluted 1:1 in saline and injected at 10 cc/s for 2 s (Figure 5).

Despite the different low-dose injection protocols listed above, all four groups demonstrated a consistent lack of hemodynamic perturbations in response to low-dose direct digital ventriculography. It is anticipated that this application of digital subtraction angiography will allow safer examinations of a variety of patients including those with pre-existing renal disease; diabetes, multiple myeloma, aortic stenosis, unstable angina or poor ventricular function. Furthermore, Tobis *et al.* [32] have demonstrated that such low-dose digital ventriculography techniques can be used to advantage when attempting to assess the effects of interventions, such as atrial pacing, on global and regional ventricular function. It should be realized, however, that if one were to use repeated doses of greatly diluted contrast material for such studies, the volume load of the diluent may be detrimental in patients with impaired ventricular function.

Clinical assessment of regional wall motion

Although regional left ventricular function is of great importance in the assessment of coronary disease and although digital ventriculography lends itself readily to the quantitative assessment of this parameter, it is surprising how little attention has been focused on the quantitation of regional wall motion by this new technique. Instead, most studies have analyzed wall motion on a qualitative basis and compared the results from digital ventriculograms to similar analyses of direct contrast left ventriculograms. The interobserver variability of such assessments is known to be quite marked [33, 34]. No method of quantitative wall motion assessment is presently accepted universally, because there are known limitations of each specific method of wall motion analysis [35–37]. However, an

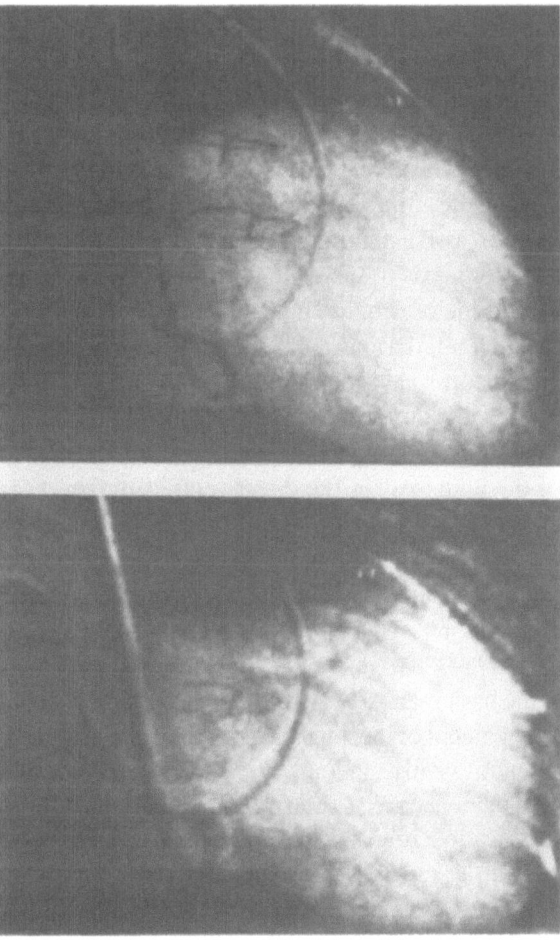

Figure 5. End-diastolic (upper) and end-systolic (lower) frames of a direct left ventriculogram obtained with a 50% solution of sodium meglumine diatrizoate delivered at 10 cc per second for 2 s in a cardiac transplantation candidate. The patient experienced no discomfort or dyspnea despite a greatly elevated end-diastolic pressure prior to ventriculography. No significant hemodynamic changes ensued. The ejection fraction of the patient was 6%. (Reproduced with permission from Mancini, New concepts in cardiac imaging, G.K. Hall Medical Publishers, in press.)

attempt at objective quantitation is of particular importance if interventions are to be accurately studied and digital ventriculography is well suited for such assessments on a rapid and routine basis.

Nichols *et al.* [30] analyzed quantitative wall motion by measuring percent chordal shortening of hemiaxes in 28 patients. They compared low-dose, intra-ventricular digital left ventriculograms and direct contrast left ventriculograms on a regional basis. The percent chordal shortening obtained by these two methods correlated moderately well ($r = 0.81$), however, the analysis was impaired by an effective framing rate of only ten frames per second for the digital studies, a rate that is inadequate for accurate assessment of regional wall motion.

Mancini *et al.* [38] studied regional wall motion in 45 patients by a radial shortening technique applied to digital intravenous ventriculograms and direct left ventriculograms. Because the digital left ventriculogram was obtained from the levophase of the intravenous contrast injection, the left atrium, the basal portion of the LV and the aorta were simultaneously opacified and, therefore, the ususal landmarks for assignment of the major axis of the LV were obscured. Consequently, the long axis of the digital ventriculogram was taken as the line joining the apex and the centroid of the end-diastolic frame. For analysis of the direct left ventriculogram, the long axis of the end-diastolic frame was taken from the mid-point of the aortic valve plane to the apex. Furthermore, because of the difficulties in defining the mitral and aortic valve planes, the computer-generated centroid of the end-diastolic image was generally located closer to the apex than the midpoint of the long axis for the direct ventriculogram. For these reasons, normal ranges for radial shortening were expected to be different for the two techniques and thus were established for each technique. Using these quantitative criteria to define normal or abnormal wall motion, agreement in assessing wall motion was found in 87% (274 of 315 segments). Disparities in wall motion assessment occurred in 13% (41 of 315 segments). Eighteen of these 41 discrepancies occurred in the basilar and apical radii which are known to be quite variable, are sensitive to assignment of the long axis and which are obscured (basal radii) in the digital intravenous ventriculogram.

Nissen *et al.* [25] demonstrated a similar concordance rate (91%) in quantitative wall motion classification from intravenous digital ventriculograms and direct ventriculograms. This group used a regional area reduction method of objective wall motion analysis.

Quantitative wall motion analyses of time-interval-difference images were reported by Engels *et al.* [26]. Although the specific method of analysis was not stated, a high correlation for quantitative assessment of the anterior and apical walls ($r = 0.89$) was reported, whereas inferior wall motion from the digital images correlated poorly ($r = 0.62$) with the direct cineventriculograms. This problem was attributed to difficulty in separating this region from the diaphragm [39], but the reason why this should be a problem was not clearly stated.

Aside from the geometric approach to wall motion analysis outlined above, parametric images of the LV can be produced in which the relative amplitude of contraction of the pixels making up the LV region can be displayed at video gray levels proportional to the amplitude of contraction. For these images, amplitude is derived from the first harmonic of the Fourier analysis of the X-ray transmission vs. time curve for each pixel of the left ventricular region of interest. Similarly, parametric images can be generated in which phase of contraction of various segments relative to each other can be displayed [40, 41]. These images provide a measure of the phase angle between onset of contraction of a specific pixel and the QRS complex of the ECG. The phase analysis images show the synchronicity of contraction of the LV. Since myocardial depression and ischemia are associated with loss of synchrony, these images may be useful in quantitating the severity of LV dysfunction. A series of phase images from a normal patient is shown in Figure 6. A similar series from a patient with occlusion of the left anterior descending coronary artery is shown in Figure 7.

Widmann *et al.* [41] were able to identify quantitative, regional differences in the standard deviation of the phase angle histograms obtained from anterior, apical and inferior left ventricular regions of interest determined from digital intravenous ventriculograms. Ischemic segments showed a higher standard deviation (greater asynchrony) than normal segments.

The optimal method of quantitative analysis of such images and the value and accuracy of these images has not yet been defined [42]. Furthermore, both amplitude and phase analysis images are critically dependent on homogeneous ventricular opacification which cannot be achieved with direct contrast injection. For complete mixing, contrast must be injected proximal to the left ventricle in the right-sided circulation.

Ventricular function in response to ischemic stress

Mask mode digital ventriculography does not lend itself readily to assessments of ventricular function during exercise because of patient motion and consequent misregistration artifacts. Some workers, however, have reported that this is feasible [43, 44]. Time-interval-difference imaging [6, 26] is less affected by patient motion and, thus, might appear more suitable for this purpose; however, no experience with this method of exercise assessment has been published.

Induction of ischemia by atrial pacing is ideally suited to digital techniques because of lack of patient motion. Several groups have studied this approach with excellent results [32, 38, 45, 46]. Mancini *et al.* [45] demonstrated that in most coronary patients pacing caused a more severe regional contraction abnormality or unmasked a new contraction abnormality. Twenty-two patients (5 normal and 17 CAD patients) had DSA studies of the left ventricle at a control stage and after atrial pacing until the onset of angina or a maximal rate of 160 beats/min [38, 45]. Cessation of pacing was timed to coincide with the appearance of the intravenous bolus of contrast in the left atrium. The digital ventriculogram was obtained within four to seven beats post-pacing when the ischemic response was most likely to be maximal [44–49]. Ninety-one percent of patients with normal resting wall motion showed a quantitative deterioration in regional wall motion, while a smaller number showed deterioration in ejection fraction (Figures 8, 9). Thus, assessment of regional function during stress increased the sensitivity of digital intravenous ventriculography for detection of patients with significant coronary disease. Similar results were reported by Tobis *et al.* [32] and Johnson *et al.* [46].

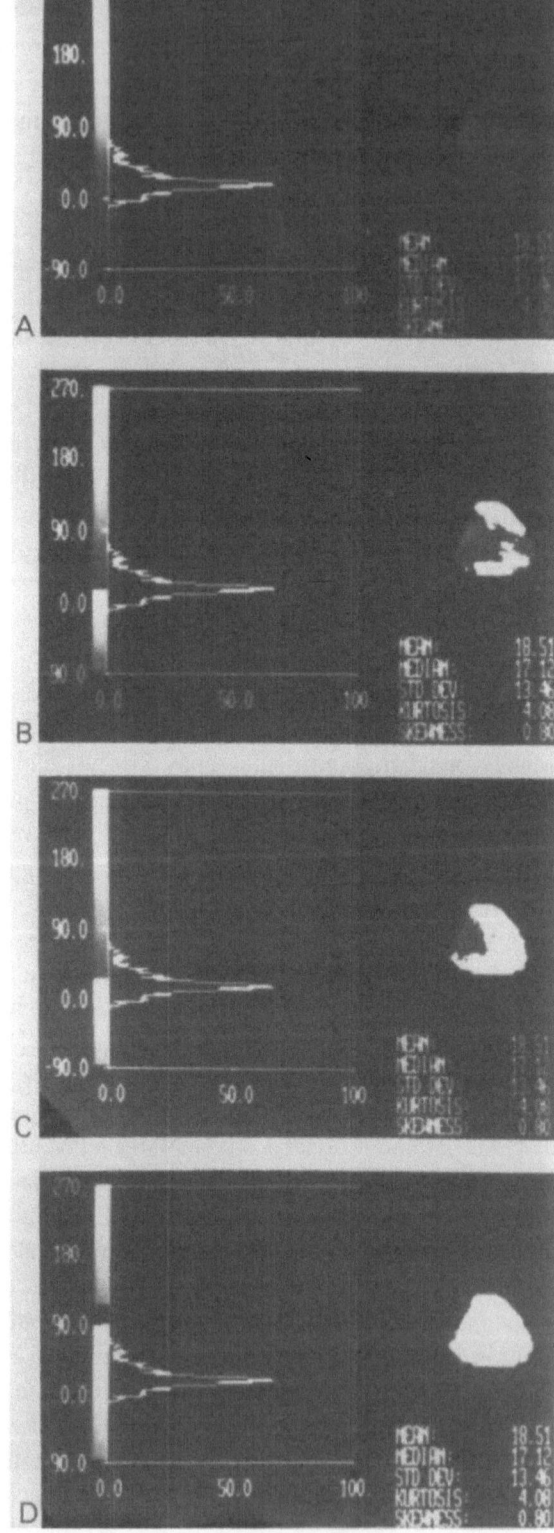

Figure 6. Phase images and quantitative phase histogram in a normal patient. Images correspond to an area of interest at end-diastole (A), early systole (B), midsystole (C), and end-systole (D). Onset of contraction is relatively synchronous in the various left ventricular segments. (Reproduced with permission from Mancini *et al.,* Cardiovasc Intervent Radiol 6: 252–262, 1983.)

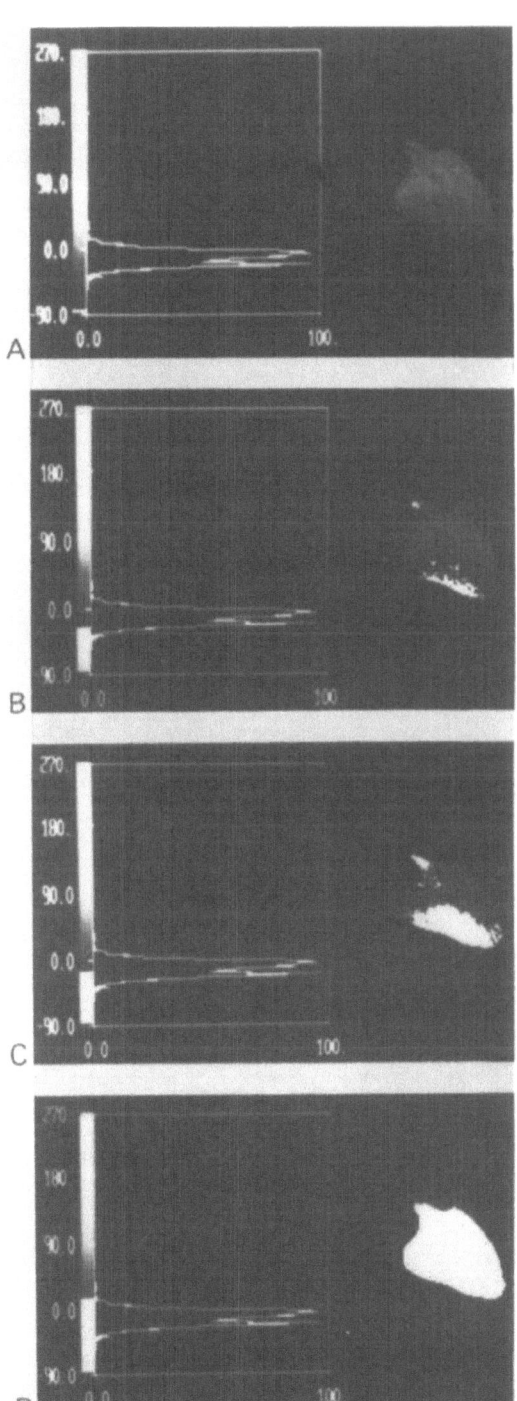

Figure 7. Phase images and quantitative phase histogram in a patient with a high-grade stenosis of the left anterior descending coronary artery. Format of images is the same as in Figure 8. There is delayed onset of contraction in the ischemic anterolateral segment. (Reproduced with permission from Mancini *et al.*, Cardiovasc Intervent Radiol 6: 252–262, 1983.)

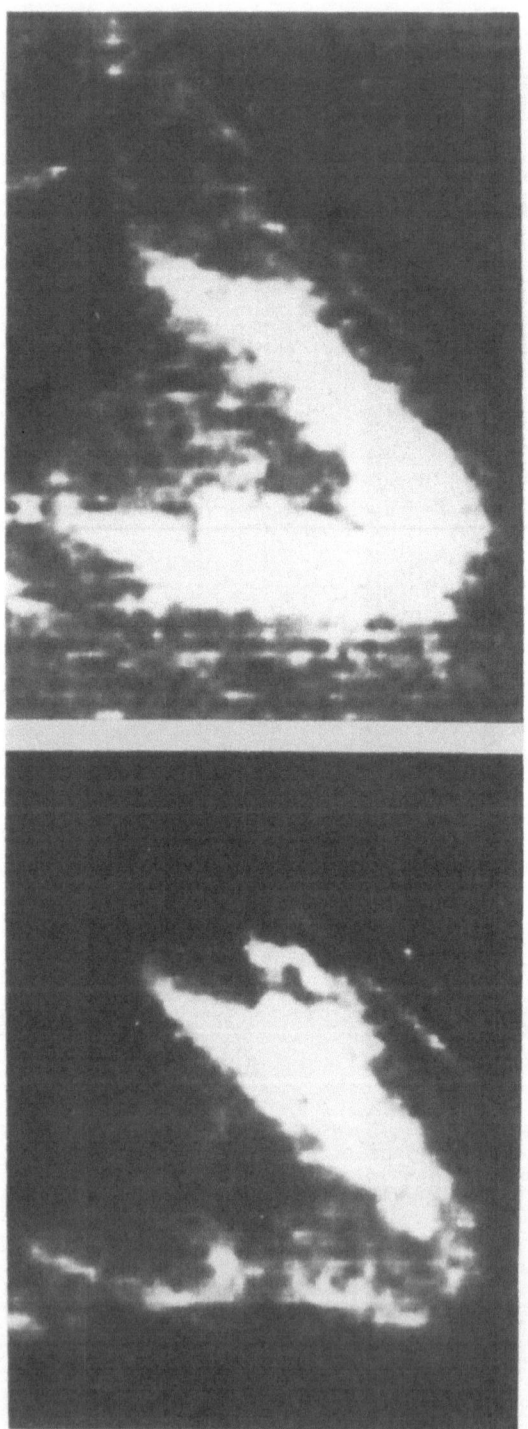

Figure 8. Control (upper) and post-pacing (lower) ejection shell images demonstrate normal wall motion at rest (uniform white rim in the anterior, apical and diaphragmatic regions), but akinesis of the diaphragmatic region (absence of white rim) after pacing induced ischemia. (Reproduced with permission from Mancini *et al.* [45].)

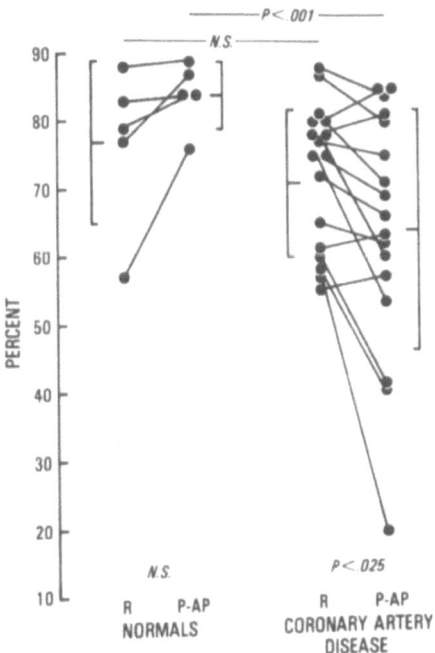

Figure 9. Ejection fraction at rest (R) and post-atrial pacing (P-AP) in normal subjects and patients with coronary disease. Coronary patients showed a significant fall in the post-pacing ejection fraction determined from mask mode, digital intravenous ventriculograms. (Reproduced with permission from Mancini *et al.* [45].)

Pharmacological methods of inducing ischemic stress, the cold-pressor test and hand-grip methods are probably also suitable alternatives to exercise (and atrial pacing), because no patient motion is involved. The results of several centers using exercise stress and post-exercise digital intravenous ventriculograms [43, 44], are also quite encouraging. These efforts, perhaps in conjunction with respiratory gating, merit further clinical trials.

Relative merits of intravenous digital ventriculography and direct, low-dose digital ventriculography

The primary advantages of digital intravenous ventriculography over direct low-dose digital ventriculography are the avoidance of arterial cannulation, virtual absence of arrthythmias during the left ventricular imaging phase of contrast transit and relatively homogeneous opacification of the left ventricle. The latter two conditions are of critical importance for wall motion analysis, generation of parametric images and potential application of videodensitometric techniques in determination of ventricular volumes. These conditions are not met when direct

LV injections are used. The relative lack of invasiveness make the method of potential use in outpatient settings, especially in conjunction with low, fluoroscopic exposure levels.

The principal advantages of direct digital ventriculography are the low doses of contrast required, the ability to safely perform repeated ventriculography and the ability to safely study cardiac patients with severe left ventricular dysfunction, atrioventricular valve regurgitation, renal insufficiency and other critical illnesses.

Both methods are inherently suited to rapid, quantitative analyses, and the spatial resolution of the images is excellent even at this early stage of implementation.

Summary

The potential clinical utility of digital ventriculography has only recently been explored, and most of the early results are extremely encouraging. At the very least, digital ventriculography can provide a powerful adjunctive imaging capacity to cardiac catheterization laboratories that gives an added measure of safety to patient studies while allowing more routine, computer-facilitated quantitation. Continuing advances in this technology, in conjunction with its potential role in assessing coronary anatomy and coronary flow reserve, should advance the diagnostic capabilities of digital subtraction angiography.

Acknowledgement

Preparation of this manuscript was supported in part by NIH grant HL 29716 and funds from the Veterans Administration.

References

1. Robb GP, Steinberg I: Visualization of the chambers of the heart, pulmonary circulation, and great blood vessels in man. AJR 1: 1–17, 1939.
2. Heintzen PH, Brennecke R, Bursch JH: Automated video-angiographic image analysis. Comp in Cardiol (IEEE) 8: 55–64, 1975.
3. Brennecke R, Brown TK, Bursch JH: Digital processing of angiocardiographic image series using a minicomputer. IEEE Computers in Cardiol 255–260, 1976.
4. Frost MM, Fisher HD, Nudelman S, Roehrig H: A digital video acquisition system for extraction of subvisual information in diagnostic medical imaging. Proc SPIE, Appl Opt Instrument Med VI, Sept 25–27, Bellingham, WA, 127: 208–215, 1977.
5. Kruger RA, Mistretta CA, Houk TL, Reiderer SJ, Shaw CG, Goodsitt MM, Crummy AB, Zweibel WZ, Lancaster JC, Rowe GG, Flemming D: Computerized fluoroscopy in real-time for non-invasive visualization of the cardiovascular system. Radiology 130: 49–57, 1979.

6. Kruger RA, Mistretta CA, Houk TL, Kubal W, Reiderer SJ, Ergun DL, Shaw CG, Lancaster JC, Rowe GG: Computerized fluoroscopy techniques for intravenous study of cardiac chamber dynamics. Invest Radiol 14: 279–287, 1979.

7. Ovitt T, Christenson PC, Fisher HD, Frost MM, Nudelman S, Roehrig H, Seeley G: Intravenous angiography using digital video subtraction: X-ray imaging system. AJR 135: 1141–1144, 1980.

8. Crummy AB, Strother CM, Sackett JF, Ergun DL, Shaw CG, Kruger RA, Mistretta CA, Turnipseed WD, Leiberman RP, Myerowitz PD, Ruzicka FF: Computerized fluoroscopy, digital subtraction for intravenous angiocardiography and arteriography. AJR 135: 1131–1140, 1980.

9. Meaney TF, Weinstein MA, Buonocore E, Pavlicek W, Borkowski GP, Gallagher JH, Sufka B, MacIntyre WJ: Digital subtraction angiography of the human cardiovascular system. AJR 135: 1153–1160, 1980.

10. Gerber KH, Tubau J, Witztum KF, Butterfield TK, Higgins CB, Ashburn WL, Hall DR: Spatial and temporal convolutions for frequency filtering of radionuclide ventriculography (RNV). Invest Radiol (abstr) 16: 371, 1981.

11. Nelson JA, Miller FJ Jr, Kruger RA, Liu P-Y, Bateman W: Digital angiography using a temporal band pass filter: initial clinical results. Radiology 145: 309–313, 1982.

12. Kruger RA, Mistretta CA, Crummy AB: Digital K-edge subtraction radiography. Radiology 125: 243–146, 1977.

13. Gerber KH, Slutsky RA, Ashburn WL, Higgins CB: Detection and assessment of severity of regional ischemic left ventricular dysfunction by digital fluoroscopy. Am Heart J 104: 27–35, 1982.

14. Carey PH, Slutsky RA, Ashburn WL, Higgins CB: The validation of cardiac output by digital intravenous ventriculography in dogs: correlation with thermodilution estimates. Radiology 143: 623–626, 1982.

15. Slutsky RA, Mancini GBJ, Norris S, Ashburn WL, Higgins CB: Digital intravenous ventriculography: comparison of volumes from mask-mode and non-subtracted images with thermodilution and sonocardiometric measurements. Invest Radiol 18: 327–334, 1983.

16. Vas R, Diamond GA, Forrester JS, Whiting JS, Swan HJC: Computer enhancement of direct and venous-injected left ventricular contrast angiography. Am Heart J 102: 719–728, 1981.

17. Kronenberg MW, Price RR, Smith CW, Robertson RM, Perry JM, Pickens DR, Domanski MJ, Partain CL, Freisinger GC: Evaluation of left ventricular performance using digital subtraction angiography. Am J Cardiol 51: 837–842, 1983.

18. Goldberg HL, Borer JS, Moses JW, Fisher J, Cohen B, Skelly NT: Digital subtraction intravenous left ventricular angiography: comparison with conventional intraventricular angiography. J Am Coll Cardiol 1: 858–862, 1983.

19. Sasayama S, Nonogi H, Kawai C, Eiho S, Kuwahara M: Automated method for left ventricular volume measurement by cineventriculography with minimal doses of contrast medium. Am J Cardiol 48: 746–753, 1981.

20. Radtke W, Bursch JH, Brennecke R, Hahne HJ, Meissner L, Heintzen PH: Visualization of the left ventricular wall by digital angiocardiography. Eur Heart J 2: 135–142, 1981.

21. Slutsky RA, Gerber KH, Higgins CB: Digital intravenous ventriculography: analysis and validation of wall thickness changes during ischemia and inotropic stimulation in dogs. Am J Cardiol 50: 874–880, 1983.

22. Tobis J, Nacioglu O, Johnston WD, Seibert A, Iseri LT, Roeck W, Elkayam U, Henry WL: Left ventricular imaging with digital subtraction angiography using intravenous contrast injection and fluoroscopic exposure levels. Am Heart J 104: 20–27, 1982.

23. Norris SL, Slutsky RA, Mancini GBJ, Gregoratos G, Ashburn WL, Peterson KL, Higgins CB: Comparison of digital intravneous ventriculography with direct left ventricuography for quantitation of left ventricular volumes and ejection fractions. Am J Cardiol 51:1399–1403, 1983.

24. Felix R, Eichstadt H, Kempter H, Kewitz A, Banzer D, Schmutzler H, Marhoff P: A comparison of conventional contrast ventriculography and digital subtraction ventriculography and digital subtraction ventriculography. Clin Cardiol 6: 265–276, 1983.

25. Nissen SE, Booth D, Waters J, Fassas T, DeMaria AN: Evaluation of left ventricular contractile pattern by intravenous digital subtraction ventriculography: comparison with cineangiography and assessment of interobserver variability. Am J Cardiol 52: 1293–1298, 1983.
26. Engels PHC, Ludwig JW, Verhoeven LAJ: Left ventricular evaluation by digital video subtraction angiography. Radiology 144: 471–474, 1982.
27. Higgins CB: Effects of contrast materials on left ventricular function. Invest Radiol 15 (suppl): S220–S231, 1980.
28. Mancini GBJ, Ostrander DR, Slutsky RA, Shabetai R, Higgins CB: Comparative effects of ionic contrast agents injected intravenously or directly into the left ventricle: implications for digital angiography. AJR 140: 425–430, 1983.
29. Fujita M, Sasayama S, Kawai C, Eiho S, Kuwahara M: Automatic processing of cineventriculograms for analysis of regional myocardial function. Circulation 63: 1065–1074, 1981.
30. Nichols AB, Martin EC, Fles TP, Stugensky KM, Balancio LA, Casarella WJ, Weiss MB: Validation of the angiographic accuracy of digital left ventriculography. Am J Cardiol 51: 224–230, 1983.
31. Tobis JM, Nalcioglu O, Johnston WD, Seibert A, Roeck W, Iseri LT, Elkayam U, Henry WL: Correlation of 10-milliliter digital subtraction ventriculograms compared with standard cineangiograms. Am Heart J 105: 946–952, 1983.
32. Tobis J, Nalcioglu O, Johnston WD, Seibert A, Iseri LT, Roeck W, Henry WL: Digital angiography in assessment of ventricular function and wall motion during pacing in patients with coronary artery disease. Am J Cardiol 51: 668–675, 1983.
33. Chaitman BR, DeMoto H, Bristow JD, Fosch J, Rahimtoola SH: Objective and subjective analysis of left ventricular angiograms. Circulation 52: 420–425, 1975.
34. Vas R, Diamond GA, Forrester JS, Whiting JS, Pfaff MJ, Levisman JA, Nakano FS, Swan HJC: Computer-enhanced digital angiography: correlation of clinical assessment of left ventricular ejection fraction and regional wall motion. Am Heart J 104: 732–739, 1982.
35. Clayton PD, Jeppson GM, Klausner SC: Should a fixed external reference system be used to analyze left ventricular wall motion. Circulation 65: 1518–1521, 1982.
36. Gelberg JH, Brundage BH, Glantz S, Parmley WW: Quantitative left ventricular wall motion analysis: a comparison of area chord and radial methods. Circulation 59: 991–1000, 1979.
37. Karsch KR, Lamm U, Blanke H, Rentrop KP: Comparison of nineteen quantitative methods for assessment of localized left ventricular wall motion abnormalities. Clin Cardiol 3: 123–128, 1980.
38. Mancini GBJ, Norris SL, Peterson KL, Gregoratos G, Widmann T, Ashburn WL, Higgins CB: Quantitative assessment of segmental wall motion abnormalitis at rest and after atrial pacing using digital intravenous ventriculography. J Am Coll Cardiol 2: 70–76, 1983.
39. Engels PHC, Ludwig JW, Bruschke AVG, Plokker HW: Cardiac digital video subtraction angiography emphasizing left ventriculography. In: Heintzen PH, Brennecke R (eds), Digital imaging in cardiovascular radiology: international symposium Kiel 1982. Thieme-Stratton, New York, 1983, pp 192–204.
40. Norris SL, Widmann T, Mancini GBJ, Slutsky RA, Gregoratos G, Peterson KL, Einsidler E, Ashburn WL, Higgins CB: Assessment of wall motion by regional phase analysis of digital intravenous ventriculograms. Circulation 66 (suppl II): II-190, 1982.
41. Widmann TF, Ashburn WL, Higgins CB, Peterson KL: Assessment of left ventricular wall motion by regional phase analysis of digital intravenous contrast fluoroangiography. IEEE Computers in Cardiol 105–108, 1982.
42. Bacharach SL, Green MV, Bonow RD, de Graaf CN, Johnston GS: A method for objective evaluation of functional images. J Nucl Med 23: 285–290, 1982.
43. Tobis JM, Nalcioglu O, Johnston WD, Seibert JA, Henry WL: Exercise digital subtraction angiograms in patients with coronary artery disease. Circulation (abstr) 66 (suppl II): II-228, 1982.
44. Yiannikas J, Simpfendorfer C, Detrano R, Salcedo EE, Sheldon WC: Stress digital subtraction

angiography to assess presence of coronary artery disease in patients without myocardial infarction. Circulation 68 (suppl III): III–41, 1983.

45. Mancini GBJ, Peterson KL, Gregoratos G, Higgins CB: The effects of atrial pacing on global and regional left ventricular function in coronary heart disease assessed by digital intravenous ventriculography. Am J Cardiol 53: 456–461, 1984.

46. Johnson RA, Wasserman AG, Leibhoff RH, Katz RJ, Bren GB, Varghese J, Ross AM: Intravenous digital left ventriculography at rest and with atrial pacing as a screening procedure for coronary artery disease. JACC 2: 905–910, 1983.

47. Tomoike H, Franklin D, Ross J Jr: Detection of myocardial ischemia by regional dysfunction during and after rapid pacing in conscious dogs. Circulation 58: 48–56, 1978.

48. Sasayama S, Takahashi M, Nakamura M, Ohyagi A, Yamamoto A, Shimada T, Kawai C: Effects of diltiazem on pacing induced ischemia in conscious dogs with coronary stenosis: improvement of post-pacing deterioration of ischemic myocardial function. Am J Cardiol 48: 460–467, 1981.

49. Ricci DR, Orlick AE, Alderman EL, Ingels NB, Daughters GT, Kusnick CA, Reitz BA, Stinson EB: Role of tachycardia as an inotropic stimulus in man. J Clin Invest 63: 695–703, 1979.

50. Ross J Jr, Linhart JW, Braunwald E: Effects of changing heart rate in man by electrical stimulation of the right atrium: studies at rest, during exercise, and with isoproterenol. Circulation 32: 549–558, 1965.

51. Mahles F, Yoran C, Ross J Jr: Inotropic effect of tachycardia and post-stimulation potentiation in the conscious dog. Am J Physiol 22: 569–575, 1974.

52. Ricci DR, Orlick AE, Alderman EL, Ingels NB, Daughters GT, Stinson EB: Influence of heart rate on left ventricular ejection fraction in human beings. Am J Cardiol 44: 447–451, 1979.

8. Digital radiographic assessment of coronary flow reserve

ROBERT A. VOGEL

Although the accurate measurement of coronary blood flow by electromagnetic flow meter [1] and myocardial perfusion by radionuclide tagged particles [2] are relatively easy techniques to perform under experimental conditions, the clinical assessment of these important physiologic parameters is both considerably more difficult and inaccurate. Current methods for measuring human coronary blood flow or myocardial perfusion include thermodilution coronary sinus flow [3], inert gas washout [4], thallium-201 scintigraphy [5], doppler catheter [6] and coronary videodensitometry [7, 8]. In general, these techniques usually employ exercise, cardiac pacing, or hyperemic stimuli to provide additional information on the ability of the coronary circulation to respond to increased myocardial oxygen demands. Thallium scintigraphy has been the most widely used technique and has provided the clinician with a relatively simple, non-invasive tool for visualizing myocardial perfusion. The accuracy of this test has usually been judged using coronary arteriography as the standard [9], although the latter measures coronary anatomy rather than physiology. This fact underscores the continued use of selective coronary arteriography as the definitive standard for the assessment of human coronary disease. Much of this dependence is based upon experimental data showing a close correspondence between percent luminal narrowing and alterations in coronary flow reserve [10, 11]. More recently, this correspondence has been challenged by the failure of coronary arteriography to predict intra-operative doppler probe measurements of coronary flow reserve [12], directly measured translesional pressure gradients [13], and transcatheter determined translesional pressure gradients [14]. These findings, coupled with the data from large-scale patient studies which demonstrated that individuals with coronary disease but without physiologic evidence of myocardial ischemia have excellent prognoses [15, 16], have renewed interest in measuring coronary blood flow and myocardial perfusion.

The use of arteriography to measure coronary blood flow in addition to anatomy was first described by Rutishauser et al. [7, 8] and Smith et al. [17, 18] more than ten years ago. These investigators used videodensitometric determinations of contrast media transit times along a coronary artery segment of known diameter and length to measure absolute blood flow. Confirmation of the validity of this method has been recently reported by Spiller *et al.* [19]. Although highly accurate, this technique is both laborious and generally limited to proximal, non-circuitous arterial segments. A simpler method for measuring coronary flow reserve (i.e. relative blood flow) using radiographic arterial videodensitometry was reported by Foerster *et al.* [20]. Precise arterial diameter and length determinations are not required by this method. An alternative approach to the assessment of regional blood flow was first proposed by Robb *et al.* [21] who demonstrated that contrast media could be visualized in its microcirculation phase by use of digital radiographic subtraction. As this increasingly utilized method for enhancing low concentrations of contrast media have become more widely available, several digital radiographic techniques for measuring regional coronary flow have been proposed. In general, these methods utilize either washin or washout densitometric determinations. Washin analysis is more dependent on contrast medium injection technique, but washout phenomena do not closely reflect basal physiology due to the intrinsic vasodilation properties of the contrast medium, itself. Substantial similarities exist between the two approaches, however, and the clinical accuracy for measuring blood flow ratios by the two techniques apears to be similar [22].

During the last three years, our laboratory has developed a method for measuring relative changes in regional blood flow using digital radiographic enhancement of selective coronary arteriography [23–28]. Coronary flow reserve is measured in individual arterial distributions using the washin ratio of contrast appearance time under baseline and hyperemic conditions. Information is quantitatively presented in functional (parametric) image format. These images, termed contrast medium appearance pictures (CMAP), depict the transit of contrast through the arterial, myocardial and early venous stages. This process can be divided into three general phases: data acquisition, CMAP formation and CMAP analysis. The technique has evolved over its development period from a cine film-based technology which required substantial processing time to a real-time digital radiographic technique.

Image acquisition

Application of digital radiographic image enhancement is dependent upon precise inter-frame correspondence. Patients undergoing intravenous contrast administration peripheral arteriography are required to remain motionless during the radiographic acquisition to prevent motion-induced artifact. This basic requirement of digital radiographic image enhancement is complicated in its cardiac application by the cyclical cardiac motion. As first demonstrated by Robb *et al.* [21], and confirmed by our early work [29], ECG-gated frame acquisition is required to produce acceptable visualization of contrast medium myocardial perfusion. Either patient motion (especially respiration) or use of non-ECG correspondent frames can significantly degrade final image quality. Additionally, contrast medium administration, itself, can alter inter-frame correspondence both directly by changing ventricular geometry due to its negative inotropic effect and indirectly through alterations in cycle length. The latter can be substantially reduced using atrial pacing.

The CMAP technique operates on a set of frames, acquired under fixed-parameter radiographic conditions, obtained at the same period within consecutive cardiac cycles. The first frame is acquired just prior to contrast medium administration which is performed using ECG-gated power injection so as to standardize the volume, flow rate and timing of the contrast medium bolus. Image acquisition is usually performed over a five cardiac cycle interval (six total frames), which is generally sufficient to follow the contrast bolus transit up to its early appearance within the coronary sinus. Occasionally, additional frames are required in instances of very slow coronary flow. Early image acquisition was accomplished using 128×128 digitization of cine film frames on which the patient's ECG signal was photographically recorded. Currently, frames in 512×512 resolution are directly recorded on a live-time digital disk using automated ECG gating. Initially, pre-A wave end-diastolic frames were chosen to provide the best frame-to-frame correspondence, but current technology allows frames to be acquired from any period within the cardiac cycle. The methodology has continued to evolve so that presently a series of CMAPs, obtained at 33 ms intervals throughout the cardiac cycle, can be acquired, formed and replayed in endless loop fashion, allowing visualization of the phasic passage of contrast medium appearance.

Digital enhancement was first accomplished using serial frame subtraction (i.e. gated time interval differencing at an interval of one cardiac cycle). This method provides the best bolus transit separation into arterial, myocardial and venous phases. At 512×512 image resolution, however, it was found to produce images with insufficient signal-to-noise ratios. Currently, contrast enhancement is performed using gated maskmode subtraction of the pre-contrast administration frame from each of the subsequent frames.

CMAP Formation

As performed by either enhancement method, the resultant subtracted images depict the temporal passage of contrast media through the coronary circulation. The myocardial phase is an enhanced form of the 'myocardial blush' evident faintly on standard cine films. Measurement of relative regional blood flow by the CMAP technique is based upon assessment of the time from the onset of contrast injection until it reaches the specific region of myocardium under investigation.

This is determined using individual pixel densitometric criteria. At first, this was accomplished in time interval differencing mode using maximum pixel value to define arrival time. More recently, in mask mode, contrast medium arrival is determined using a threshold criterion. The threshold is generally chosen as low as possible, but high enough to exclude background noise. Application of either criteria to the set of images results in determination of individual pixel myocardial contrast appearance times expressed in cardiac cyle units. This information is color coded into the CMAPs so as to allow visual or computer recognition of regional appearance time in a pixel-by-pixel fashion. There is no need for subjective assignments of regions of interest as the entire image is processed as a whole.

Contrast medium density is also coded into the functional images to allow differentiation of high concentration arterial structures from low concentration myocardial regions. Thus, the resultant CMAPs contain four dimensions of data: two spatial, transit time (color coded) and contrast medium density (intensity coded). Examples of normal and abnormal CMAPs are shown in Figures 1 and 2.

CMAP analysis

In practice, arteriograms are obtained under both baseline conditions (at least three minutes after prior contrast administration) and during reactive hyperemia. Hyperemia has been induced using either an additional ten-second prior injection of contrast medium or 5–10 mg of intracoronary papaverine. Whereas, contrast is more readily available, papavarine produces a greater increase in blood flow. Baseline and hyperemic arteriograms are obtained at the same heart rate (using atrial pacing) and in the same projection. Identical regions of interest, selected through use of the arterial anatomy, are computer analyzed to determine the mean arrival times within the equivalent regions. The same threshold criterion is used for creation of both the baseline and hyperemic images. This is necessary due to the variation in mean arrival time depending on the threshold value used. Baseline-to-hyperemic appearance time ratios are less subject to such variation as long as the same reasonable threshold value is used for both images. Averaging the pixel values within the region of interest reduces the imprecision caused by the infrequent temporal sampling. As several thousand pixels are included in each region of interest, arrival time precision is increased by statistical averaging. This method makes the assumption that transit time within a region is inversely proportion to the coronary blood flow to that region. This is true if the distributional volume of the region remains roughly constant between baseline and hyperemic states. Relative changes in regional blood flow are calculated by dividing the regional baseline arrival time by the hyperemic arrival time. During the animal validation phase of investigation, it was determined that a small interval (approximately 0.5 s) should be subtracted from both the baseline and

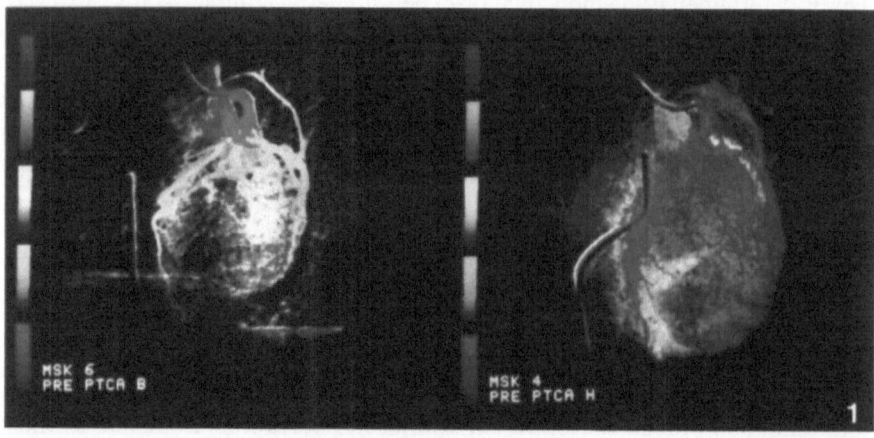

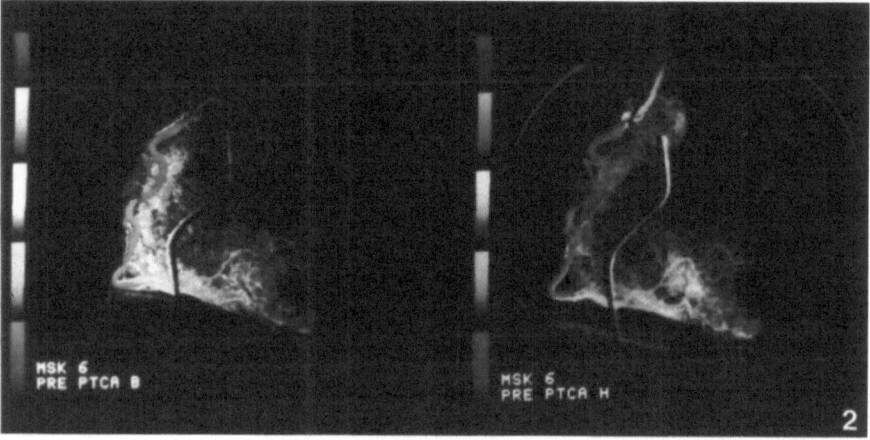

Figure 1. A normal left coronary artery in the left anterior oblique projection is seen under baseline (left) and hyperemic (right) conditions. The time of individual pixel appearance is coded from red (first cardiac cycle following contrast administration) to blue (fifth cardiac cycle). Earlier regional myocardial contrast medium appearance is noted following induction of hyperemia throughout both the left anterior descending and circumflex coronary artery perfusion beds.

Figure 2. A right coronary artery with a high-grade stenosis is shown in the left anterior oblique projection. Baseline (left) and hyperemic (right) studies depict an absence of hyperemia. This study was obtained from the same patient as Figure 1, just prior to coronary angioplasty.

hyperemic arrival times to correct for the actual duration of contrast administration. Subtraction of this interval from both the baseline and hyperemic contrast medium arrival times does not significantly alter low coronary flow reserves in the range of 1.0, but does increase the normal higher values from approximately 1.9 to 2.5 for contrast-induced hyperemia. For reasons of simplicity, we continue to express clinical coronary flow reserves without this correction, although it should be remembered that this leads to a systematic underestimation of high flow reserves.

Validation of method

Three phases of validation have been accomplished: (1) determination of the reproducibility of individual regional contrast medium appearance times and of hyperemic-to-baseline appearance time, (2) correlations of pacing-induced changes in human coronary sinus and great cardiac vein blood flow with changes in regional appearance time ratios, and (3) correlations of hyperemia-induced changes in dog electromagnetic coronary flow with changes in regional appearance times. Repetitive measurements of regional appearance times in right, left anterior descending, and circumflex coronary perfusion beds have demonstrated that the paired determinations obtained under the same conditions vary by a mean of 12% [24]. The same reproducibility value as found for paired determinations of regional contrast-induced hyperemia-to-baseline ratios. This value compares to the 9% value found for paired xenon-133 washout blood flow determinations. Use of an ECG-gated power injector has been found necessary to ensure reproducible arrival times.

Validation of human myocardial contrast appearance time ratio correlation with underlying changes in regional blood flow was performed using coronary sinus and great cardiac vein thermodilution determinations of blood flow as the standard. Overall left coronary artery perfusion regional appearance time ratios were compared in twelve instances with changes in coronary sinus flow and left anterior descending regional appearance time ratios were compared in eight instances with great cardiac vein flow changes. Coronary blood flow was varied by atrial pacing with measurements between control (non-paced) and 80, 100, or 120 paced heart rates. Due to the different heart rates of each pair, a correction for cycle length was made in the appearance time ratios. A 0.90 linear correlation coefficient was found between regional blood flow ratios determined by the CMAP arteriographic and the thermodilution techniques ($p < 0.0001$) [24]. The linear regression equation was found to be $y = 0.79x + 5.3$ where y and x represent CMAP and thermodilution percent flow changes, respectively. The CMAP technique tended to underestimate large increases in flow, although in a linear manner. This data was, however, derived without use of the above-described correction factor which, if applied, would have returned the slope closer to unity.

Validation of dog myocardial contrast appearance time ratio correlation with directly measured left anterior descending coronary artery blood flow changes was performed using electromagnetic flow meter measurements as the standard [30]. Twenty-seven ratios of baseline-to-contrast medium-induced hyperemic flow were determined in a total of ten animals. A 0.90 linear correlation was found between directly measured flow changes and CMAP ratios for flow ratios below 3.5. Above this value, the CMAP technique underestimated flow increases. It was found that the contrast medium-induced hyperemia was fairly short-lived making the timing of the hyperemic stimulus an important technical factor. Methodologically, the timing of the contrast medium bolus was found to have substantial effect on the precision of the method.

Clinical studies

During the past three years, approximately 200 patients have undergone digital coronary arteriography using film-based processing and 100 patients have undergone direct digital disk data acquisition. About 20% of patients have been found to be unable to hold their breath or remain sufficiently motionless to allow reasonable quality digital subtraction studies to be performed. Clearly, the greatest single factor in ensuring successful diagnostic imaging is lack of patient movement, especially respiration. Often patients are more able to remain motionless if they are instructed to take in a moderate breath rather than a full breath, which often leads to a Valvalva maneuver. Some patients who cannot remain motionless are benefited by watching their own diaphragmatic motion on fluoroscopy. On the functional images, patient motion is readily evident in the form of diaphragmatic and/or rib artifact. Frame registration has been found to be only partially helpful in reducing motion artifact.

Two of three hundred patients studied by this technique had episodes of ventricular tachycardia, one of which occurred during a hyperemic contrast medium administration. Both of these patients responded to a single DC-300 joule shock. One instance of prolonged asystole occurred following a hyperemia study which responded to atrial pacing. At present, we routinely perform both baseline and hyperemic studies using atrial pacing at a rate set just above the patient's intrinsic heart rate.

Normal values

Thirty-two normal arteries have been evaluated in 21 patients during the initial period of evaluation for this technique. The mean coronary flow reserve for this group was found to be 1.9 ± 0.3 with a range from 1.4 to 2.5. These values were calculated without the above-mentioned correction factor which, if applied, would have yielded a group mean of approximately 2.5. In a subgroup of 11 normal arteries studied in patients who had significant stenoses in other arteries, the coronary flow reserve was not different from the group with all normal arteries. Although the absolute arrival times were found to be longer in the right coronary artery perfusion beds, the flow ratios for the right, left anterior descending and circumflex coronary perfusion beds studied were the same.

Four conditions have been recognized which can lower the coronary flow reserves in normal arteries.

1. *Myocardial hypertrophy*. Patients with substantial myocardial hypertrophy and normal coronary arteries have been observed to have flow reserves, as assessed by this technique, as low as 1.1. In these patients, left coronary flow reserve seemed to be more depressed than right coronary flow reserves. Depressed flow reserves in animals and humans with myocardial hypertrophy

have been reported by several different blood flow assessment techniques [31]. Although total basal flow is elevated in this situation, flow per unit tissue may be normal. The vasculature appears to be insufficient in this instance to provide additional flow increases.

2. *Total coronary occlusion.* Coronary perfusion beds adjacent to those with total coronary occlusion and associated infarction have been found to have reduced flow reserves. This is especially evident in those beds adjacent to a totally occluded left anterior descending coronary artery. The mechanism for this may be either through increased contractility demands and/or myocardial hypertrophy in the adjacent perfusion zones [32].

3. *Collaterals.* Arteries providing substantial collateral perfusion to either totally occluded or highly stenosed arteries have been found to have reduced flow reserves. In one instance of a normal right coronary artery which supplied collateral flow to a highly stenosed left anterior descending coronary artery, successful angioplasty on the latter was observed to be associated with disappearance of the collateral bed and increase in the flow reserve in the right coronary artery from 1.4 (borderline) to 1.6 (normal). This observation has also been observed in experimental animals [33].

4. *Post-angioplasty.* Following successful angioplasty in vessels without residual translesional gradients, flow reserves have been found to be less than at subsequent follow-up evaluation six months later. Whereas, this may be partly explained by continued absorption of the lesion, a more important factor is likely the high baseline flow seen in this situation. The latter can be attributed to the multiple vasodilators and coronary trauma associated with the procedure. In this instance, the baseline appearance time following angioplasty has been observed to be faster than that prior to the intervention. Slowing of myocardial contrast transit time has been observed with a prolonged Valsalva maneuver, although arrival time ratios may not be significantly affected.

These four circumstances which cause decreased coronary flow reserve in normal arterial distributions underscore a major deficiency in the use of this relative parameter to fully describe coronary hemodynamics. Under conditions of elevated basal coronary flow, hyperemic-to-baseline flow ratios may be depicted despite absence of significant coronary obstruction. It must be remembered that individual coronary artery physiology cannot be totally separated from global hemodynamics or from physiologic alterations in other coronary arteries.

Flow reserve in stenosed arteries

Forty-five arteries with caliper stenoses ranging from 15% to 100% have been investigated by this technique. The mean coronary flow reserve of arteries with greater than 70% stenoses was found to be 1.0 ± 0.15. Although the range of this group was from 0.75 to 1.35, no arteries with greater than 75% stenoses had flow reserve values above 1.1. Considerable variability was observed in the flow reserves of arteries with less than 70% stenoses, with normal values being found in arteries with as much as 60% stenosis and abnormal values being found in arteries with as little as 30% stenosis. Four of 21 arteries with stenoses greater than 75% had flow reserves below 0.90. This has been interpreted as evidence for 'coronary steal' [34] in these arterial distributions. Coronary steal was observed in three settings. The first was that of a high-grade stenosis in the mid-portion of a major artery, in which flow rates increased proximal to, but decreased distal to the lesion. Secondly, it was associated with a proximal left anterior descending or circumflex coronary stenosis, in which flow rates increased in one and decreased in the other artery. Thirdly, it was observed in a collateralized perfusion bed which was supplied by a stenosed coronary artery.

Bypass grafts

Thirty-one bypass grafts were studied by this methodology at a mean of three months post-operative. The flow reserve of these non-stenotic grafts was 1.45 ± 0.18, with a range from 1.2 to 2.1. This was less than our normal mean [28]. The reason why flow reserve in these perfusion beds did not return fully to normal levels is, as yet, unexplained. Possible reasons include the presence of residual disease not evident on angiography, myocardial hypertrophy, or chronic changes in vascular reactivity. Bypass grafts containing graft or anastomotic stenoses were found to have lower flow reserves (1.0 ± 0.10) and, therefore, did not provide substantial improvements over the pre-bypass situation.

Angioplasty

Recently, percutaneous transluminal angioplasty has gained increased use as an alternative to bypass surgery. Usually, only one or two vessels are dilated, as compared with the multiple saphenous vein grafts placed during surgery. Thus, it is helpful to be able to assess the individual artery pathophysiology prior to angioplastic intervention, so that dilation of only the arteries with significant obstruction be undertaken. During the past year, twenty arterial distributions were evaluated immediately prior to and following successful angioplasty, as defined by the NHLBI criterion of greater than 20% decrease in luminal stenosis (mean of this group 72% before to 31% after angioplasty). These arteriographically successful interventions were further divided into groups with either more or less than 16 mmHg residual translesional pressure gradients. There was no difference between the residual stenosis $(34 \pm 8\%)$ in the higher residual gradient group $(26 \pm 13 \text{ mmHg})$ and the residual stenosis $(30 \pm 11\%)$ in the lower residual gradient group $(9 \pm 5 \text{ mmHg})$. There was, however, a better coronary flow reserve achieved in the lower residual gradient arteries (1.41 ± 0.13) than in the higher residual gradient arteries (1.19 ± 0.06), despite similar flow reserves prior to dilation. Additionally, there was a close correlation between all the translesional gradients and flow reserves measured for the entire angioplasty group [27]. In our laboratory, a residual gradient of less than 16 mmHg has now become a second criterion for angioplastic success, as this has been found to return coronary flow reserve to the lower normal range. It should be remembered that the flow reserve value immediately following angioplasty may be less than the true baseline value due to the vasoactive drugs used during the procedure.

To help clarify this situation, a second group of 14 arteries was investigated at an average of 6 months following successful angioplasty (residual gradient less than 16 mmHg). The coronary flow reserve in this group was 1.55 ± 0.16, which was higher than the acute post-angioplasty value. This suggests that either increased baseline flow was present in the acute study or that continued lesional resolution had occurred. Overall, these data suggest that angioplasty provides comparable hemodynamic improvements in coronary flow reserve as compared with bypass surgery. Individual values for normal, stenosed, bypassed and dilated arteries are shown in Figure 3. The ability to determine which individual arteries have hemodynamically significant stenoses, so that they may be dilated, may prove to be the most clinically useful feature of this technique. The four factors, discussed above, which may alter individual arterial flow reserve in addition to the effect of the stenosis itself, must be considered in any pre-angioplasty patient evaluation.

Future directions

Clearly, this technique is in its early phase of development and will need to undergo additional validation and refinement. It would be advantageous to develop appearance time algorithms which have greater temporal precision, less arbitrary appearance criteria than the current threshold method and means for correcting patient motion artifact. The first goal is already under investigation in the form of a real-time digital acquisition system which allows 30 frame-per-second digital disk acquisition. Cyclical CMAPs which depict the continuous phasic appearances of contrast appearance within the myocardium can now be generated. It is possible that the greater temporally precision provided by this technique will prove helpful, especially if the phasic flow information can be utilized.

Other approaches to the arteriographic measurement of coronary flow and flow reserve are alo being investigated. Contrast medium washout using a correction for veiling-glare has been reported [35] to provide good correlation with regional perfusion and with estimations of arterial stenosis. As mentioned above, this method is less subject to contrast medium injection technique and follows

116

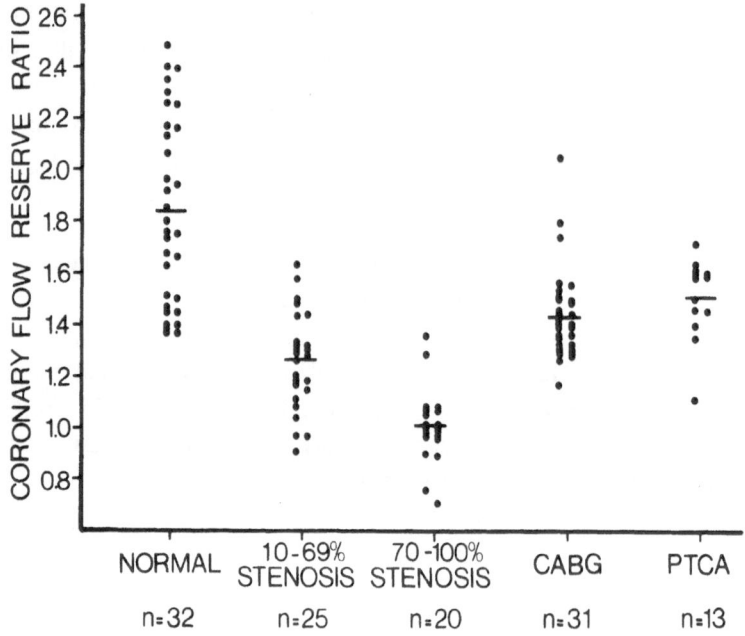

Figure 3. Group mean and individual coronary flow reserve values for normal, stenotic arteries, post-bypass surgery, and post-angioplasty arteries are shown.

more closely classic indicator-dilutional algorithms. It is, however, affected by the instrinsic vasoactivity of the contrast medium bolus, itself. This and the appearance time technique are, of course, not mutually exclusive and can be performed on the same contrast bolus transit. Arterial densitometric analysis, as first described by Rutishauser [7, 8], could be performed using the substantial efficiencies provided by current digital computer technology. A potential advantage of this approach is that absolute coronary flow is determined. Overall, there is little doubt that in the future, important clinical information on coronary blood flow physiology will be obtained through arteriographic means.

Acknowledgements

The author gratefully acknowledges the secretarial assistance of Ms Diane Bauer. This manuscript was prepared with the collaboration of: Michael T. LeFree, BS, Eric R. Bates, MD, William W. O'Neill, MD, G.B. John Mancini, MD, John McB Hodgson, MD, Joseph S. Smith, MD, Fred M. Aueron, MD, and Victor LeGrand, MD.

References

1. Westersten A, Herrold G, Assali NS: A gated sine wave flowmeter. J Appl Physiol 15: 533, 1960.
2. Heyman MA, Payne BD, Hoffman JE, Rudolph AM: Blood flow measurements with radionuclide labeled particles. Prog Cardiovasc Dis 20: 55, 1977.
3. Ganz W, Tamura K, Marcus HS, Donoso R, Yoshida S, Swan HJC: Measurement of coronary sinus blood flow by continuous thermodilution in man. Circulation 44: 181, 1971.
4. Cannon PJ, Dell RB, Dwyer EM Jr: Measurement of regional myocardial perfusion in man with [133]Xenon and a scintillation camera. J Clin Invest 51: 964, 1972.
5. Vogel RA: Quantitative aspects of myocardial perfusion imaging. Sem Nucl Med 10: 146, 1980.
6. Cole JS, Hartley CJ: The pulsed Doppler coronary artery catheter. Preliminary report of a new technique for measuring rapid changes in coronary artery flow velocity in man. Circulation 56: 18, 1977.
7. Rutishauser W, Bussman W-D, Noseda G, Meier W, Wellauer J: Blood flow measurement through single coronary arteries by roentgen densitometry. Part I. A comparison of flow measured by a radiologic technique applicable in the intact organism and by electromagnetic flowmeter. Am J Roentgenol 109: 12, 1970.
8. Rutishauser W, Noseda G, Bussman W-D, Preter B: Blood flow measurement through single coronary arteries by roentgen densitometry. Part II. Right coronary artery flow in conscious man. Am J Roentgenol 109: 21, 1970.
9. Sones FM Jr, Shirey EK: Cine coronary arteriography. Mod Conc Cardiovasc Dis 31: 735, 1962.
10. Gould KL, Lipscomb K, Hamilton GW: Physiologic basis for assessing critical coronary stenosis: instantaneous flow response and regional distribution during coronary hyperemia as measures of coronary flow reserve. Am J Cardiol 33: 87, 1974.
11. Gould KL, Lipscomb K: Effects of coronary stenoses on coronary flow reserve and resistance. Am J Cardiol 34: 48, 1974.
12. Wright CB, Doty DB, Eastham CL, Marcus ML: Measurement of coronary reactive hyperemia with a Doppler probe. Intra-operative guide to hemodynamically significant lesions. J Thorac Cardiovasc Surg 80: 888, 1980.
13. Bateman T, Gray R, Raymond M, et al.: Physiologic limitation to stress scintigraphic detection of coronary stenoses. Circulation (abstr) 68 (suppl III): III–138, 1983.
14. Banka VS, Agarwal JB, Bodenheimer MM et al.: Determination of the severity of coronary stenoses in man: correlation of angiography and hemodynamics. Circulation (abstr) 64 (suppl IV): IV–108, 1981.
15. Varnauskas E, Olsson SB, Carlstrom E, et al.: Long-term results of prospectively randomized study of coronary artery bypass surgery with stable angina pectoris. Lancet 11: 1173, 1982.
16. Jones RH, Floyd RD, Auston EH, et al.: The role of radionuclide angiocardiography in the preoperative prediction of pain relief and prolonged survival following coronary artery bypass surgery. Ann Surg 197: 743, 1983.
17. Smith HC, Frye RL, Donald DE, Davis GD, Pluth JR, Sturm RE, Wood EH: Roentgen videodensitometric measurement of coronary blood flow. Determination from simultaneous indicator-dilution curves at selected sites in the coronary circulation and in coronary artery-saphenous vein grafts. Mayo Clin Proc 46: 800, 1971.
18. Smith HC, Sturm RE, Wood EH: Videodensitometric system for measurement of vessel blood flow, particularly in the coronary arteries, in man. Am J Cardiol 32: 144, 1973.
19. Spille P, Schmiel FK, Politz B, et al.: Measurement of systolic and diastolic flow rates in the coronary artery system by X-ray densitometry. Circulation 68: 337, 1983.
20. Foerster J, Link DP, Lantz BMT, Lee G, Holcroft JW, Mason DT: Measurement of coronary reactive hyperemia during clinical angiography by video dilution technique. Acta Radiol 22: 209, 1981.
21. Robb RA, Wood EH, Ritman EL, Johnson SA, Sturm RE, Greenleaf JF, Gilbert BK, Chevalier

118

PA: Three-dimensional reconstruction and display of the working canine heart and lungs by multiplanar X-ray scanning videodensitometry. IEEE Computers in Cardiol 151, 1974.

22. Nivatpumin T, Vas R, Pfaff J, *et al.*: Changes in myocardial perfusion due to reactive hyperemic measured by digital angiography. Circulation (abstr) 68 (suppl III): III-42, 1983.

23. Vogel R, LeFree M, Pitt B: Visualization of myocardial perfusion using application of digital radiographic techniques to selective coronary arteriography. Am J Cardiol (abstr) 49: 935, 1982.

24. Vogel R, LeFree M, Bates E, O'Neill W, Foster R, Kirlin P, Smith D, Pitt B: Application of digital techniques to selective coronary arteriography: use of myocardial contrast appearance time to measure coronary flow reserve. Am Heart J 107: 153, 1984.

25. LeFree MT, Vogel RA: Digital radiography of the heart. Diagn Imaging 5: 62, 1983.

26. LeFree MT, Vogel RA, Smith DN, Pitt B: A digital radiographic technique for visualizing and quantitating regional myocardial perfusion. IEEE Computers in Cardiol 153–156, 1983.

27. O'Neill WW, Vogel RA, Walton JA, Colfer HT, Bates ER, Aueron FM, LeFree MT, Pitt B: Quantitative changes in coronary flow reserve after successful coronary angioplasty. J Am Coll Cardiol (abstr) 1 (2): 724, 1983.

28. Bates ER, Vogel RA, LeFree MT, O'Neill WW, Kirlin PC, Pitt B: Digital coronary radiographic determination of the coronary flow reserve provided by nonstenotic saphenous vein bypass grafts. J Am Coll Cardiol (abstr) 1 (2): 619, 1983.

29. Vogel R, LeFree M, Foster R, Smith D, Pitt B: Integral signed ECG-synchronized difference (ISED): a new technique for performing digital left ventriculography. Circulation (abstr) 64 (suppl IV): IV–220, 1981.

30. O'Neill W, Vogel R, LeFree M, Bates E, Kirlin P, Beauman G, Pitt B: Digital coronary radiographic assessment of relative regional coronary blood flow. Circulation 66 (abstr) (suppl II): II–229, 1982.

31. Pichard AD, Gorlin R, Smith H, Ambrose J, Meller J: Coronary flow studies in patients with left ventricular hypertrophy of the hypertensive type. Am J Cardiol 47: 547, 1981.

32. Schwartz JS, Cohn JN, Bache RJ: Effects of coronary occlusion on flow in the distribution of a neighboring stenotic coronary artery in the dog. Am J Cardiol 52: 189, 1983.

33. Schaper W, Flameng W, Winkler B, *et al.*: Quantification of collateral resistance in acute and chronic experimental coronary occlusion in the dog. Circ Res 39: 371, 1976.

34. Bates ER, Vogel RA, LeFree MT, *et al.*: Demonstration of intra- and inter-coronary steal by digital coronary radiography. Circulation (abstr) 68 (suppl III): III–42, 1983.

35. Whiting JS, Pfaff JM, Drury JK, *et al.*: A new reproducible and sensitive method for quantifying myocardial perfusion using digital angiography. Circulation (abstr) 68 (suppl III): III–89, 1983.

9. Quantitative coronary arteriography

NATHAN LAUFER and ANDREW J. BUDA

Introduction

The clinical objective of coronary arteriography is to demonstrate the anatomic basis for the patient's clinical presentation and to provide information necessary to guide therapy. Coronary artery disease has classically been determined by estimates of percent stenosis from cineangiograms. However, this method has been shown to be characterized by large interobserver and intraobserver variability. As a result, recent attempts have been made to quantitate coronary luminal dimensions more precisely.

This chapter will focus on the problems with current methods of angiographic analysis of coronary lesions. We will address technical considerations necessary to obtain high quality cineangiograms that are essential for objective quantification of coronary lesions. Finally, we will review past attempts at quantitative analysis of coronary arteriograms and current techniques that are presently being developed.

Technical aspects of coronary arteriography

Certain technical details are particularly important for obtaining high quality arteriograms that are suitable for precise clinical diagnosis and adequate for quantitative analysis. Careful consideration must be given to the combination of film type, X-ray tube voltage, and cineframe exposure time. At the University of Michigan we currently use angiographic equipment which delivers a maximum of 120 kV, 21 millirads per frame, 6–8 ms per frame pulse width, and a maximum of 550 mA. If higher tube voltages are used, then image contrast decreases due to loss of differential absorption. With longer exposure times, motion blurring becomes evident.

A sufficiently small image intensifier field must be used in order to provide enough initial magnification so that the arterial size to film grain size is optimized.

Sharper edge resolution when viewed at high magnification can be accomplished by using film of small grain size. Large areas of lung field should be screened out with the aid of an adjustable lead or lucite shield in order to prevent overpenetration of radiolucent structures that can result in cardiac underpenetration due to the automatic brightness control.

An important determinant of vessel edge resolution is the concentration of angiographic contrast medium. The contrast medium must be injected rapidly enough to fill the entire artery. This can be confirmed by observing contrast medium refluxing in the coronary cusp both in diastole and in systole.

X-ray sources of error

There are certain problems inherant in all cardiac angiographic systems used. These problems must be overcome for precise quantitation of coronary lesions to be accomplished.

Pincushion distortion describes the selective magnification of objects viewed near the edges of the angiographic field, compared with objects viewed at its center. When using a 10 inch angiographic field, as much as 35% greater magnification may occur at the periphery [1]. However, with the five and six inch fields commonly used for coronary arteriography, only 5–8% maximum pincushion distortion is present [1–3].

Differential magnification describes another form of image distortion that occurs due to the fact that objects closest to the X-ray tube are being selectively magnified. The differential in magnification for two objects located along the X-ray beam axis is about 1.5% for each centimeter that separates the objects axially [4]. This problem is particularly important in quantitative programs that use the angiographic catheter as a scaling device. These programs all assume that the catheter and coronary artery lie in the same plane.

The above two forms of image distortion may introduce maximum errors in diameter estimates of 5–10%. These inaccuracies are not trivial when compared to the 16–18% luminal diameter narrowing due to the vasoconstrictor effects of ergonovine, or a 10–12% average vasodilator effect of nitroglycerin [4].

Quantum mottle [5] is another source of image degradation. Because each cine frame is generated by an X-ray pulse of short duration and low energy, relatively few X-ray photons are generated by each pulse. These effects result in a statistical uncertainty as to the amount of X-ray energy absorbed in any given region. The image intensifier accentuates the mottling effect yielding an image which is degraded. This phenomenon is not usually observed when coronary arteriograms are viewed with standard cine projectors but can be easily observed at higher magnification. This mottling may be coarse enough to considerably degrade the margins of coronary arteries.

Coronary artery alignment

Because coronary atherosclerosis often results in short segments of focal luminal narrowing, visualization of the lesion is best achieved by viewing the involved arterial segment in a projection that is nearly perpendicular to the vessel axis. The projection must avoid superimposition of multiple vessels that may interfere with the clear definition of the individual arteries. Since coronary stenosis often occurs at arterial branching, each major bifurcation should be visualized in a projection that is perpendicular to its epicardial plane.

Variability in interpretation of coronary arteriograms

Numerous studies document the presence of significant interobserver and intra-observer variability in determining the percent stenosis of coronary arteries by routine cineangiography [6–11]. As well, there is poor correlation between the anti-mortem coronary arteriogram and the corresponding post-mortem coronary artery specimen, often with significant underestimation of actual disease [12–14].

DeRouen *et al.* [7] studied the interpretation of 10 cinefilms by 11 readers. The average standard deviation for any segmental stenosis was 18%. Disagreement about the number of major vessels with a 70% stenosis occurred in one third of cases.

This problem was well outlined by the Coronary Artery Surgery Study (CASS) investigators [10]. The quality control procedures in cardiac catheterizations provided a large amount of information with which to evaluate the variability and interpretation of coronary angiograms. In the 870 arteriograms read independently by observers at different centers, there was an absolute difference in percent stenosis of between 5 and 10% depending on the arterial segment involved. Table 1 gives an estimate of the percent of the time a second reader would record no lesion given that the first reader records a lesion of a fixed amount (greater than 50% or greater than 70%). As can be seen, stenosis of the proximal and mid right coronary artery (RCA) are read more reproducibly than lesions of the distal RCA. For the posterior descending coronary artery, one reader will not identify a lesion in 28.5% of patients whereas the other reads a lesion of 50% or more. Of more importance clinically, is the substantial variation in reading presence or absence of disease in the left main coronary artery (LMCA). When a single reader reads a lesion of greater than 50% in the LMCA, 15.7% of the time the second reader will fail to identify a lesion. Likewise, the proximal and mid-left anterior descending arteries (LAD) are read well, whereas the distal LAD is read relatively less consistently. In 94.7% of the films, the number of significantly diseased vessels (greater than 70% stenosis) was the same for both readers (72.1%) or differed by one vessel (22.6%).

The CASS Study found, as well, that the intra-reader variability was approximately one-half of the inter-reader variability when evaluating percent stenosis. This difference was statistically significant. The left hand panel of Figure 1 shows the intra-reader scatter plot for percent stenosis in the proximal LAD artery. The right hand panel shows the scatter comparing the readings between readers. As might be expected, if comparisons about other aspects of the disease process, including the presence or absence of collaterals, morphology of the lesion, morphology of the distal vessel, size of the distal vessel, and presence or absence of disease of the distal vessel, are made, the variability between readers increases. It is obvious from this discussion that if meaningful statements about coronary artery pathology, progression, or regression are to be made, then a more objective method of quantitating coronary artery lesions is necessary.

Percentage stenosis as an index of coronary artery disease

Another current source of error in the interpretation of coronary arteriograms is the method of grading lesions by determining the percentage stenosis. Percentage stenosis is a relative estimate of luminal diameter reduction, whereas the hemo-dynamic significance of a stenosis depends largely on its minimal diameter [4]. The nearby normal vessel whose diameter forms the denominator of the percent stenosis estimate, may be dilated by aging or by post-stenotic turbulence [15] or narrowed by diffuse proliferative thickening of the intimal smooth muscle layer. An example of this concept is illustrated in Figure 2. The top panel represents serial lesions of 50% and 75% diameter stenosis. If the atherosclerotic process subsequently diffusely involves the entire arterial segment, reducing the 'normal' diameter by 50%, then a subjective angiographic interpretation may not detect

Table 1. Likelihood of reader number 1 recording zero stenosis when reader number 2 reads a stenosis of 50% or more, and 70% or more. (From: Clinical diagnosis of atherosclerosis: quantitative methods of evaluation, Springer-Verlag Inc., 1983, p 482, reproduced with permission.)

Segment	≥50%	≥70%
Proximal RCA[a]	2.2	2.1
Mid RCA	1.9	0.9
Distal RCA	10.5	8.6
PDA[b]	28.5	25.6
LMCA[c]	15.7	11.6
Proximal LAD[d]	2.9	1.5
Mid LAD	0.9	0.5
Distal LAD	10.2	6.4
Proximal Circumflex	3.0	2.4

[a] Right coronary artery.
[b] Posterior descending artery.
[c] Left main coronary artery.
[d] Left anterior descending coronary artery.

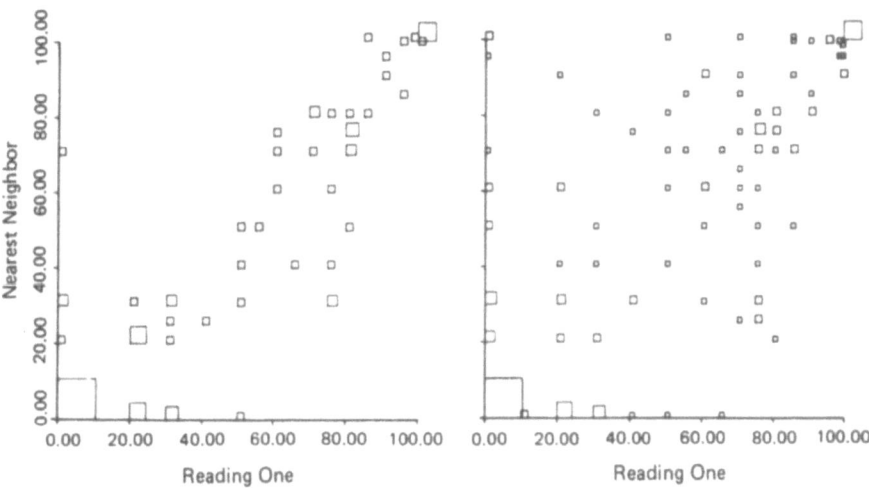

Figure 1. Inter- and intrareader variability in reading the percent stenosis in the proximal LAD. (From: Clinical diagnosis of atherosclerosis: quantitative methods of evaluation Springer-Verlag Inc., 1983, p 484; reproduced with permission.)

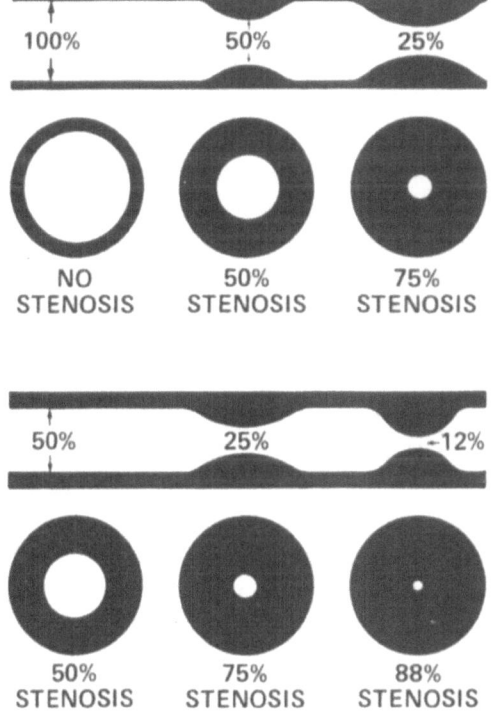

Figure 2. The top panel represents serial lesions of 50% and 75% stenosis, resulting in 50% and 25% of the original lumen remaining patent. With diffuse progression of the entire segment by 50% (bottom panel), the resulting diameters are only 25% and 12% of the original. Hence, interpretation of percent intimal narrowing of 50% and 75% in this situation would be misleading.

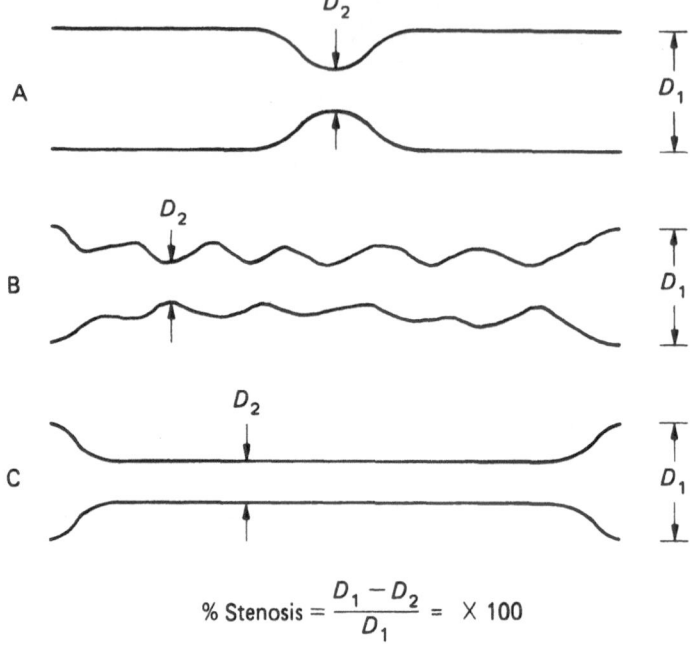

$$\% \text{ Stenosis} = \frac{D_1 - D_2}{D_1} = \times 100$$

Figure 3. Identical values for stenosis are given to arteries with varying amounts of disease. (From: Clinical diagnosis of Atherosclerosis: quantitative methods of evaluation Springer-Verlag Inc., 1983, p 45; reproduced with permission.)

any progression and continue to interpret this arterial segment as having a 50% and 75% stenosis, rather than the true progression of 75% and 88% when compared to the original diameters. Progression would therefore be evident only if the absolute cross-sectional diameter were determined rather than just the percent stenosis. Among film readers, variation in selecting the 'normal' referenced area has been identified as a major cause of interobserver error [6].

Stenosis length is another variable that is not used in the current estimate of disease severity. The effect of length on moderate stenosis has been demonstrated experimentally [16]. As seen in Figure 3, arterial segments with vastly different amounts of atherosclerosis are described by the same stenosis value.

In summary, the present standard for clinical assessment of coronary disease severity is the subjective visual estimate of percent stenosis. This method lacks accuracy and reproducibility. Because of the variability of the nearby 'normal' arterial diameter, it may not be the best method for gauging coronary artery pathology.

Quantitative analysis of coronary artery lesions

Quantitation of atherosclerosis should ideally be concerned with four related, but

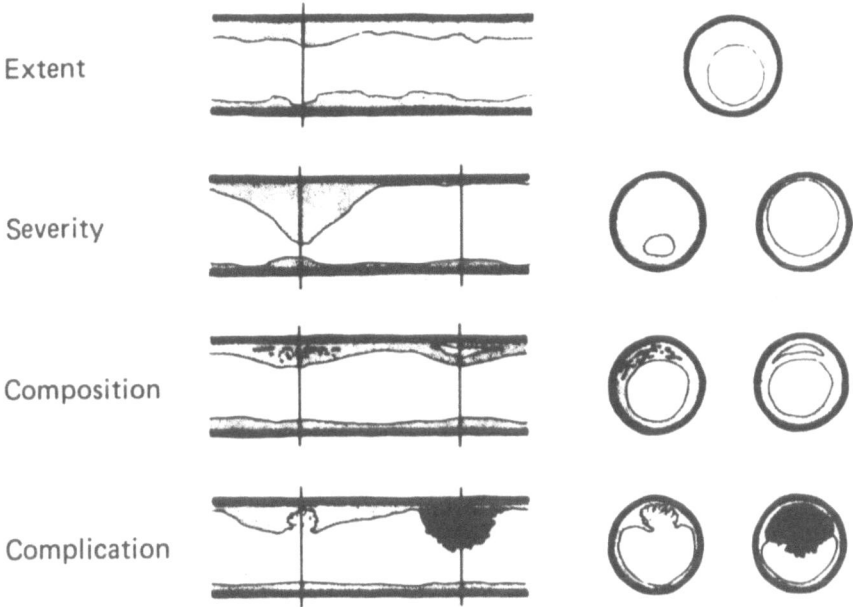

Figure 4. Diagram of quantifiable aspects of atherosclerosis. Vertical lines identify levels of transverse cross-sections shown at right. (From: Clinical diagnosis of atherosclerosis: quantitative methods of evaluation Springer-Verlag Inc., 1983, p 13; reproduced with permission.)

distinguishable, anatomic manifestations of lesions. These include extent, severity, lesion composition, and complications of atherosclerosis. Figure 4 illustrates this diagramatically. 'Extent' is a measure of the bulk of atherosclerotic intimal tissue in a specified arterial segment. 'Severity' is an evaluation of the degree to which the lumen is narrowed. This should commonly be expressed as minimal lumen diameter. 'Composition' deals with differences in concentration and distribution of the cellular and matrix constituents of lesions. Lesions could be dense, hard and calcific, or soft and semi-solid. 'Complication' is concerned with secondary disruptions which are manifested as plaque hemorrhages, ulcerations, and thrombosis [17]. Most methods of quantification currently under study involve determination of the extent and severity of atherosclerosis.

In order to directly measure vessel change from serial images, the following conditions would have to exist: (1) replicable exposure geometry, (2) controllable vasospasm and vasodilation, (3) correction for arterial pulsation effects, and (4) discrete and symmetric lesions. Conditions 1 and 2 can be achieved by careful angiographic techniques. If pulsation size changes are significant, then phasic matching or cardiac gating of serial frames can be used. The necessity of lesion symmetry can be overcome by radiographic methods based on quantitative densitometry of iodine X-ray absorption that makes it possible to compute true arterial cross-sectional area and thus incremental lumen volume changes [18–25].

Methods using direct measurements of arterial images

For over ten years, investigators have attempted to more precisely quantitate coronary artery lesions. MacAlpin *et al.* [3] used calipers to make direct measurements of projected arteriographic coronary images and of a calibrating object filmed at the level of the left ventricle. The mean accuracy of known object dimensions was ± 0.2 mm. Feldman and associates [26, 27] used a comparable technique and reported 0.5 mm of variability in the measurement of projected dimensions. Gensini *et al.* [28] used a viewing telescope that projects cross-hairs into film images. The margin of error was found to be 0.08 mm or 2–3% of the vessel diameter. Rafflenbeul *et al.* [29, 30] reported a vernier estimate of coronary arterial dimension taken directly from the projected screen at about three times magnification. Post-mortem validation determined the correlation coefficient to be 0.85 [30]. Feldman *et al.* [2] subsequently combined high quality 105 mm photospot arteriographic images with a magnifying vernier having 0.1 mm graduations. The catheter tip was used as a scalling device. The standard deviation of repeated dimension estimates was 0.1 mm.

The above descriptions of direct measurements of projected arterial dimensions have several limitations. These methods are quite time consuming and are therefore not applicable to routine coronary arteriographic analysis. No attempt was made to overcome the technical problems of pincushion distortion, diffential magnification, and quantum mottle. These problems are all accentuated by increasing the magnification of the coronary arteriograms. As well, these methods assume that the diseased coronary lumen is circular. However, it is well known that the measured severity in one arteriographic projection may differ from that in another projection. One way to compensate for this would be to average measurements from as many different projections as possible.

Measurements from computer assisted image reconstruction

Because of the difficulties with direct measurement of image border information, Brown and associates [1, 4, 31] developed a method using digital computation to compensate for distortion of the arteriographic image in order to create a true scale three-dimensional representation of a diseased arterial segment. Cineframes are selected for lesion clarity at comparable points in the cardiac cycle in each view of a perpendicular projection pair (e.g. 40° LAO, 50° RAO) in which the lesion of interest is best seen. These frames are projected at approximately five fold magnification. The borders of the image of the diseased arterial segments are traced from the proximal 'normal' portion, through the stenosis, to the distal 'normal' portion. A segment of catheter of known dimensions is traced as a scaling factor. These tracings are digitized into a PDP 11/45 digital computer where they are converted to true scale by compensating for pin cushion distortion, X-ray beam divergence, and magnification (Figure 5). Figure 6 shows a hard

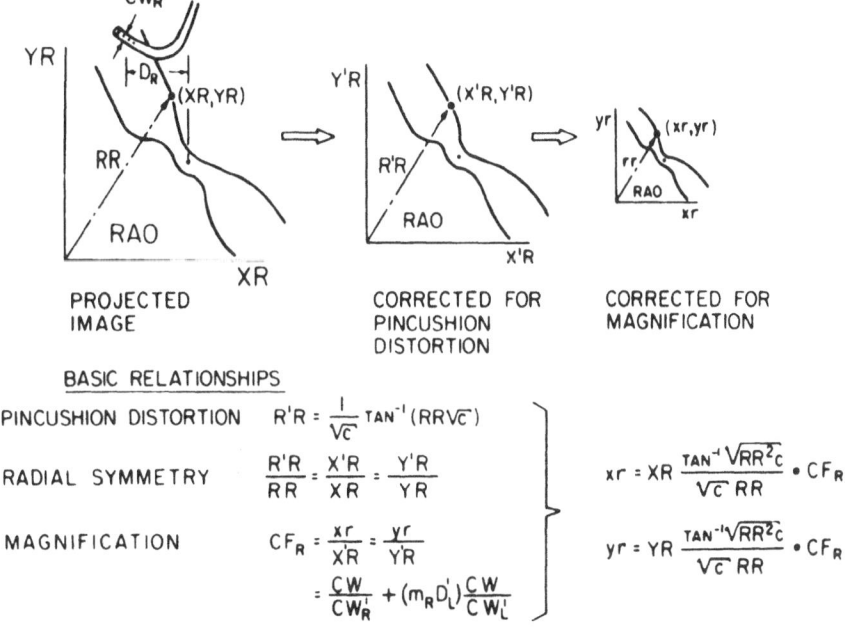

Figure 5. Coordinate systems in computer-assisted lesion analysis and the transformations relating to them. On the left is the image plane of the projected cine frame. The image is digitized and corrected for pincushion distortion and for magnification to arrive at a true-scale representation of the diseased lumen. The catheter of known width CW and projected width CW_R serves as a scaling device. CF_R is the dimensional correction factor which converts projected dimensions to true dimensions. (From reference 4, reproduced with permission.)

copy computer printout of this analysis in which the LAO and the RAO images are combined into a three-dimensional characterization of the diseased segment. From this data the vessel diameters and cross-sectional areas are computed for the 'normal' ends and for the point of greatest narrowing. Other computations are lesion length, estimated atheroma mass, and stenosis flow resistance. These formulas can be found elsewhere [1, 31].

Brown's method has been shown to be accurate to within an average of 0.1 mm for measurements of known dimensions. The standard deviation of variability averages 3% in estimates of percent stenosis and 0.1 mm for estimates of minimum lesion diameter, when compared to brass phantoms with known minimum diameters [1, 31].

There are practical limitations to this technique. It is presently time-consuming and tedious. As well, it requires subjective interpretation in the tracing of the lumen border. However, Brown argues [4] that with high quality arteriograms, border definition is less of a problem than might be expected. The human eye is an image processor that appears to perform functions such as edge detection, border interpolation, and longitudinal smoothing remarkably well.

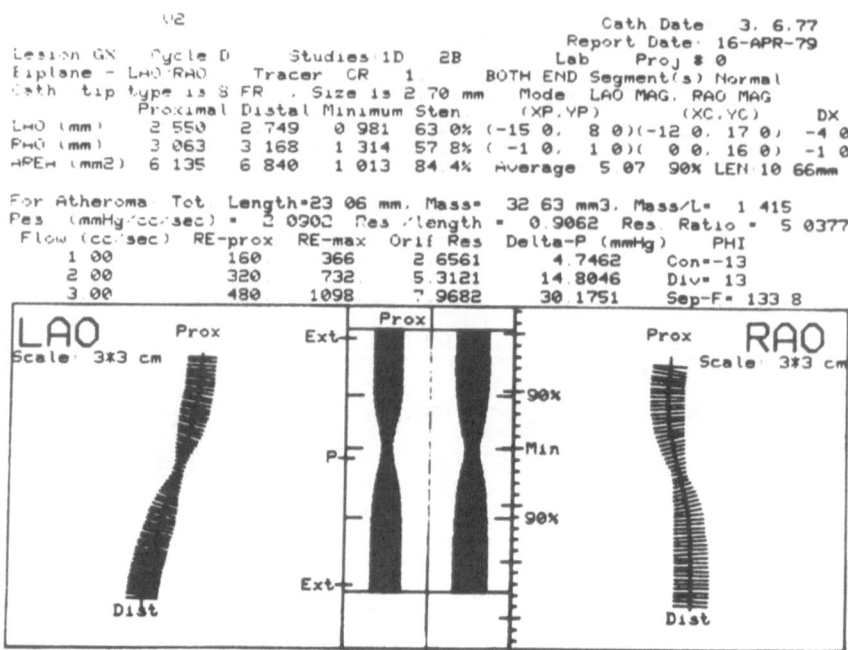

Figure 6. Computer printout of the Brown and Dodge analysis of a coronary stenosis. The two perpendicular views of the diseased segment are reduced to true scale in the 3 × 3 cm panels. These images are matched at the point of greatest narrowing and combined to form a three-dimensional representation, which is stretched mathematically to true length in the center panels. (From reference 4, reproduced with permission.)

Computerized edge detection techniques

As noted above, current approaches are laborious and require operator assistance to locate the coronary lumen boundary. The rapid progress in the field of image processing by digital techniques and parallel developments in computer design offer the opportunity for investigating additional alternative approaches to the analysis of coronary arteriograms.

Investigators at our institution have developed a new image processing technique for evaluation of coronary arteriograms [32, 33]. This technique uses a special purpose computer, the cytocomputer, that was developed at the Environmental Research Institute of Michigan. A cytocomputer is a serial pipeline of identical processing stages where each stage in the pipeline does a single image transformation on the entire image using neighborhood pixel operations. Standard clinical contrast coronary arteriograms obtained from 35 mm film in our catheterization laboratory are digitized into 256 × 256 × 8 bit image array at an effective magnification of seven times. Figure 7 shows the original 35 mm cine film image. Figure 8 demonstrates the digitized version. The location of the artery

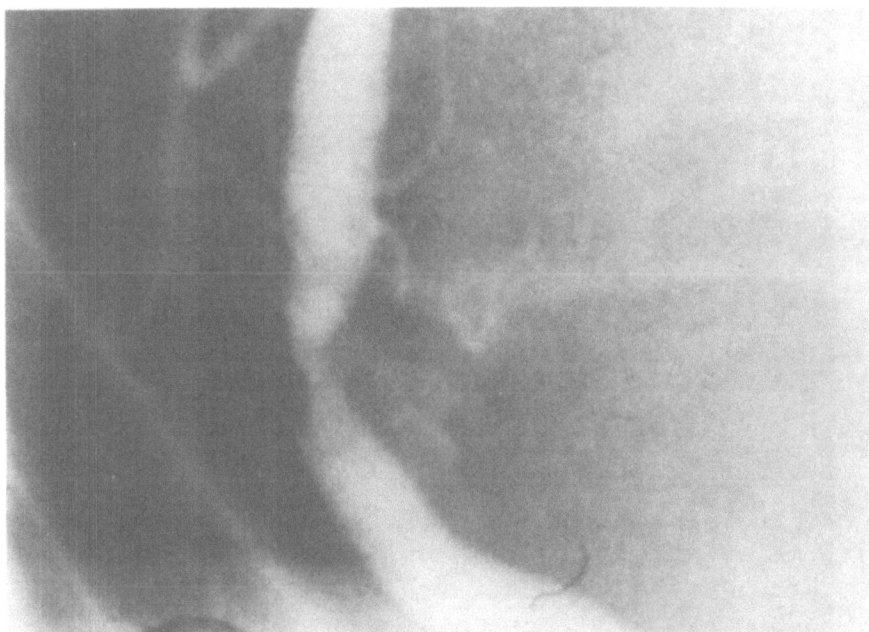

Figure 7. Original 35 mm cine film image of a right coronary lesion.

is reasonably well defined in profile; however, there is no single threshold value that identifies the vessel boundary. Also the jagged appearance of the profile indicates a fair degree of high frequency noise in the image.

The first step in the algorithm is to eliminate the high frequency noise using what amounts to a low pass filter. This is done by generating a structuring element in the shape of a small sphere that in effect rolls or slides over and under the surface of the image, smoothing it with respect to the size of the sphere. The resultant image is seen in the right hand panel of Figure 8. The next operation removes the non-coronary background. This spatially varying background prohibits the location of a global threshold value to determine the coronary boundary. This background can be removed effectively by performing a high pass filter which is done by sliding a larger sphere underneath the surface of the image. If the diameter of the sphere is chosen specifically to be larger than the diameter of the artery, only the low frequency background component will be isolated by the transformation. This is diagramatically presented in Figure 9. This low frequency image can then be subtracted to provide a background corrected (normalized) image (left hand panel of Figure 10). A single threshold level that defines the border of the artery is now easily determined from the background corrected image. Figure 10 demonstrates the background corrected image prior to and after the threshold operation. Through further processing a center line of the vessel is created (Figure 11.)

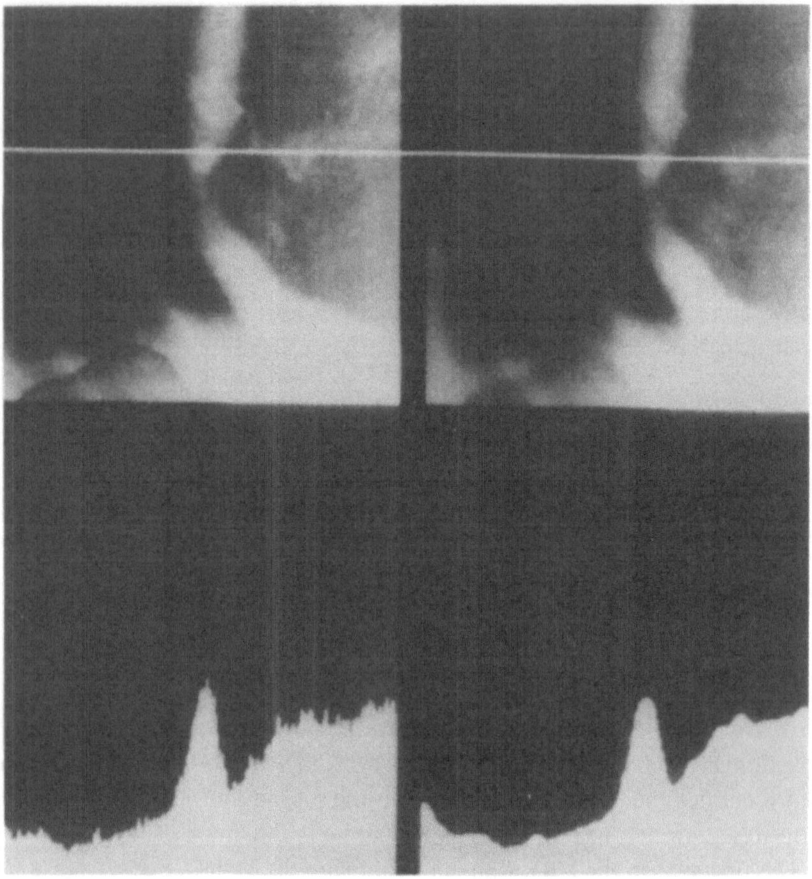

Figure 8. Digitized (left panel) and smoothed (right panel) image.

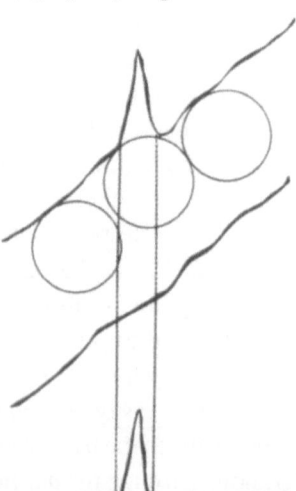

Figure 9. Diagram of high pass filter technique to remove background.

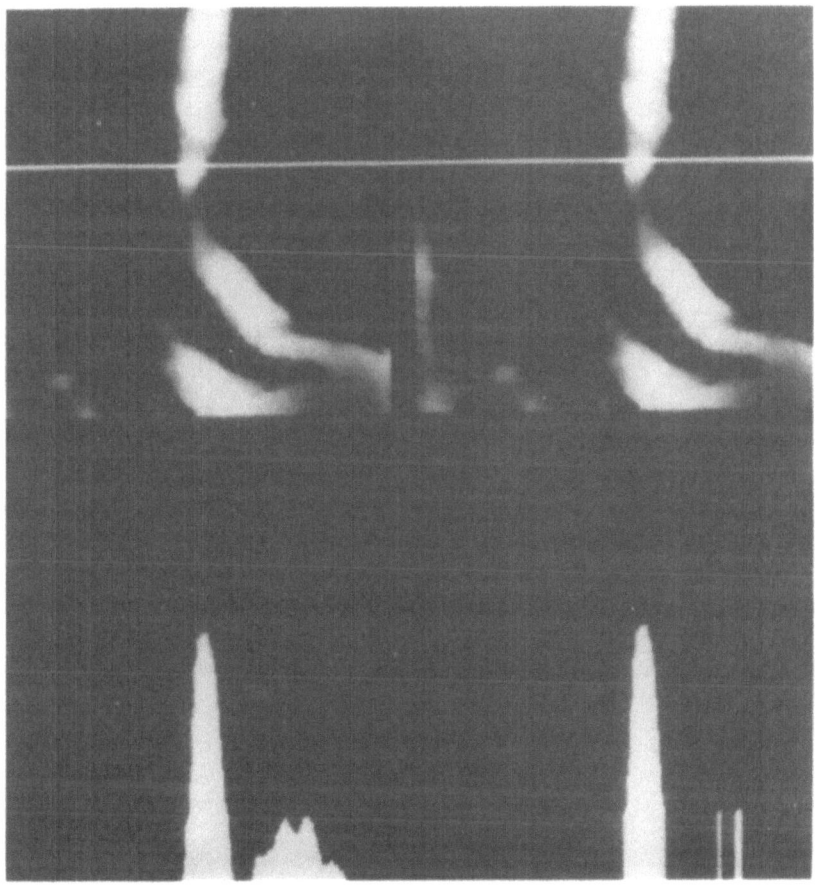

Figure 10. Background corrected (left panel) and thresholded (right panel) images.

Because of differences in X-ray geometry and digitization magnification for successive images, it is impossible to obtain actual lesion diameters without using a known scaling device. We have chosen to use the angiographic catheter as the scaling device since its diameter is known, it is usually in close proximity to the vessel under study, and its image can be obtained from the same film frame as the affected coronary artery. In order to obtain a magnification correction factor, a section of catheter is digitized and processed in an identical fashion to the artery processing just described.

The catheter and artery images are then entered into a non-cytocomputer program to calculate actual lesion parameters and generate a final report (Figure 12). Superimposed on the catheter and artery images are the cytocomputer generated edges and center line. The proximal and distal 'normal' segments are chosen to be the maximum diameters proximal to and distal to the area of stenosis. These locations may be manually adjusted if desired. The upper right

132

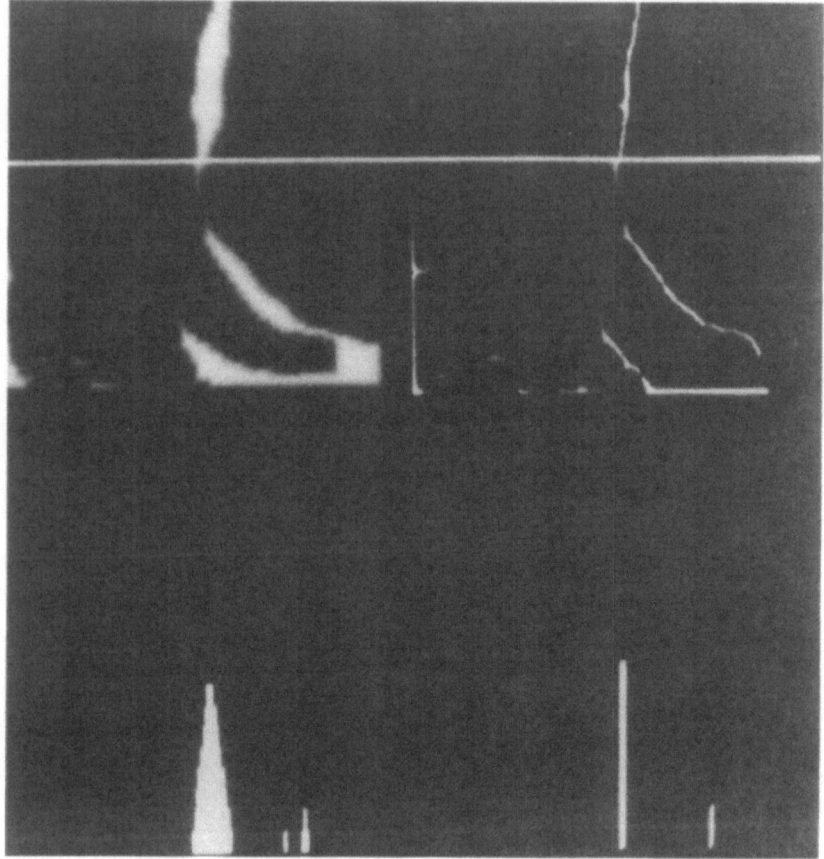

Figure 11. Creation of vessel center line.

hand image shows the reconstructed radius image that has been straightened and the segments of interest chosen. Both the cued edges and the straightened artery images serve as visual quality control checks for proper program operation. The lesion length is calculated as the distance between the segments where the diameter decreases to 90% of its normal value. The area calculations are derived by assuming a circular vessel lumen.

This algorithm has been validated with a brass arterial phantom (average error 0.04 mm), and against the hand traced method of Brown *et al.* [1] (r = 0.96). The intraobserver error from repeated processing of the same cineangiographic film was ±0.150 mm and serial measurements on the same patient produced correlations of 0.97. These results indicate that this digital image processing approach has a small estimate of error and requires less time than most other methods of arterial quantification.

Limitations of this technique include an inability to provide three-dimensional

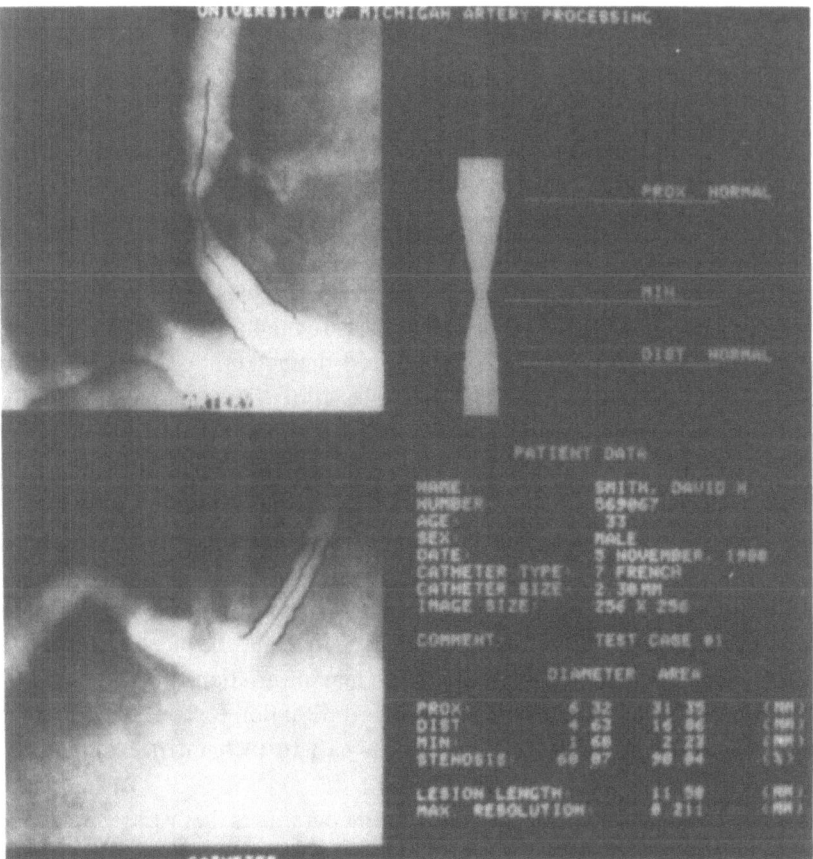

Figure 12. Final report. The cytocomputer generated edges and center lines are superimposed on the artery and catheter images (top left and bottom left respectively). The upper right hand image shows the reconstructed radius image that has been straightened and the segments of interest chosen.

reconstruction of coronary anatomy, and the necessity for operator selection of a threshold that prevents full automation of the analysis. At present, images are entered into the cytocomputer in line scan format from digital disk storage. However, the line scan format is ideally suited to the real time processing of video information that is found in most catheterization laboratories.

Other groups of investigators are currently developing algorithms that automatically detect the edges of digitized coronary cineangiograms. Reiber *et al.* [34, 35] have described an edge detection algorithm that depends on the difference of average grey scale (intensity gradation) values in the digitized image. However, an operator must determine a tentative center line for the artery. The variability of the method in determining the contours and calculating the percent stenosis was found to be 1.84% (standard deviation). The accuracy of this algorithm was verified against brass phantoms with various known percentage diameter narrowing. The correlation coefficient was 0.99 with a standard error of the estimate of 2.33%.

Sanders *et al.* [5] have combined the work of Blankenhorn [22] for automatic edge detection based on the grey scale (intensity gradation) first derivative, with the work of Brown and Dodge [1, 31] to construct a three-dimensional model of a coronary artery segment from two serial biplane views. In Sander's program, the center line is defined by calculating a line which is the average of the two lines defining the margins. The diameter of the segment is measured at each point along the center line by constructing a line perpendicular to the center line and intersecting each margin. All subsequent measurements are based on the center line and the corresponding set of measured diameters. A three-dimensional reconstruction technique is used to construct a three-dimensional model of the coronary artery segment from two perpendicular views. This model consists of a string of elliptical disks, with the center of each disk being along the three-dimensional center line. The major and minor diameters of the ellipse are obtained from the two perpendicular views. With this model, the true length of the vessel is obtained, eliminating foreshortening due to the relative angle of the vessel with respect to the plane of the projection in any single view. The assumption of an elliptical cross-section rather than a circle may be more accurate. This method yielded a standard deviation of 0.05 mm in variation of measurements of a series of 60 images. However, the standard deviation for measured diameter was 7.5% of the diameter, attributable in part to incomplete elimination of quantum mottle.

It is not generally widely appreciated by angiographers that vessel images have edge gradients rather than sharply demarcated edges (Figure 13). Accurate diameter measurements are dependent on precise localization of the anatomic vessel edge within the edge gradient. A mathematical algorithm that detected the true edge within the edge gradient was recently validated using cylindrical phantoms filled with contrast [36].

Videodensitometry of arteriographic images

Videodensitometry performed on a scanning trajectory that crosses the arteriographic lumen image, is theoretically very useful. Points at which optical density changes abruptly along the trajectory mark the borders of the arteriographic lumen. This concept forms the basis for the edge detection algorithms previously described.

Under defined conditions, the optical density of each arterial segment recorded on the angiographic frame, is a specific function of the volume of contrast medium within the arterial lumen, which represents the volume of the arterial segment. The optical density profile can thus provide an estimate proportional to the cross-sectional area of the vessel. Thus, three-dimensional information is extracted from a two-dimensional image [18–25]. Luminal density analysis from densi-

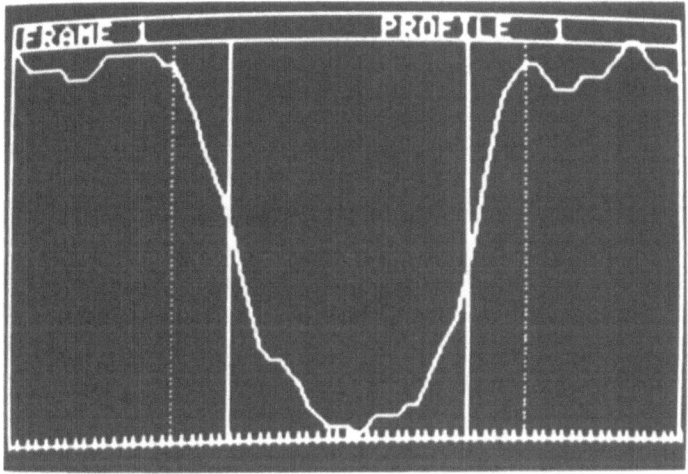

Figure 13. Transverse densitometric scan across phantom vessel image. Film optical density on the ordinate is plotted against distance across the vessel image on the abscissa. Note the gradient of density at the vessel edges. (From reference 36, reproduced with permission of American Heart Association.)

tometric profiles performed across the vessel image at the 'normal' segment compared to a point of greatest narrowing, may be used to estimate the percent area reduction by the stenosis.

Nichols *et al.* [24] recently validated a cinevideodensitometric method for quantitating coronary arteries. The digital grey scale was found to be linearly related to the film density. The cinevideodensitometric signal was found to vary linearly with the concentration of contrast medium. The integrated videodensitometric signal measured over contrast filled cylinders correlated linearly with the cross-sectional areas of the cylinders over a wide range of contrast concentrations. In phantom experiments of eccentric stenosis, the relative reduction in the cinevideodensitometric signal correlated highly with the actual reduction in cross sectional area. Videodensitometric analysis of coronary cineangiograms resulted in comparable values for relative stenosis of eccentric lesions in different angiographic projections. The percent relative stenosis measured by this method correlated well with percent reduction of cross-sectional area measured histologically in post-mortem hearts ($r = 0.97$).

This technique is promising in dealing with irregularly shaped stenosed lumina because the densitometric profile is a function of luminal area, independent of its cross-sectional shape. The need for border recognition is eliminated. The operator simply positions a rectangular region of interest across the arterial lumen with the ends of the rectangle extending well beyond the vessel margin. The average background density is then calculated and subtracted to yield a video signal that is proportional to the amount of contrast in the vessel. The simplicity of this approach considerably reduces the time required for each analysis. Unfortunately, this technique is still significantly complicated by X-ray scatter and veiling glare within the image intensifier.

Methods that combine border information and videodensitometry

Investigators at the University of Southern California – Jet Propulsion Laboratory have used computer based image scanning videodensitometry of cut film femoral arteriograms to estimate vessel edge roughness and lumen volume irregularity [36]. Several indices derived from such digital pattern data have correlated well with the measured arterial cholesterol content and with visual grading of atherosclerosis in the opened vessel. Although the primary focus of this group has been the radiographic analysis of the femoral artery, this approach appears to be particularly useful for the angiographic analysis of early atherosclerosis in coronary arteries. Figure 14 is a computer processed image of the right coronary artery. The computer was programmed to find the edges of the artery as those points along a line perpendicular to the vessel image where the film density change was greatest. A smooth tapered cylinder designed to simulate the normal arterial lumen, was 'best fit' to the detected edges and the average difference between the cylinder and the edges computed. This difference was found to correlate with amount of atherosclerosis within the vessel wall [37].

Conclusion

This chapter emphasized the necessity for close attention to the technical aspects of coronary arteriography as a prerequisite for computer assisted quantitative coronary measurements. Current computer programs are attempting to overcome the problems of pincushion distortion and differential magnification. The problems of inter- and intraobserver variability and the use of percentage stenosis as an index of coronary atherosclerosis limit standard approaches. Investigators are currently working on automatic edge detection algorithms in order to determine a minimal cross-sectional diameter of coronary stenosis. Others are developing algorithms based on videodensitometry that, with the use of a scaling device, can determine an absolute cross-sectional area from the cine frame. A potentially exciting area of development, still in its infancy, is the absolute quantitation of atherosclerosis by combining videodensitometry and edge detection techniques. These techniques may gradually change our concepts of coronary artery disease. These methods of precise quantitation are essential if risk factor interventions that potentially reverse coronary artery disease are to be appropriately evaluated.

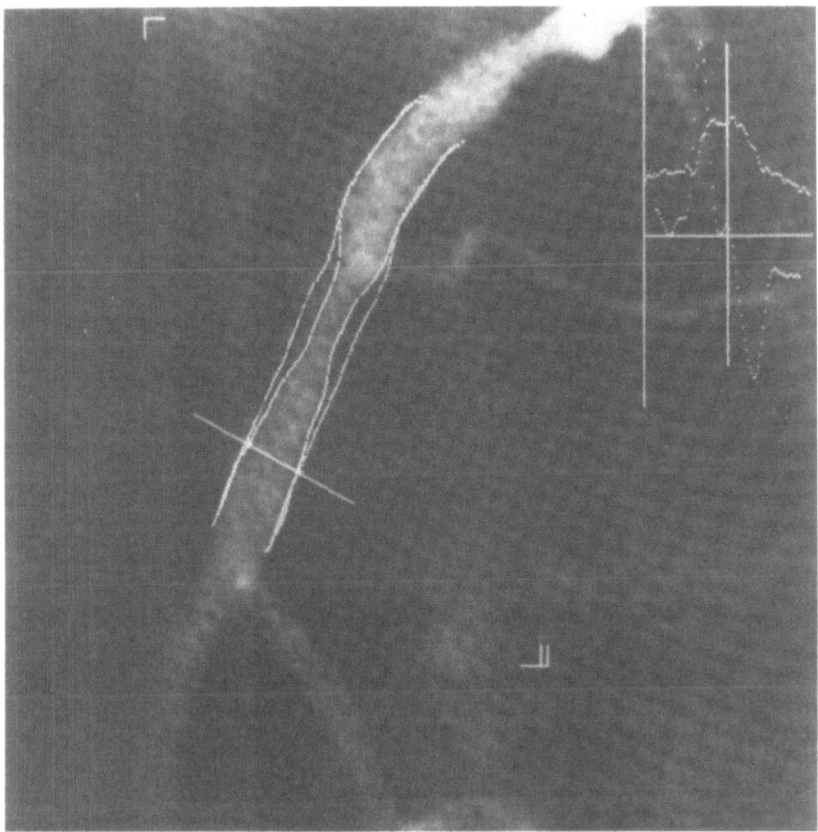

Figure 14. Computer processed image of right coronary artery. A sample intensity profile line and the computer gradient curve are shown in the upper right hand corner of the frame. (From: Clinical diagnosis of atherosclerosis: quantitative methods of evaluation, Springer-Verlag Inc., 1983, p 54; reproduced with permission.)

Acknowledgements

We wish to thank Dave Smith, Michael LeFree, and Harry Colfer, MD for their helpful suggestions. As well, we wish to thank Judy Seeger for her expert typing assistance.

Support in part for the preparation of this manuscript under funding from NIH grant HL 29716 is gratefully acknowledged.

References

1. Brown BG, Bolson E, Frimer M, Dodge HT: Quantitative coronary arteriography: estimation of

138

dimension, hemodynamic resistance, and atheroma mass of coronary artery lesions using the arteriogram and digital computation. Circulation 55: 329–337, 1977.

2. Feldman RL, Pepine CJ, Curry RC, Conti CR: Quantitative coronary arteriography using 105 mm photospot angiography and an optical magnifying device. Cathet Cardiovasc Diagn 5: 195, 1979.

3. MacAlpin RN, Abbasi AS, Grothman JH, Eber L: Human coronary artery size during life. Radiology 108: 567, 1973.

4. Brown BG, Peterson RB, Pierce CD, Bolson EL, Dodge HT: Arteriographic assessment of coronary disease: advantages, limitations, and clinical uses of a computer-assisted method. In: Rappaport E, Kouchoukos NT, Oparil S, Pitt B, Popp RL, Scheinman MM (eds), Cardiology update 1982 edition. Elsevier Biomedical, New York, 1982, pp 67–98.

5. Sanders WJ, Alderman EL, Harrison DC: Coronary artery quantitation using digital image processing techniques. IEEE Computers in Cardiol 15–20, 1979.

6. Zir LM, Miller SW, Dinsmore RE, Gilbert JP, Harthorne JW: Interobserver variability in coronary angiography. Circulation 53: 627–632, 1976.

7. DeRouen TA, Murray JA, Owen W: Variability in the analysis of coronary arteriograms. Circulation 55: 324–328, 1977.

8. Sanmarco ME, Brooks SH, Blankenhorn DH: Reproducibility of a concensus panel in the interpretation of coronary angiograms. Am Heart J 96: 430–437, 1978.

9. Detre KM, Wright PH, Murphy ML, Takaro T: Observer agreement in evaluating coronary angiograms. Circulation 52: 979–986, 1975.

10. Kennedy JW, Fisher LD, Killip T: Coronary angiography quality control in the Cass Study. In: Bond MG, Insull W, Glagov S, Chandler AB, Cornhill JF (eds), Clinical diagnosis of atherosclerosis: quantitative methods of evaluation. Springer-Verlag, New York, 1983, pp 475–491.

11. Galbraith JE, Murphy ML, DeSoyza N: Coronary angiogram interpretation: interobserver variability. J Am Med Assoc 240: 2053–2056, 1978.

12. Schwartz JN, Kong Y, Hackel DB, Bartel AG: Comparison of angiographic and post-mortem findings in patients with coronary artery disease. Am J Cardiol 36: 174–178, 1975.

13. Vlodaver Z, Frech R, Van Tassel RA, Edwards JE: Correlation of anti-mortem coronary arteriogram and the post-mortem specimen. Circulation 47: 162–169, 1973.

14. Zarins CK, Zatina MA, Glagov S: Correlation of post-mortem angiography with pathologic anatomy: Quantitation of atherosclerotic lesions. In: Bond MG, Insull W, Glagov S, Chandler AB, Cornhill JF (eds), Clinical diagnosis of atherosclerosis: quantitative methods of evaluation. Springer-Verlag, New York, 1983, pp 284–306.

15. Roach MR: Changes in arterial distensibility as a cause of post-stenotic dilatation. Am J Cardiol 12: 802, 1963.

16. Feldman RL, Nichols WW, Pepine CJ, Conti CR: Hemodynamic significance of the length of a coronary arterial narrowing. Am J Cardiol 41: 865, 1978.

17. Glagov S, Zarins CK: Quantitating atherosclerosis: problems of definition. In: Bond MG, Insull W, Glagov S, Chandler AB, Cornhill JF (eds), Clinical diagnosis of atherosclerosis: quantitative methods of evaluation. Springer-Verlag, New York, 1983, pp 11–35.

18. Sandor T, Als AV, Paulin S: Cinedensitometric measurement of coronary arterial stenosis. Cathet Cardiovasc Diagn 5: 229–245, 1979.

19. Kishan Y, Yerushalmi S, Deutsh V, Neufeld HN: Measurement of coronary arterial lumen by densitometric analysis of angiograms. Angiology 30 (5): 304–312, 1979.

20. Hoornstra K, Hanselman JMH, Holland WPJ, DeWey Peters GW, ZWamborn AW: Videodensitometry for measuring blood vessel diameter. Acta Radiol Diagn 21: 155–164, 1980.

21. Sandor T, Sridharb, Paulin S: Remote densitometric analysis of stenotic lesions. Int J Bio Med Comp 10: 15–22, 1979.

22. Crawford DW, Brooks SH, Barndt R, Blankenhorn DH: Measurement of atherosclerotic

luminal irregularity and obstruction by radiographic densitometry. Invest Radio 12: 307–313, 1977.

23. Kruger RA: Estimation of the diameter of an iodine concentration within blood vessels using digital radiography devices. Med Phys 8 (5): 652–658, 1981.

24. Nichols AB, Gabrich CFO, Fenoglio JJ, Esser PD: Quantification of relative coronary arterial stenosis by cinevideodensitometric analysis of coronary arteriograms. Circulation 69: 512–522, 1984.

25. Buis B, Endlick B, Amtzenius AC: A technique for measuring the diameter of coronary arteries and venous bypass grafts from 70 mm spot films. In: Lichtlen PR (ed), Coronary angiography and angina pectoris. George Thieme Verlag, Stuttgart, 1976, pp 265–272.

26. Feldman RL, Pepine CJ, Curry RC, Conti CR: Case against routine use of glyceryl trinitrate before coronary arteriography. Brit Heart J 40: 992, 1978.

27. Feldman RL, Pepine CJ, Curry RC, Conti CR: Coronary arterial responses to graded doses of nitroglycerin. Am J Cardiol 43: 91, 1979.

28. Gensini GG, Kelly AE, DaCosta BCB, Huntington PP: Quantitative angiography: the measurement of coronary vasomobility in the intact animal and man. Chest 60: 522–530, 1971.

29. Rafflenbeul W, Heim R, Dzeuiba M, Henkel B, Lichtlen P: Morphometric analysis of coronary arteries. In: Lichtlen P (ed), Coronary angiography and angina pectoris, Symp of the Eur Soc of Cardiol. Georg Thein Verlag, Stuttgart, 1976 pp 255–265.

30. Rafflenbeul W, Smith LR, Rogers WJ, Mantle JA, Rackley CE, Russell RO: Quantitative coronary arteriography: coronary anatomy of patients with unstable angina pectoris reexamined 1 year after optimal medical therapy. Am J Cardiol 43: 699–707, 1979.

31. McMahon MM, Brown BG, Cukingnan R, Rolett EL, Bolson E, Frimer M, Dodge HT: Quantitative coronary angiography: measurement of the 'critical' stenosis in patients with unstable angina and single vessel disease without collaterals. Circulation 60: 106–113, 1979.

32. Smith DN, Colfer H, Brymer JF, Pitt B, Kliman SH: A semiautomatic computer technique for processing coronary angiograms. IEEE Computers in Cardiol 325–328, 1981.

33. Smith DN, Colfer HT, Delp EJ, Walton JA, Pitt B: Cellular image transformation with an application to quantitative coronary arteriography. IEEE J Biomed Eng (in press).

34. Reiber JHC, Booman F, Tan HS, Slager CJ, Schuurbiers JCH, Gerbrands JJ, Meester GT: A cardiac image analysis system: objective quantitative processing of angiograms. IEEE Computers in Cardiol 239–242, 1978.

35. Booman F, Reiber JHC, Gerbrands JJ, Slager CJ, Schuurbiers JCH, Meester GT: Quantitative analysis of coronary occlusions from coronary cineangiograms. IEEE Computers in Cardiol 177–180, 1979.

36. Spears JR, Sandor T, Als AV, Malagold M, Markis JE, Grossman W, Serur JR, Paulin S: Computerized image analysis for quantitative measurement of vessel diameter from cineangiograms. Circulation 68: 453–461, 1983.

37. Selzer RH: Atherosclerosis quantitation by computer image analysis. In: Bond MG, Insull W, Glagov S, Chandler AB, Cornhill JF (eds), Clinical diagnosis of atherosclerosis: quantitative methods of evaluation. Springer-Verlag, New York, 1983, pp 43–45.

10. Clinical applications of cardiac CT

BRUCE H. BRUNDAGE

During the past decade a new diagnostic imaging technology, X-ray transmission computed tomography, has established itself as a valuable diagnostic tool. In the course of the latter half of the 1970's several investigators [1, 2] recognized the potential for computed tomography to become an important imaging device for evaluating the cardiovascular system and they reported preliminary observations in humans with heart disease. More recently other clinical investigators have documented the diagnostic use of CT scanning of the heart and great vessels in several important cardiovascular diseases. This chapter will summarize the clinical utility of this new imaging modality as it is applied using currently available body scanners. The future of the technique will also be discussed in the context of development of new ultrafast CT scanners which are now commercially available.

First generation CT scanners were limited to the imaging of the head because of slow scanning times. As technology progressed scanning became faster and imaging of other body organs was possible. Continuing advances in scanner technology resulted in even greater reduction in scan time so that many currently available body scanners are capable of obtaining images in 2–4 s. Although cardiac motion still blurs images of the heart at such speeds, it is possible to obtain images of adequate quality to provide useful assessment of certain cardiovascular diseases.

There are two scanning protocols that are currently employed for evaluation of the cardiovascular system with computed tomography. One, commonly called conventional scanning, is performed by obtaining cross-sectional images of the body at 0.5 to 1.0 cm increments in the region of interest. The longitudinal extent of the heart and great vessels can usually be covered by obtaining 8–12 one cm adjacent scans. The conventional scanning protocol is usually employed to evaluate the spatial relationships of cardiac anatomy. Dynamic scanning, the other commonly employed scanning protocol obtains repetitive scans at the same anatomic level with each scan being interrupted by a 1–3 s delay. Dynamic scanning is often employed to study rapidly changing cardiovascular phenomena such as blood flow.

Contrast enhancement is required for most cardiac CT scanning because the density of the myocardium and blood are nearly identical. Therefore, in order to differentiate the various cardiac structures it is necessary to increase the density of the blood pool with conventional contrast agents. Contrast enhanced cardiac CT is usually performed using contrast agents with an iodine concentration of 370 mg/ml or greater. The contrast is delivered by gravity-drip infusion or bolus injection into a superficial arm or neck vein. During conventional scanning gravity-drip contrast enhancement is usually preferred. Rapid hand injection of a contrast bolus is often employed in conjunction with dynamic scanning. Usually a bolus of 20–25 ml of contrast is adequate for dynamic scanning and an infusion of 1.5 ml/kg body weight provides satisfactory enhancement for conventional scanning.

The cross-sectional demonstration of cardiac anatomy by CT scanning provides the clinician with a good description of three-dimensional relationships (Figure 1A). Coupling this excellent spatial resolution with the tenfold greater density resolution of CT compared to conventional roentgenography makes CT a unique method for evaluating cardiovascular disease. Currently most tertiary care hospitals have body scanners with scanning speeds of 2–5 s and many of these scanners have software packages that make dynamic scanning feasible. These body scanners are capable of being clinically useful in the evaluation of cardiovascular disease [3].

The aorta, compared to the heart, moves much less during cardiac contraction and therefore it is not surprising that relatively artifact free images can be obtained with CT scanning. Also, the pathology of aortic disease is often intraluminal and the cross-sectional imaging format of CT makes it uniquely valuable for the assessment of aortic pathology. Already there is considerable clinical experience with CT for the evaluation of patients suspected of having aortic dissection [4]. Usually a conventional scanning protocol is employed in conjunction with contrast enhancement to define the false lumen created by the intimal flap which is characteristic of aortic dissection. Often blood flow is present in both the true and false lumen so the intimal flap is well identified during contrast enhancement (Figure 1B). The excellent density resolution of computed tomography often permits detection of any associated peri-aortic hematoma. Scanning at adjacent 1 cm intervals from the top of the aortic arch to the abdomen often makes it possible to define the proximal and distal extent of the dissection. On occasion, conventional scanning with drip infusion of contrast may not demonstrate the intimal flap adequately. In these cases, scanning is repeated using the dynamic protocol in conjunction with a hand injection of an intravenous bolus of contrast. The denser enhancement of the aortic lumen on arrival of the contrast bolus in the aorta will usually define the intimal flap. Dynamic scanning can also determine the temporal relationship of blood flow in the true and false lumens. In most cases, the true lumen enhances prior to the false lumen. If there is no blood flow in the false lumen, then it is more difficult to demonstrate the intimal flap. However, the excellent density resolution of CT scanning may detect

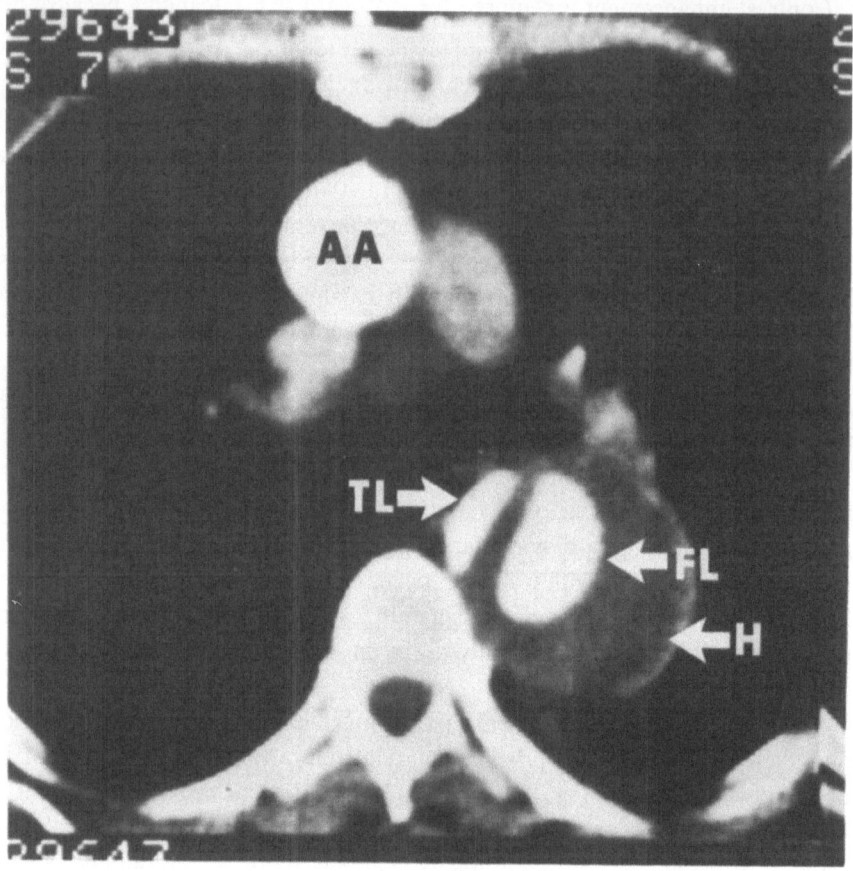

Figure 1A. This contrast enhanced CT scan shows a type III aortic dissection. The true lumen (TL) is separated from the false lumen (FL) by the intimal flap. The excellent density resolution of CT also defines the associated periaortic hematoma (H). AA = ascending aorta.

the density differences between the thrombosed false lumen and a true lumen. Very occasionally the excellent density and spatial resolution of CT may permit detection of the intimal flap without contrast enhancement if there is any calcification of the intima. The minimally invasive nature of contrast enhanced CT makes it an ideal diagnostic technique for evaluating the unstable and often critically ill patient suspected of having aortic dissection. Although further experience is necessary to determine the sensitivity and specificity of CT for identifying aortic dissections, there is little uncertainty about the diagnosis when an intimal flap is identified. It is premature to delegate specific roles for CT and aortography in the diagnosis of aortic dissection. However, some centers with extensive experience with cardiac CT do use the CT information to make therapeutic decisions and on occasion proceed to surgery without invasive aortography [5]. CT also appears to be a good method for the follow-up evaluation of patients

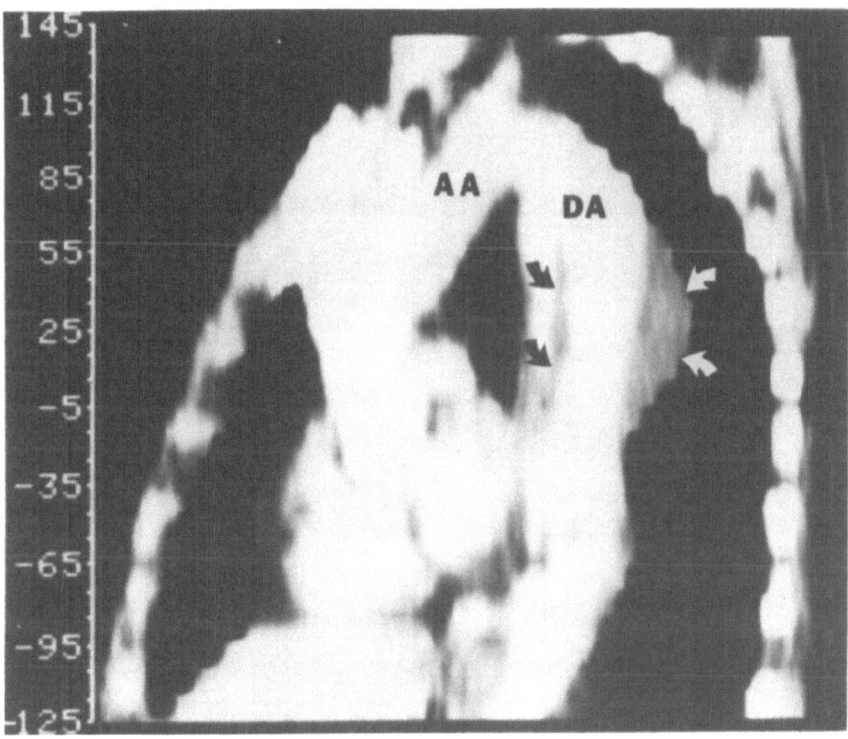

Figure 1B. Computer 'stacking' of the scan in Figure 1A and adjacent scans permits redisplay of the images in an oblique parasagittal format. The intimal flap (black arrows) and the periaortic hematoma (white arrows) are well defined. AA = ascending aorta; DA = descending aorta.

with aortic dissection by detecting any further enlargement or extension of the dissection.

CT can be used to image other types of thoracic and abdominal aortic aneurysms. However, aortography remains the standard method of diagnosis and in many cases abdominal ultrasound provides useful information. There are instances where CT can be used as a screening method for evaluating patients with masses of unknown origin on chest roentenogram and pulsatile abdominal masses found by physical examination. As with aortic dissection, the cross-sectional representation of CT images coupled with the excellent density resolution of the technique often leads to detection on any thrombus associated with the aneurysm.

Contrast enhanced CT has been used to detect proximal pulmonary artery thrombosis [6] (Figure 2). In most cases of pulmonary artery embolism the thrombus resolves over a period of several weeks. However, in some patients for unknown reasons, instead of dissolving the thrombus becomes organized and fibrosed. These events produce chronic obstruction to pulmonary blood flow and resultant pulmonary hypertension. Recently, surgical removal of this form of

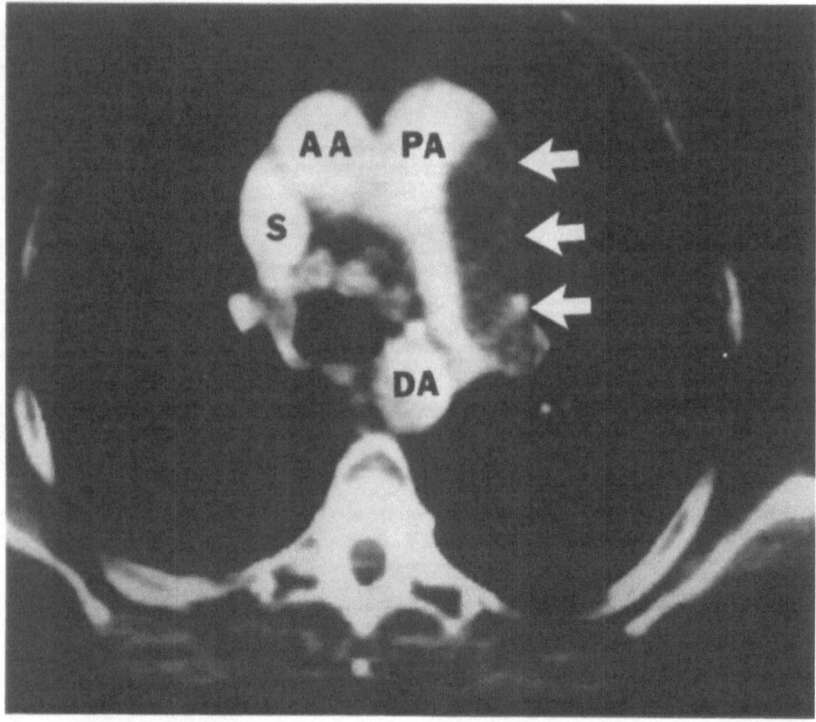

Figure 2. A large old organized thrombus (arrows) is clearly outlined by contrast enhancement of the pulmonary artery (PA). AA = ascending aorta; DA = descending aorta; S = superior vena cava.

chronic pulmonary artery obstruction has been reported to be successful in effecting permanent reduction of the pulmonary hypertension and ameliorating symptoms [7]. Therefore, recognition of this uncommon entity becomes of great importance. The patients with chronic obstruction and severe pulmonary hypertension are often seriously ill and therefore physicians are reluctant to perform pulmonary angiography. Consequently the chronic obstructive process is not diagnosed and the patient is labeled as primary pulmonary hypertension. Contrast enhanced CT, because of its minimally invasive nature should provide for the more frequent detection of this potentially correctable cause of pulmonary hypertension. On occasion the cross-sectional format of computed tomography may provide better definition of the proximal extent of the chronic pulmonary embolism. This information is of critical importance to the surgeon, because it determines whether or not surgical extraction of the thrombosis is feasible. Should the thrombus not extend far enough into the proximal portions of the right and left pulmonary artery, the surgeon may be frustrated in attempts to grasp the proximal portion of the thrombosis necessary for successful extraction. Current image resolution of available body scanners is inadequate for detecting the smaller more commonly encountered pulmonary emboli which occlude peripheral pulmonary branches.

More than 150 000 coronary artery bypass operations were performed in the United States in 1981 [8] and more than one million patients have undergone this procedure since it was first employed in 1967. Approximately 1/3 of bypass patients develop recurrence of anginal symptoms within three years of operation and 2/3 within ten years [9]. Therefore, any diagnostic technique which could determine graft patency in a simple and accurate manner would be of great clinical utility. Contrast enhanced CT offers great promise as such a tool. In 1978 contrast enhanced CT was shown to be capable of detecting patent bypass grafts using a relatively slow five second body scanner [10]. Subsequent studies with faster body scanners employing a dynamic scanning protocol have demonstrated that this technique can determine graft patency with a predictive accuracy of greater than 90% [11]. Utilizing a dynamic scanning protocol in conjunction with an intravenous bolus injection of contrast into a superficial vein, patent coronary bypass grafts can be detected by a characteristic enhancement that coincides with peak aortic enhancement (Figure 3). Usually, occluded grafts are not visualized on contrast enhanced CT scans unless they are densely fibrosed or calcified. In any case, occluded grafts do not show the progressive increase and decrease in density as seen with patent grafts during dynamic scanning. The multiple images provided by rapid dynamic scanning increases the diagnostician's confidence in detecting the characteristic progressive graft enhancement. When dynamic scanning capability is not available, graft patency can be determined by initially obtaining a single scan prior to contrast injection and a second at the estimated time of peak aortic enhancement which is usually 10–13 s after injection. This technique has been reported to be accurate enough to be clinically useful [12]. As with any other diagnostic technique, there is the potential for interpretative error. On occasion occluded grafts will have a residual diverticulum protruding from the anterior wall of the aorta. If the chosen scanning plane includes the region of the persistent diverticulum this can be misconstrued as a patent graft. However, repeat scanning at one or more levels caudal to the initial level will differentiate this entity from a patent graft. Occasionally, the native coronary arteries or pulmonary veins may be confused with patent bypass grafts. A thorough knowledge of cardiovascular anatomy as represented in the transverse plane will minimize this interpretative problem. The major limitation of computed tomography for the assessment of coronary bypass graft patency is the inability to detect the presence of significant graft stenosis. When dynamic scanning is employed, time-density curves can be constructed and preliminary observations indicate that the presence of significant stenosis may produce alterations in the height and contour of these time-density curves (Figure 4). Presumably these changes are due to reduced graft flow [13]. The development of CT scanners capable of scanning in 30–50 ms coupled with simultaneous multiple slice capability offers real promise as a minimally invasive means for evaluating

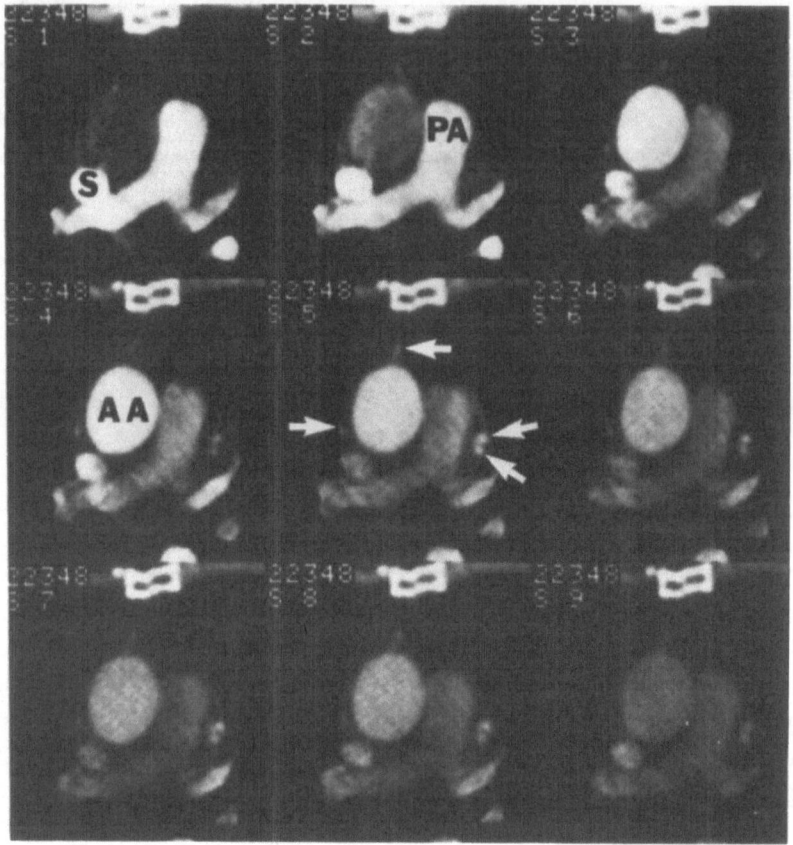

Figure 3. Four patent coronary artery bypass grafts (arrows) are demonstrated with contrast enhancement and dynamic scanning. AA = ascending aorta; PA = pulmonary artery; S = superior vena cava.

graft patency and measuring graft flow. If these new scanners meet expectations, then a truly accurate minimally invasive method for evaluating the more than one million patients with coronary artery bypasses will exist.

Echocardiography is an extremely useful non-invasive tool for evaluating left ventricular aneurysm and detecting associated left ventricular thrombus. Several investigators have compared the relative sensitivity and specificity of contrast enhanced CT to echocardiography for detection of left ventricular thrombus. Reported results indicate that computed tomography is as sensitive as echocardiography and slightly more specific [14] (Figure 5). However, the completely non-invasive nature of echocardiography makes it the procedure of choice for screening patients with suspected left ventricular thrombus and contrast enhanced CT is reserved for evaluating those patients where interpretation of the echocardiogram is equivocal for the presence of apical thrombus.

The antemortem or preoperative detection of left atrial thrombus has always

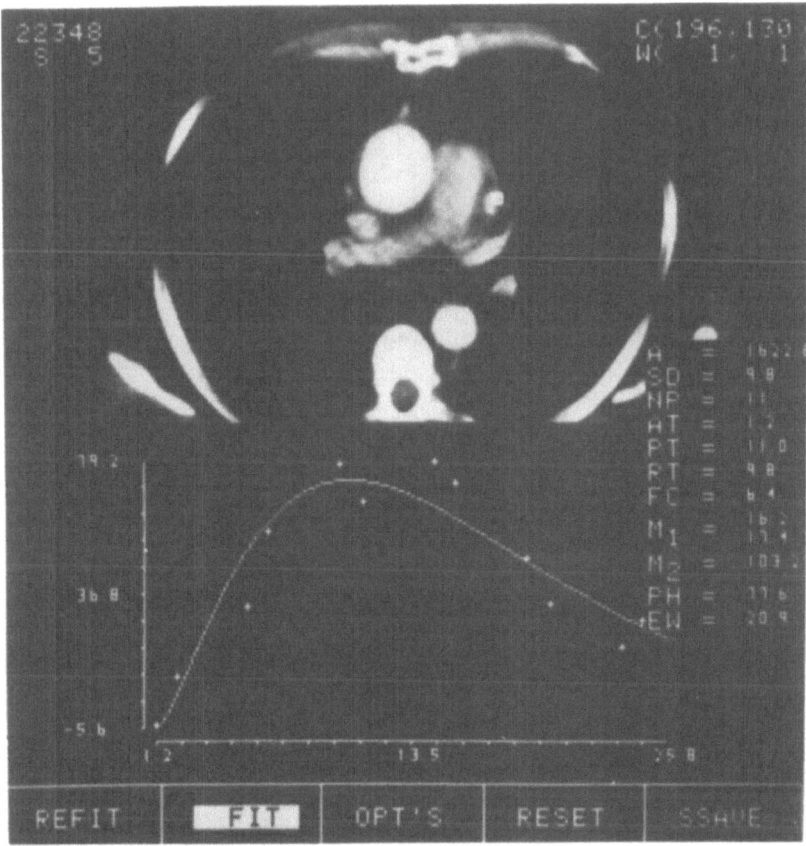

Figure 4. A time-density curve for one patent bypass (◆) demonstrated in Figure 3 is constructed. The peak height (PH) of 77.6 suggests good graft flow.

been very difficult. Echocardiography and contrast angiography have proven to be too insensitive. Recently Tomada *et al.* [15] reported a 100% sensitivity and 91% specificity for computed tomography in the detection of left atrial thrombus in 28 patients with mitral valve disease. Echocardiography had a sensitivity of 60% and a specificity of 68% and angiocardiography had a sensitivity of 70% and a specificity of 88% in the same group of patients. These results suggest that contrast enhanced CT is the diagnostic method of choice for evaluating patients suspected of left atrial thrombus.

Tomographic representation of anatomic relationships coupled with a excellent density and spatial resolution of computed tomography makes this technique particularly good for the evaluation of cardiac tumors. Most cardiac tumors are metastases from tumors arising in other organs. Commonly, these are the nearby breast or lung. Computed tomography not only identifies the cardiac involvement but also defines the relationship of this involvement with other thoracic struc-

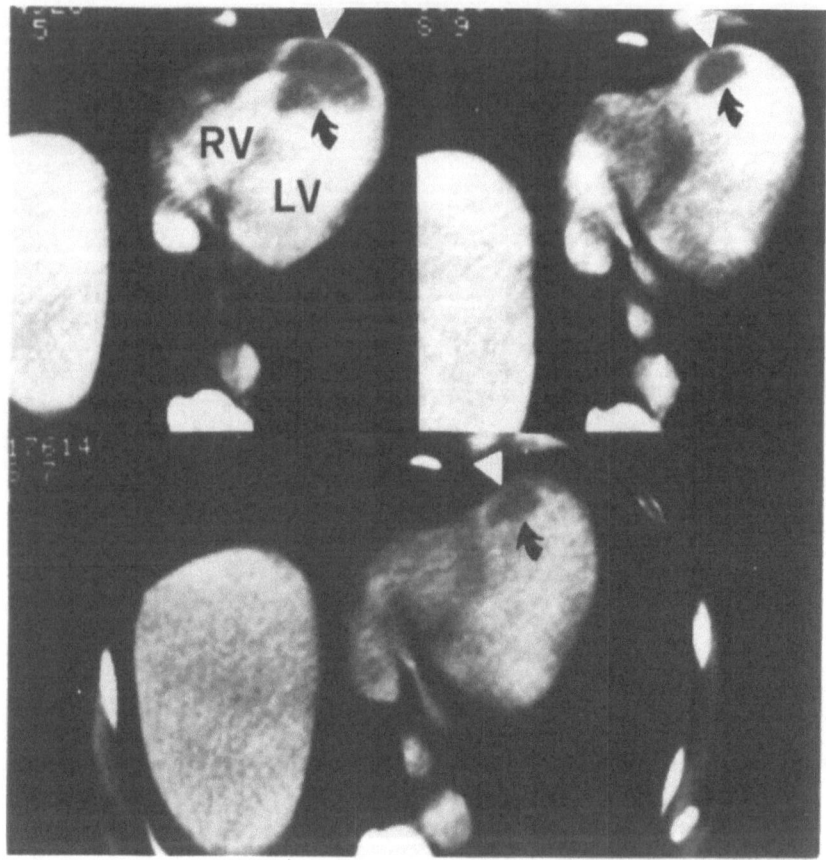

Figure 5. Three CT scans of the left ventricle (LV) obtained over a 6 month period show gradual resolution of an apical thrombus (arrows). RV = right ventricle.

tures. CT can also be used to follow the effects of radio- or chemotherapy on the tumor. Although cardiac myxoma has been diagnosed by computed tomography [16], the currently available relatively slow body scanners may not detect a very mobile myxoma. Echocardiography is still the diagnostic method of choice for the detection of pedunculated cardiac tumors.

Echocardiography has proven to be an important diagnostic modality for evaluating pericardial disease and is particularly useful for the detection and assessment of pericardial effusion. However, pericardial constriction may be missed by echocardiography and the differention of constriction from myocardial restriction may be impossible even after complete cardiac catheterization. Computed tomography offers a new diagnostic approach to this problem and appears to be capable of providing accurate measurement of pericardial thickness (Figure 6). When trying to determine whether a patient's symptoms and hemodynamic

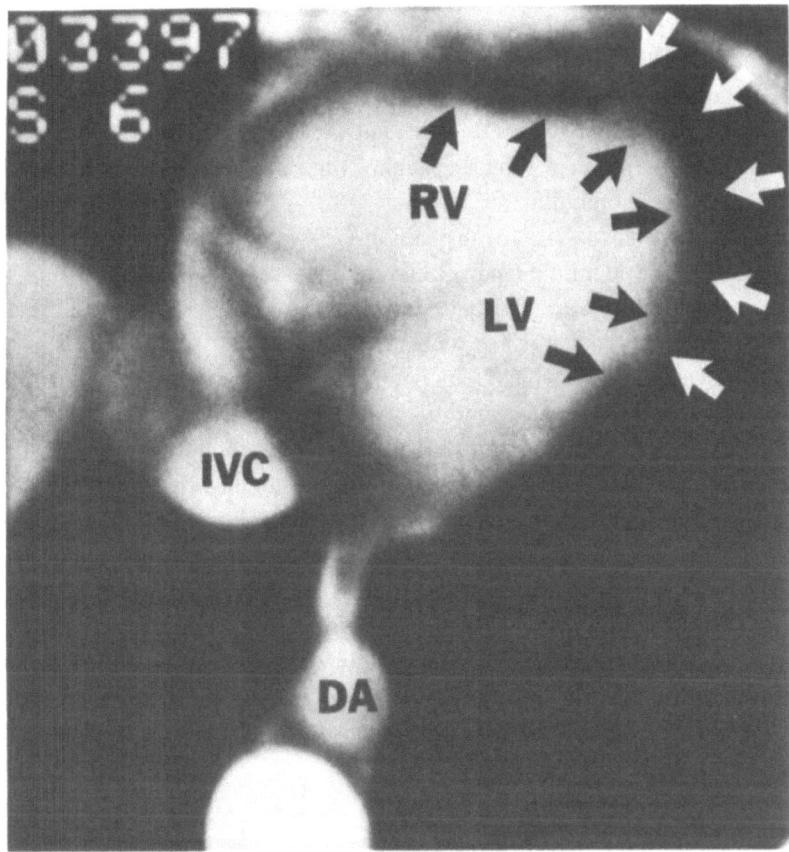

Figure 6. Marked thickening of the pericardium (arrows) over the right ventricle (RV) and left ventricle (LV) are demonstrated on this scan. IVC = inferior vena cava; DA = descending aorta.

findings are the result of pericardial constriction or myocardial restriction, measurement of the pericardial thickness by computed tomography may assist in the differentiation. Disease capable of causing contriction usually causes pericardial thickening of 4 mm or more [17]. Normal pericardium is usually 1–2 mm thick. Computed tomography is also capable of detecting and defining pericardial effusion and has been employed to diagnose pericardial cyst [18]. The method has also been reported to be useful for the diagnosis of partial absence of the left hemipericardium [19].

Although CT shows real promise as a diagnostic tool for the evaluation of cardiovascular disease, its application continues to be limited because of the degree of cardiac motion that occurs during the 2–5 s scanning period. The resultant artifact significantly degrades the images produced. Several investigators have employed retrospective and/or prospective ECG gating of the CT X-ray data. Gating does reduce motion artifact and the multiple images produced per cardiac cycle do permit some assessment of cardiac volume, wall motion and wall thickening [20, 21]. Although the images produced by gated CT are superior to those obtained without gating, the radiation dose received during gated CT scanning sequences may be up to eight times that obtained during conventional scanning. Furthermore, a longer scanning time is required and often greater amounts of contrast medium are necessary.

A new approach to X-ray transmission CT scanning has recently been developed which may eliminate many of the problems associated with current body CT scanners. Boyd *et al.* [22] have developed a non-mechanical CT scanner capable of scanning speeds as fast as 33 ms. This ultrafast CT scanner generates a powerful electron beam which is magnetically steered to strike a series of four tungsten target rings that surround the patient's thorax. When the beam strikes the target rings it is converted into X-radiation which then traverses the chest at right angles and strikes an array of detectors opposite the target rings (Figure 7). The electron beam can be swept back and forth on any one of the four tungsten rings at high speeds. Furthermore, the electron beam can be split into two adjacent fan beams producing two scans simultaneously. By steering the electron beam to cascade across four tungsten rings in rapid succession, eight adjacent scans can be obtained in 200 ms. This new type of CT scanner has a resolution better than 2 mm which is comparable to current body scanners (Figure 8). The ultrafast scanning speed eliminates motion artifact and makes it an ideal tool for

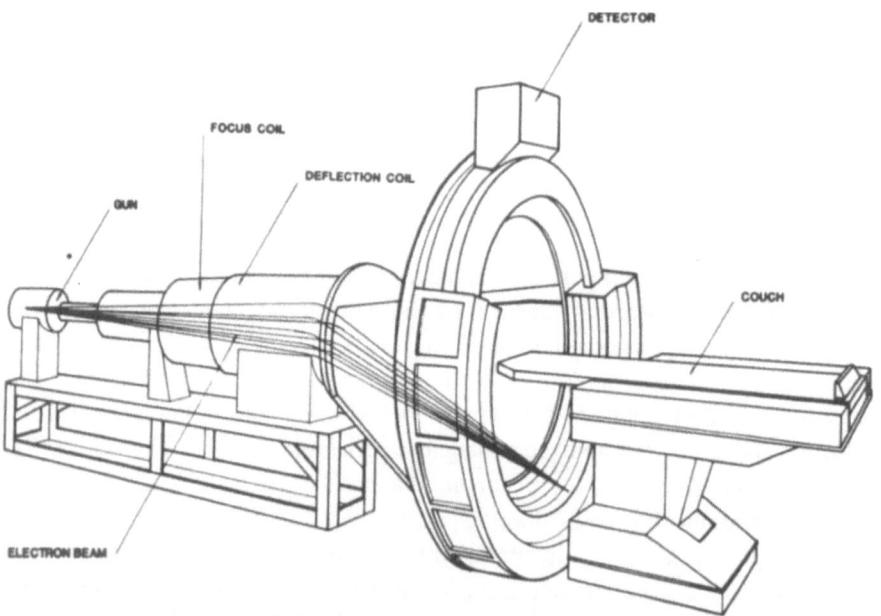

Figure 7. This drawing of the Imatron TM ultrafast CT scanner demonstrates the magnetic deflection of the scanner's electron beam causing it to strike the tungsten target ring.

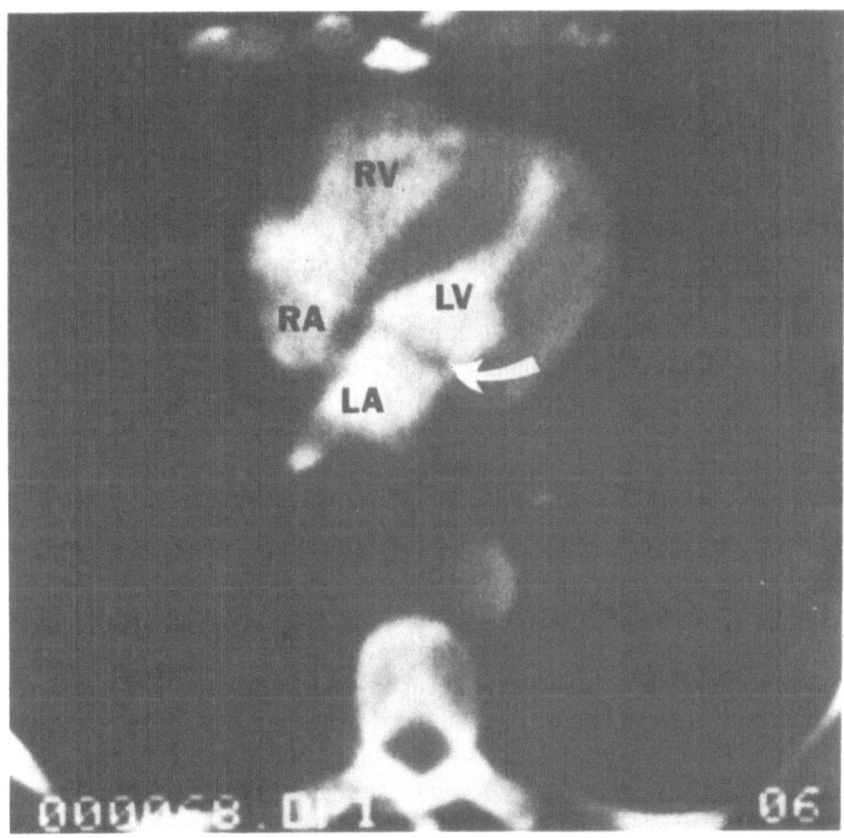

Figure 8. A single scan from a patient with hypertrophic cardiomyopathy obtained with the Imatron TM ultrafast CT scanner shows that resolution comparable to conventional body scanners is obtained. LV = left ventricle; LA = left atrium; RV = right ventricle; RA = right atrium; arrow = mitral valve.

imaging the heart. The ability to obtain two adjacent scans simultaneously in 50 ms or better creates the feasibility of making quantitative measurements of regional myocardial blood flow [23].

To compare the radiation dose received from computed tomography with that received from cineradiography is difficult because of the differences in dose distribution [24]. The skin entry dose received from CT is approximately 1 rad per slice and is limited to an area determined by the thickness of the CT slice. Conventional planar roentgenography exposes many more adjacent areas than CT scanning because of scatter. So, for example, if 12 adjacent CT scans are obtained at 1 cm intervals over the chest area, the total dose to the thorax would be one rad. Most cardiovascular studies require 20–30 scans. The new non-mechanical scanners will deliver approximately the same X-ray dose as conventional scanners. It is quite possible, however, that these scanners will result in an increased number of scans because of their ability to assess cardiovascular dynamics. The total patient dose per study would be 3–8 rads. The new ultrafast scanners should increase the diagnostic capability of CT for the evaluation of cardiovascular disease.

Cardiologists continue to search for a accurate method to size myocardial infarction. Precordial mapping, measurement of CPK release, myocardial scintigraphy, and echocardiography have been employed but do not provide sufficiently accurate measurements of infarct size. Contrast enhanced CT of transmural anterior myocardial infarction has produced excellent images of infarcted myocardium (Figure 9). But image degradation caused by cardiac motion still precludes accurate measurement of transmural inferior and small subendocardial infarctions. Ultrafast CT scanning will eliminate motion artifact and offers real promise as a method for accurately assessing infarct size. With the current enthusiasm for thrombolysis to reduce infarct size, clinicians may find that this method provides a means of quantifying the amount of myocardium salvaged. Ultrafast CT will also provide a simultaneous evaluation of regional wall motion and thickening for determining the immediate functional impact of acute infarction.

The many methods now available for imaging left ventricular aneurysm have led to increased understanding of this cardiac abnormality. However, all methods have either relied on projection imaging or have not provided adequate anatomic landmarks so there is confusion about what image represents true ventricular aneurysm. The excellent spatial resolution of CT and the artifact-free imaging possible with the new ultrafast CT scanners should make the method ideal for evaluating ventricular aneurysm. Furthermore, the simultaneous assessment of wall motion and wall thickness should assist in carefully delineating the extent of this contraction abnormality.

Myocardial mass is directly related to any stimulus of cardiac hypertrophy. Therefore, an accurate measurement of myocardial muscle mass should be a very sensitive way of detecting any hemodynamic state which stimulates hypertrophy. However, to date, there are no good diagnostic means for accurately measuring cardiac muscle mass. Traditionally, electrocardiography, because of its simplicity and low cost, is used to assess severity of cardiac hypertrophy. However, the inadequacies of this method for measuring myocardial mass are well-known. In recent years, echocardiography has been employed to assess ventricular wall thickness in multiple regions. From these measurements extrapolations are made to estimate the total amount of heart muscle. However, sampling errors, limitations of resolution and the interstudy variation of serial echocardiograms makes it difficult to detect the small serial changes in hypertrophy that occurs in the clinical course of systemic hypertension. Animal studies indicate that CT can accurately measure left ventricular mass [25]. The improved image resolution of ultrafast CT scanning should make it an even better tool for the accurate measurement of cardiac muscle mass in humans and should provide a means for assessing the effects of therapeutic interventions such as long-term treatment of hypertension or valve replacement on myocardial mass.

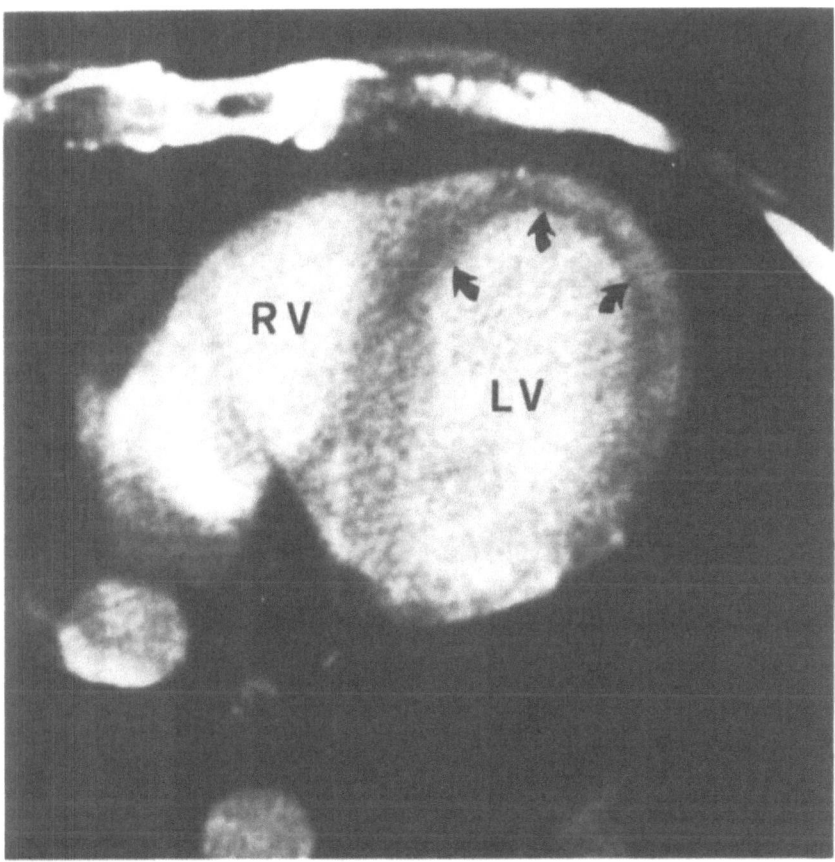

Figure 9. A anterior subendocardial myocardial infarction (arrows) is defined by its low density during contrast enhancement on this CT scan. RV = right ventricle; LV = left ventricle.

The new ultrafast CT scanners will provide images up to a rate of 24 cross-sectional slices per second. The high speed, high resolution cross-sectional images will provide an excellent method for measuring cardiac chamber size and measurements of left ventricular function by determining ejection fraction, chamber stroke volume and indices of ejection and filling. Very accurate measurements of segmental wall motion and systolic wall thickening will also be possible with this technique. Of particular value will be the three-dimensional representation of the heart and chest cavity during all phases of the cardiac cycle which should help to clarify the continuing confusion about what type of wall motion represents true ventricular dyskinesia. Furthermore, ultrafast CT's capability of imaging two adjacent myocardial regions simultaneously should provide quantitative assessment of regional myocardial blood flow. These observations coupled with evaluation of regional wall motion and regional wall thickening will make computed tomography an ideal methodology for the study of ischemic heart disease.

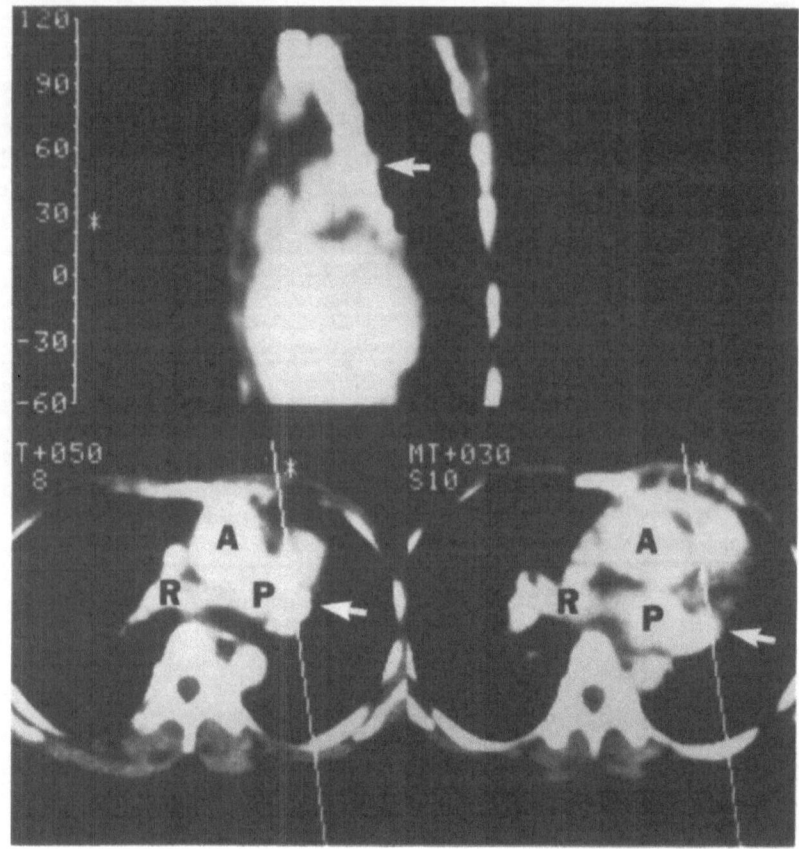

Figure 10. The parasagittal reformating of 18 transverse scans in the plane indicated by the dashed line fails to demonstrate any left pulmonary artery (arrows). The main pulmonary artery (P) and the right pulmonary artery (R) are seen on both transverse scans. A = ascending aorta.

Quite possibly, ultrafast CT scanning may revolutionize the evaluation of congenital heart disease. Small children and infants with congenital heart disease have not been evaluated by current body CT scanners because of the slow scan time and the inability of these patients to remain motionless and control breathing during scanning. However, the very limited experience in a few adults with complex congenital heart disease suggests that computed tomography with its excellent spatial and density resolution will provide superb definition of pathologic anatomy. Several clinical reports have indicated that conventional CT body scanners are useful for imaging coarctation of the aorta and for detection of true pulmonary artery tissue in pulmonary atresia [26] (Figure 10).

Contrast enhanced CT can provide limited images of the proximal portion of the right and left coronary atery. It is likely that ultrafast CT scanning will provide even better images by eliminating motion artifact. However, as current image resolution is limited to 1.5 mm, images of the coronary arteries will not be satisfactory for making clinical decisions. If predicted advances in detector technology improve the resolution to 0.2–0.3 mm then contrast enhanced high speed CT may provide minimally invasive clinically useful images of the coronary arteries.

The future of cardiac CT is indeed bright because of the development of millisecond CT scanners. One can expect that this imaging modality will find increasing usefulness in cardiology. However, currently available CT body scanners can be used in some clinical situations to provide unique and useful information about coronary bypass graft patency, aortic dissection, intracardiac thrombus, cardiac tumors and some types of pericardial disease.

References

1. Abrams HL, McNeil BJ: Medical implications of computed tomography ('cat scanning'), part two. N Engl J Med 298: 310–318, 1978.
2. Carlsson E, Lipton MJ, Brundage B, Doherty P, Berninger WH, Redington RW: The diagnostic potential of cardiac computed tomography. Appl Radiol 7: 105–108, 1978.
3. Brundage BH: Computed tomography: a new view of cardiovascular disease. Prim Cardiol 9: 57–72, 1983.
4. Godwin JD, Herfkens RJ, Skioldebrand CG, Federle MP, Lipton MJ: Evaluation of aortic dissections and aneurysms by conventional and dynamic CT scanning. Radiology 136: 125–133, 1980.
5. Turley K, Ullyot DJ, Godwin JD, Wilson JM, Lipton MJ, Carlsson E, Ebert PA: Repair of dissection of the thoracic aorta: evaluation of false lumen utilizing computed tomography. J Thor Cardiovasc Surg 81: 61–68, 1981.
6. Keriakes DJ, Herfkens RJ, Brundage BH, Gamsu G, Lipton MJ: Computerized tomography in chronic thromboembolic pulmonary hypertension. Am Heart J 106: 1432–1436, 1983.
7. Moser KM, Spagg RG, Utley J, Daily PO: Chronic thrombotic obstruction of major pulmonary arteries. Ann Int Med 99: 299–305, 1983.
8. CASS principle investigators, Coronary artery surgery study (CASS): A randomized trial of coronary artery bypass surgery: survival data. Circulation 68: 939–950, 1983.
9. Hall RJ, Elazada MA, Gray A, Mathur VS, Garcia E, DeCastro CM, Massumi A, Cooley DA: Coronary artery bypass: long-term follow-up of 22 284 consecutive patients. Circulation 68 (II): 20–26, 1983.
10. Brundage B, Lipton M, Berninger W, Redington R, Dougherty P, Chatterjee K, Carlsson E: The use of contrast enhanced computerized axial tomography to assess coronary bypass graft patency. Circulation 58: II–26, 1978.
11. Brundage BH, Lipton MJ, Herfkens RJ, Berninger WH, Redington RW, Chatterjee K, Carlsson E: Detection of patent coronary bypass grafts by computed tomography: a preliminary report. Circulation 61: 826–831, 1980.
12. Moncada R, Salinas M, Churchill R, Love L, Reynes C, Demos T, Hale D, Schrieba R: Patency of saphenous aortocoronary – bypass grafts demonstrated by computed tomography. N Engl J Med 303: 503–505, 1980.
13. Goldstein J, Brundage B, Herfkens RJ, Lipton MJ, McKay C: Evaluation of coronary bypass graft flow by contrast enhanced computed tomography. Circulation 64 (IV): 182, 1981.
14. Tomada H, Mitsumoto H, Furuya H, Kuribayaski S, Ootaki M, Matsuyama S, Koide S, Kawada

S, Shotsu A: Evaluation of intracardiac thrombus with computed tomography. Am J Cardiol 51: 843–852, 1983.

15. Tomada H, Hoshiai M, Furuya H, Shotsu A, Ootaki M, Matsuyama S: Evaluation of left atrial thrombus with computed tomography. Am Heart J 100: 306–310, 1980.

16. Huggins T, Huggins M, Schnopf D, Brott W, Sinnott R, Shawl F: Left atrial myxoma: computed tomography as a diagnostic modality. J Comput Assist Tomogr 4: 253–255, 1980.

17. Isner JM, Carter BL, Bankoff MS, Pastore JO, Ramaswamy K, McAdam K PWJ, Salem DN: Differentiation of constrictive pericarditis from restrictive cardiomyopathy by computed tomographic imaging. Am Heart J 105: 1019–1025, 1983.

18. Moncada R, Baker M, Salinas M, Demos TC, Churchill R, Love L, Reynes CHD, Cardoso M, Pifarre R, Gunnar R: Diagnostic role of computed tomography in pericardial heart disease: congenital defects, thickening, neoplasms, and effusions. Am Heart J 103: 263–282, 1982.

19. Bain RS, MacDonald IL, Wise DJ, Leakei SC: Computed tomography of absent left pericardium. Radiology 135: 127–128, 1980.

20. Johnson GA, Godwin JD, Fran EK: Gated multiplanar cardiac computed tomography. Radiology 145: 195–197, 1982.

21. Mancini GBJ, Peck WW, Slutsky RA, Mattrey RF, Higgins CB: Pharmacologically induced changes in wall thickening dynamics and mid-ventricular volumes in dogs assessed by prospectively gated computed tomography. Am J Cardiol 51: 1739–1743, 1983.

22. Boyd D, Gould R, Quinn J, Sparks R, Stanley R, Hermannsfeldt W: A proposed dynamic cardiac 3-D densitometer for easy detection and evaluation of heart disease. IEEE Trans Nucl Sci NS 26: 2724, 1979.

23. Bassingthwaighte JB: Physiology and theory of tracer washout techniques for the estimation of myocardial blood flow: flow estimation from tracer washout. Prog Cardiovasc Dis 20: 165–189, 1977.

24. Carlsson E, Palmer RG, Masuda Y: Cardiac computed tomography. Am J Cardiol 49: 1362–1365, 1982.

25. Skioldebrand CG, Ovenfors CO, Mavroudis C, Lipton MJ: Assessment of ventricular wall thickness in vivo by computed transmission tomography. Circulation 61: 960–965, 1980.

26. Sondheimer HM, Oliphant M, Schneider B, Kavey REW, Blackman MS, Parker FB Jr: Computerized axial tomograophy of the chest for visualization of 'absent' pulmonary arteries. Circulation 65: 1020–1025, 1982.

11. Digital two-dimensional echocardiography

ANDREW J. BUDA and EDWARD J. DELP

Over the past two decades, echocardiography has emerged as an essential diagnostic tool in clinical cardiology. This is related to the fact that it is entirely non-
invasive, can be readily performed at the bedside, and can provide accurate and
reproducible information at no known risk to the patient. M-mode echocardiography was initially used to provide a unidimensional view of the heart, and
although it contributed to our knowledge of many important physiologic and
pathophysiologic relationships, it remains limited in capability because of the lack
of spatial orientation. The development of two-dimensional echocardiography in
the early 1970's has allowed real-time, tomographic imaging of several planes
through the heart. The speed of developments in the electronic industry has
resulted in dramatic improvements in transducer design and instrumentation over
the past decade which has contributed to major improvements in this cardiac
imaging modality so that good spatial and temporal resolution are now possible.

Several excellent monographs [1–3] and atlases [4, 5] related to M-mode and
two-dimensional echocardiography (2-D echo) are available. This chapter will
focus on and summarize many of the exciting newer developments related to 2-D
echo particularly those related to digital acquisition with computer processing for
quantitative analysis. We will review technical considerations related to digital
2-D echo, approaches to computer processing and edge detection, quantitative
analysis of cardiac function, contrast 2-D echo studies, and echocardiographic
tissue characterization.

Technical considerations related to digitization

The 2-D echo video chain

An understanding of specific technical factors related to 2-D echo is necessary to
comprehend methods related to digital acquisition and processing. The piezoelectric transducer is used for first transmitting the ultrasonic beam through the

heart and then receiving the echoes returning from structures along its path. The most common transducer presently used are mechanically steered elements or electronically phased arrays. The ultrasonic energy emitted by these transducers obeys the laws of geometric optics regarding reflection, transmission, and refraction. Specular reflections occur when the intercardiac reflectors are large relative to the wavelength of the ultrasonic pulse and have a smooth serface (e.g. ventricular walls) whereas backscattering occurs when a sound wave strikes a structure that is comparable to or smaller than its wavelength (e.g. myocardial fibers).

The 2-D echo video chain processing of reflected ultrasound from the transducer to the final images seen by the viewer is illustrated in Figure 1. The ultrasonic signals received from cardiac tissues are converted into oscillatory electrical signals termed RF, or radio frequency, signals. The RF signal is initially received and amplified by the RF amplifier in the echocardiograph. Because there is a hundred thousand-fold variation in the intensity of returning echoes, linear amplification, or dynamic compression, must be performed during this amplification process. A component of the amplifier chain is the time-gain compensation (TGC), or gain as a function of depth. The TGC compensates for the relative decrease in amplitude of echoes from more distant cardiac structures which occur as a result of the attenuation of the ultrasonic beam as it passes through the body.

The RF signal is transformed to a video signal by displaying only the envelope of its positive components. At this step of signal processing, the signal represents both the amplitude and duration of the pulse train. Following rectification and conditioning amplification, the video signal is converted from analog to digital data in the digital scan converter. This microprocessor built into most commercial units allows for image smoothing, temporal and spatial filtering, and gray scale enhancement, but is not user programable. The video signal is subsequently reconverted to analog television video signals by a digital to analog converter for viewing on a video monitor.

Limitations of signal processing

This complex video chain that is standard on most commercial 2-D echocardiographs has several technical problems. The overall dynamic range, defined as the ratio of the largest signal that can be detected before signal saturation to the smallest signal amplitude that can be detected above the systems noise, is in excess of 100000 to 1 (100 db) at the acoustic transducer. However, present imaging systems cannot display simultaneously this entire dynamic range and commercial units use some form of dynamic range compression with resulting cardiac images with varying shades of gray depicting the various echo amplitudes. These display video monitors only display an intensity range of approximately 64 to 1 (36 db). Thus, more than 50 db of data must be compressed to 36 db by

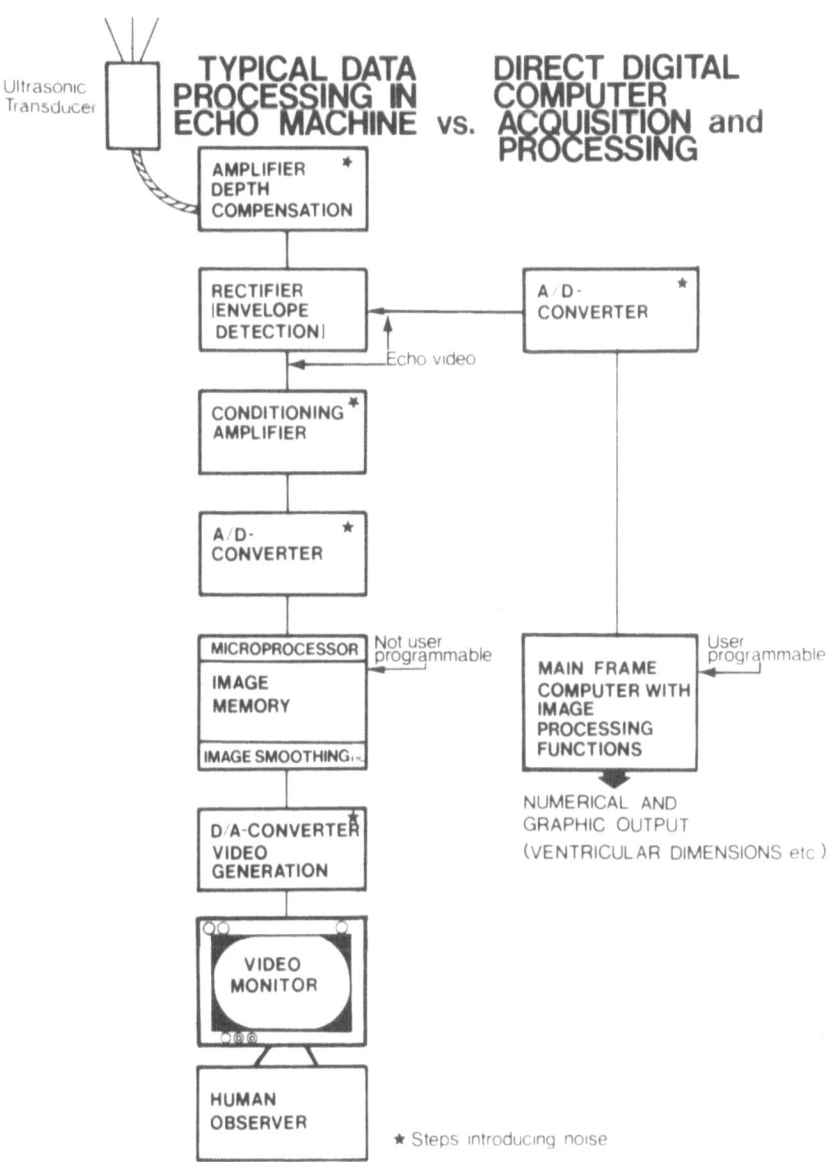

Figure 1. The processing steps in a commercial sector scanner and our method of direct digitization of the envelope-detected signal. Several steps of noise introduction are avoided by the direct digitization. (From reference 14, with permission of the American Journal of Cardiology.)

dynamic range compression. In addition, the steps of signal processing in the video chain, outlined above, are associated with at least four steps of noise introduction which further degrades the signal to noise ratio (Figure 1).

RF digitization

In view of these considerations, data acquisition for more sophisticated processing and analysis would be better performed by acquiring the signals as close to the raw RF signal as possible. However, the magnitude of ultrasound data generated by 2-D echo is staggering. A typical commercial 2-D echo unit uses 100 to 150 discrete scan lines to build up one single frame of a 2-D echo image. This is repeated usually 30 times per second (or 30 frames/s) to create a flicker free real-time display for viewing on a standard video monitor. Assuming that the dynamic range of the echo data as they are received from the transducers is 100 db, at least 16 bits would be necessary to represent a single value within this dynamic range. If the data were digitized at a sampling rate of 20 million samples per second into 16 bit words at 30 frames per second in the 130 lines per frame, the storage requirements for one second of data (approximately one cardiac cycle at a heart rate of 60/min) of a 10 cm field depth would be 20 280 000 bytes. Thus, 20 megabytes of data would have to be transmitted and stored in the computer. To record four seconds of data, 80 megabytes would have to be transmitted and stored. The transmission and storage of this volume of data is exceedingly difficult with even the most sophisticated of today's technologies.

Computer processing of 2-D echo

Digitization of analog records or recordings

Initial techniques of digitizing single frames of 2-D echo information included using video cameras pointed at still frame [6], flying spot scanners [7], contour digitizers [8], and video disc recorders [9]. However, these techniques were unsatisfactory because of the lengthy time required for digitizing a single frame of data which eliminated any real-time capability. Furthermore, there was significant deterioration of the image as it was transferred through several optical systems into the computer memory.

Subsequently, interfaces between the video output of the 2-D echo unit, or its videotape recorder, and a standard medical imaging computer were developed for analog digitization [10, 11]. Although this approach has clear advantages over previous digitization techniques, this method of digitization has several problems. First, the resampling process required to form a video image from the line-mode data tends to produce undersampling of data in the near field and over-sampling in the far field. Second, the ultrasound frame generation may not match the video frame rate. Third, the scan converter within the echo unit maps the information into a range of gray values with the dynamic range matched to the human visual system; however, the usable dynamic range of the data is significantly greater. Fourth, the averaging technique for speckle reduction is usually not under user control. Fifth, the video image data depends on the processing performed by the technician who varies the control settings on the echo unit to achieve an image that looks best to the human observer; however, this image may not necessarily be best for computer processing. For all of these reasons, digitization of analog recordings is not optimal and direct digitization techniques are preferable.

Direct digitization of line-mode data

Methods in which the RF signal, or the envelope-detected signal are directly fed to an analog to digital (A/D) converter are termed direct digitization [12]. The term 'line-mode data' has been applied to data digitized along the ultrasonic line of sight with positional information [13]. This form of digitization is preferable to analog digitization in view of the considerations discussed previously. Our laboratory [14–16] has implemented direct line-mode digitization of 2-D echo data (Figure 1). To perform this, we modified our computer's A/D converter for horizontal and vertical synchronization by external digital signals. We rebuilt the analog section of our 2-D echocardiograph to adapt to the post-TGC envelope-detected RF signal and used a sampling rate along each line of 2 MHz. The evelope-detected signal was amplified and transmitted directly to the A/D converter through a coaxial cable and the signal sector rays were mapped into a rectangular matrix of 256 × 128 pixels. Since all 128 sector lines were digitized, there was no data loss within the sector field. However, the digital transfer rate of the whole frame to digital disk was too slow to begin acquisition of the next sector frame. Thus, only every other sector frame was digitized. The data were hardware buffered and then transferred to disc via direct memory access transfer under software control. Due to limited direct memory access transfer rate and buffered capacity, approximately 15 to 25 s of data could be saved on disk for one run.

Robinson and Williams [13] indicated that direct digitization is superior to other methods of digitization for 2-D echo processing. This direct method has several advantages over digitization of analog recordings. First, the ultrasound frame generation rate is equal to the A/D frame conversion rate; this condition is not necessarily fulfilled by conventional video image digitization. Second, the envelope-detected signal is independent of all control settings on the echo unit except for gain control. Third, the dynamic range of the eight bit line-mode data significantly exceeds that of the typical four- to six-bit output of the digital scan converter used for video data acquisition. For these reasons, we believe that line-mode data digitization is presently the preferred method of ultrasound data acquisition for computer processing.

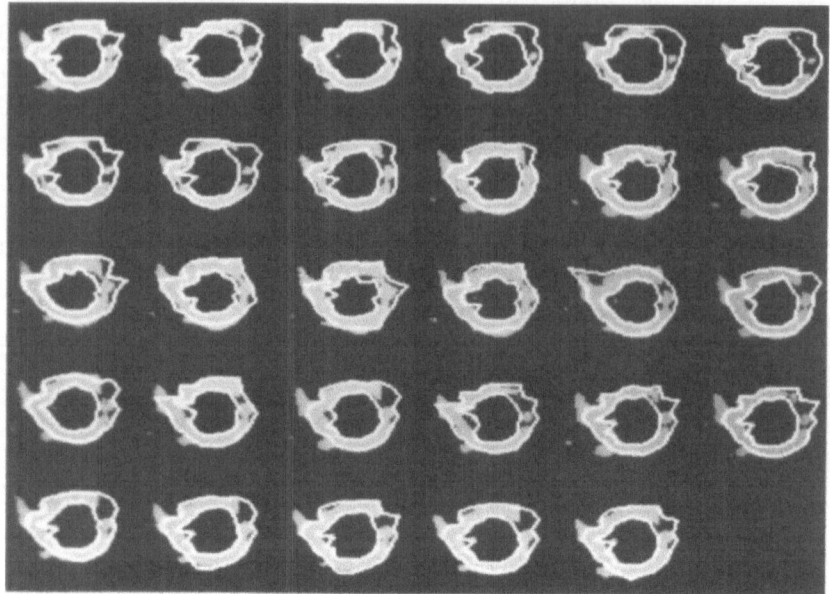

Figure 2. A parasternal, left ventricular, short-axis, video output-acquired 2-dimensional echocardiographic image after processing with superimposition of endocardial and epicardial edges. (From reference 14, with permission of the American Journal of Cardiology.)

Edge detection algorithms

Following digitization of the echo image, the next task is edge detection for determination of endocardial and epicardial boundaries or other intracardiac structures. Prior to image processing, most investigators [10, 11] have utilized some form of preprocessing, usually involving spatial and temporal smoothing. Following this step, various classical edge detection routines, usually employing thresholding and linear total gradients, are available and have been used for 2-D echo images. These include: the Sobel operator, a 2-D gradient operator which identifies the presence of an edge based on absolute differences in gray level measured across each pixel in vertical and horizontal directions; the Laplacian operator, a standard algorithm which is a digital approximation to a second derivative function; and gray level thresholding which attempts to determine a threshold in the image which defines an edge. Despite good results by several investigators [10, 11, 17, 18] using these classic edge operators, application of these edge detectors does not typically provide continuous closed contours of the ventricular walls and many edge artifacts are generated. Furthermore, these traditional edge detectors do not correct for echo dropout which require operator editing [18].

We have found classical edge detectors such as Laplacian, Sobel, trapezoidal, and high-pass filtering techniques to be unsatisfactory for edge detection of in-vivo canine or human studies. Difficulties with echo dropout, noise, and other ultrasonic artifacts produce unsatisfactory edge detection. We have had more success with a relatively simple axial gradient edge detector [11] for detection of endocardial and epicardial definition in the left ventricular short axis (Figure 2). This algorithm uses 12 radial chords spaced 30 degrees apart and originating at the center of the left ventricular cavity to detect local boundaries of the ventricular wall using a combined thresholding and first derivative approach. More recently, dynamic scene analysis [19] has been developed for various applications to problems of images with moving targets. Our initial experience [16] with this form of time-varying image analysis suggests that this more sophisticated form of edge detection would be more suitable for the dynamically moving heart visualized by 2-D echo. This algorithm takes advantage of the temporal redundancy of the real-time information by analyzing adjacent frame by frame data.

Even by using video digitization and classical edge operators, recent studies [17, 18] suggest that computer processing improves variability and reliability of quantitative measures. The development of direct digitization and more sophisticated edge operators should further improve the accuracy of quantitative measurements using automatic techniques.

Quantitative analysis

Global left ventricular analysis

Several investigators have taken advantage of the 2-D echo to analyze global and regional left ventricular function. In view of the many tomographic views that are available for study, this technique is particularly well suited to left ventricular functional analysis. Despite the many advances in data acquisition computer processing described above, most investigators continue to rely on manual digitization of the 2-D echo until these newer technologies are more completely developed.

Manual digitization of 2-D echo can be performed using commercially available digitizers and microprocessors which interact with the 2-D echo video tape. Careful manual tracing and computer analysis of global and regional left ventricular function parameters using an end-diastolic and end-systolic frame usually requires approximately one to two hours of operator time. In view of the excessive time and labor required to analyze two frames of data, sequential manual digitization and analysis of the entire cardiac cycle is usually not performed in most laboratories. There is presently no standardization of tracing techniques which can contribute to variability, but most laboratories continue to use the black-white interface despite the known problems related to leading-edge considerations [20]. However, careful manual digitization can be performed accurately and reproducibly at the expense of time. Newer methods of automatic computer processing of 2-D echo for edge detection [14, 18] are designed to avoid the excessive time, labor, and subjectivity of manual tracing, and to improve the reliability and validity of quantitative measures.

Several quantitative validation studies of left ventricular mass and function have been reported in the recent literature [21–31]. A number of mathematical models, analogous to those used for left ventricular angiographic studies, have been used for 2-D echoes of the left ventricle [21–23]. The most widely accepted model is the Simpson's rule, but other algorithms for determining left ventricular volumes have proven useful including area-length methods, and the so-called 'bullet formula'. Using these measures in in-vitro and in-vivo studies, 2-D echo measures left ventricular volumes and mass with acceptable accuracy and 10 to 20% variability. These mesures are comparable to those of other imaging techniques. In general, 2-D echo tends to underestimate left ventricular volume and mass compared to angiographic studies for several possible reasons [32]. First, the angiographic outline of the left ventricle includes some area within the trabeculae carnae since the columnae carnae are surrounded by angiographic contrast medium in left ventriculography. The 2-D echo outline most likely represents the apices of these columnae because of the finite lateral resolution of the beam. Second, placement of the transducer proximal to the true anatomic apex, or orientation of the scan plane off the maximal cross-section of the ventricle, could reduce the size of the 2-D echo image representing ventricular area [33].

A unique feature of 2-D echo is circumferential estimation of left ventricular wall thickness at multiple levels of the left ventricle. These wall thickening measures and dynamics provide a mechanism for studying wall stress and patterns of hypertrophy in the left ventricle.

Regional left ventricular analysis

Manual digitization of 2-D echo images has also allowed analysis of regional function [34, 35]. This regional analysis of left ventricular function is a major strength of 2-D echo since regional function is more sensitive than global parameters in the assessment of ischemic dysfunction [35]. Regional analysis is generally performed using the left ventricular short axis images so that circumferential function can be assessed (Figure 3). Various conventions have been used in analyzing regional parameters of endocardial motion or wall thickening. All of these methods use a coordinate system usually requiring a centroid, or an imaginary center of mass towards which the left ventricle is considered to contract. This coordinate system approach assumes homogeneity and symmetry of left ventricular contraction. However, considerable data supports the concept of non-uniformity of regional left ventricular function in both normal and abnormal states [37–46]. Further, the definition of the centroid used is variable. For example, some investigators use the center of mass of the endocardial area

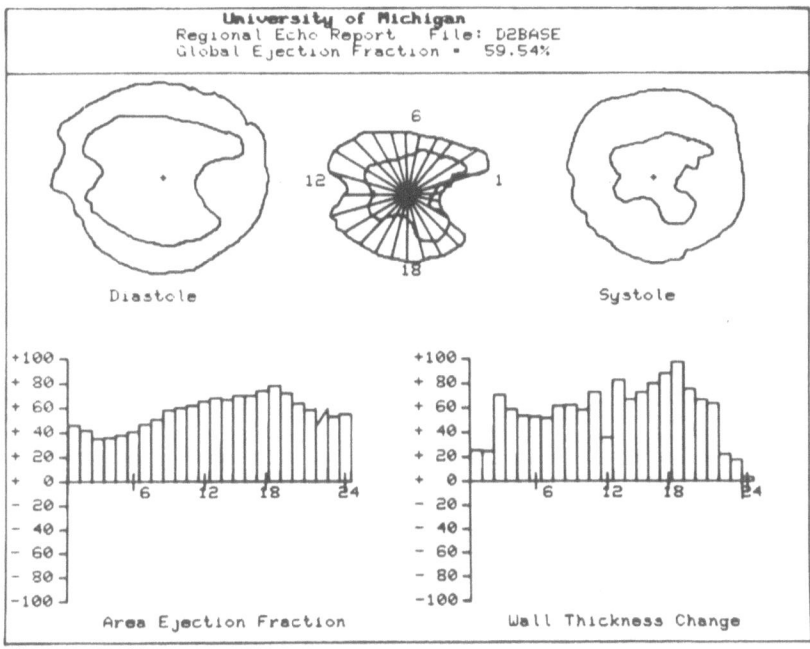

Figure 3. Typical regional analysis program used for quantitative 2-D echo studies. (From reference 14, with permission of the American Journal of Cardiology.)

whereas others use the center of mass of the epicardial outline. In addition, methods of dealing with the three-dimensional motion that occurs with left ventricular contraction, namely, translation and rotation, vary among different laboratories. Some investigators use a fixed centroid approach whereas others prefer correction of the centroid for end-systole, the floating axis approach. Furthermore, there is also variability in the anatomic landmarks used to correct for rotation. Some investigators use the posterior right ventricular – left ventricular junction whereas others use a papillary muscle as a landmark. Finally, the number of segmentations used for analysis of regional function has ranged between eight at 45° angles, to 180, at 2° intervals. There are advantages and disadvantages with both approaches; an increased number of segments analyzed tends to increase variability of results whereas fewer segments limit spatial circumferential sampling resolution.

Clearly, there are many deficiencies and great variability in the present methods of regional analysis. Our preferred method (Figure 3) presently uses a fixed diastolic center of mass defined by the endocardial area at the mid-papillary muscle level. The left ventricle is divided into 16 to 24 segments circumferentially using the apex of the lateral papillary muscle as a landmark for correction of rotation. Although we initially included the papillary muscle in the regional analysis, we now exclude it since it tends to cause spurious artifacts of regional function. Regional area ejection fraction is calculated as: diastolic area – systolic area/diastolic area × 100%. Regional wall thickening is calculated as: systolic thickness – diastolic thickness/diastolic thickness × 100%.

2-D echo studies of regional function

Since the classical studies of Tennant and Wiggers [41], the rapid appearance of myocardial contraction abnormalities has been a hallmark of myocardial isch-emia. Regional contraction abnormalities are a more sensitive indicator of ischemia than electrocardiographic ST segment changes. Although most previous animal studies have used sonomicrometer crystals to accurately measure regional myocardial function, many recent studies have relied more on M-mode [41] and 2-D echocardiography [42–51] in experimental models of myocardial ischemia. Pandian and Kerber [52, 53] compared 2-D echo to intramyocardial sonomicro-metry and found that 2-D echo was a sensitive and specific method for detecting ischemia-induced transient myocardial dyskinesis. Although there were quantita-tive discrepencies which may be related to limitations of both techniques, there was always complete qualitative concordance between the two techniques.

Several investigators [42–50] have attempted to measure the size of the ischemic and infarcted myocardium using 2-D echo. Most studies have demon-strated that the area of 2-D echo dysfunction tends to overestimate actual infarct size. This has been attributed to a tethering phenomenon of the bordering, normally perfused tissue by the infarcted myocardium [45, 46, 50]. This area of normally perfused but functionally abnormal tissue has been termed the 'func-tional border zone' and is an area of ongoing research interest.

The importance of wall thickness abnormalities during ischemia has been emphasized by several recent canine studies [54–56]. During graded coronary occlusion, systolic wall thickening decreases, and with greater decreases in coro-nary perfusion, systolic wall thinning results [54]. Lieberman et al. [45] compared wall thickening dynamics and endocardial motion in a canine model of acute infarction. They found that both measures of regional function were sensitive in detecting infarction, but that wall thickening produced better differentiation between infarcted myocardium and adjacent risk zones. In addition, they re-ported that at 48 h, the transmural extent of infarction, bore a non-linear relationship to wall motion abnormality with a thresholding phenomenon in that almost all areas that had greater than 20% transmural infarction had total dysfunction. Other investigators [48] have compared regional estimates of endo-cardial motion and wall thickening and have had similar results. However, it is clear that endocardial motion remains a valid means of identifying some degree of ischemia and infarction.

Following infarction, there is evidence that compensatory changes in wall thickness result over time and may be a significant mechanism in maintaining the level of function [46, 56]. One of the major problems in these functional-pathologic studies continues to be spatial registration between tomographic slices. Because of the complex motion of the left ventricle through the fixed tomographic beam, this is a problem that has no simple solution.

Some investigators [49, 57] have used 2-D echo to measure the area of jeopardized, or at-risk myocardium. Since the ratio of infarcted to risk region would reduce the variability of ischemic damage produced in groups of animals or patients, the measurement of this parameter is important. Pandian *et al.* [49] found that myocardial dysfunction by 2-D echo tended to underestimate in-vitro risk mass. Our laboratory [57], using left ventricular mass measured by 2-D echo and thallium-201 perfused mass by single photon emission computed tomography, found a good correlation with in-vitro measures of risk mass. However, our measurement of risk mass tended to underestimate the in-vitro risk mass but may be closer to actual, functional risk mass. Further studies using in-vivo measures of risk mass may provide a better correspondence.

There have been several recent reports using 2-D echo to assess functional recovery following coronary reperfusion [51, 58–60]. Although most reports [51, 60, 61] have suggested little or no change in regional myocardial function following coronary reperfusion, we [58, 59] have seen early changes in regional endocardial motion which appear to be related to the degree of myocardial reperfusion (Figure 4). Other investigators [51, 60, 61] have not seen active systolic thickening in animals with transient coronary occlusion until 72 h after reperfusion. Recent studies [60] have suggested that inotropic stimulation with dopamine may accelerate recovery of the stunned myocardial function.

Other 2-D echo studies of regional function have assessed the effect of pharmacologic intervention [43, 60, 62, 63] or the study of the effect of ventricular premature beats on ventricular performance [64, 65]. These studies have demonstrated the potential of 2-D echo to study the regional effects of pharmacologic potentiation during acute ischemia and infarction (Figure 5), and to map out the site of ventricular arrhythmias using regional contraction patterns.

Left ventricular shape analysis

There continues to be controversy concerning the use of specific coordinate systems in the correction of three-dimensional motion [66]. We [67] have proposed a coordinate free approach of regional analysis using shape descriptors to circumvent the need for coordinate reference systems. Fourier shape analysis and mean tensor analysis [68] are potential methods that are well suited to global and regional analysis of the left ventricle in the short axis projection. Further research into the application of new shape descriptors in the analysis of left ventricle performance should improve the variability presently related only to the choice of the axial coordinate system used for the study.

The importance of cardiac shape and geometry in the understanding of cardiac function is well recognized [69–72]. Although there is considerable knowledge

168

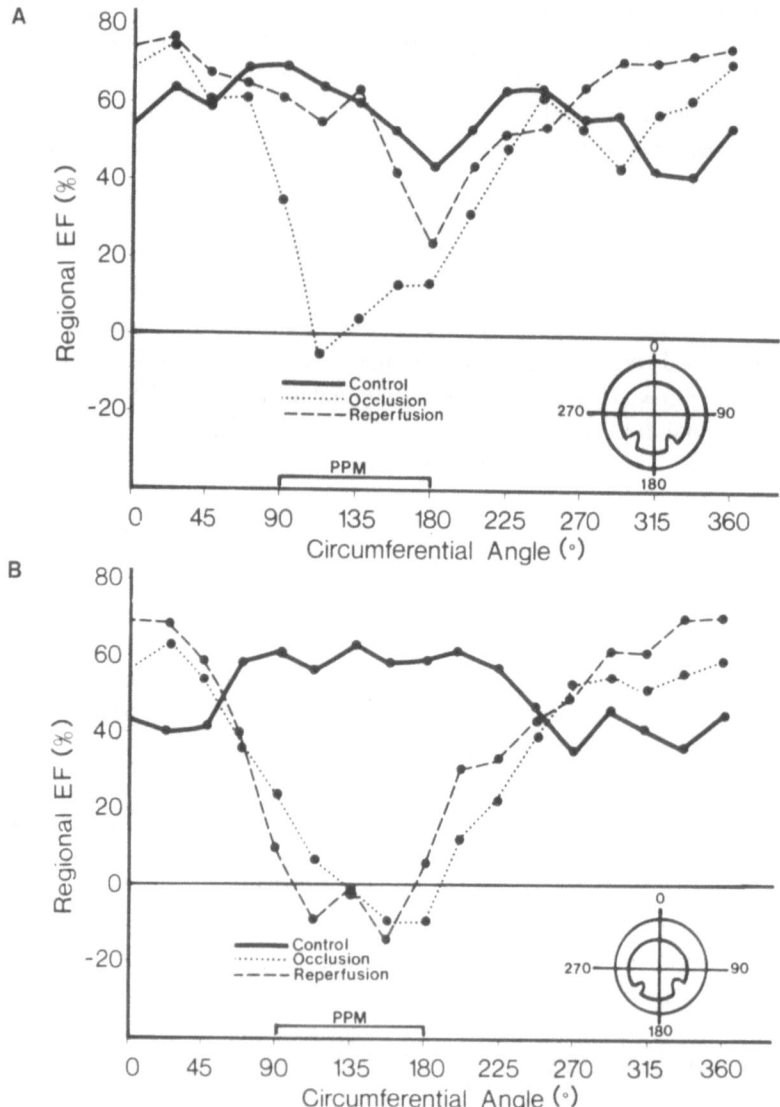

Figure 4. Regional function map from canine studies during baseline conditions, following circumflex coronary occlusion, and after circumflex coronary reperfusion. (A) This animal had good functional recovery and this correlated with significant myocardial reperfusion (49%). (B) This animal had no functional recovery following circumflex reflow and this correlated with poor myocardial reperfusion (5%), presumably because of a no-reflow phenomenon. PPM = posterior papillary muscle.

concerning dynamic geometry and shape of the heart, to date, most characterizations have resulted from experiments using sonomicrometer crystals which have established dimensional and volume descriptors. The use of sonomicrometry, however, has certain limitations related to sampling due to the limited number of crystals implanted. As a result, generalizations about two- and three-dimensional

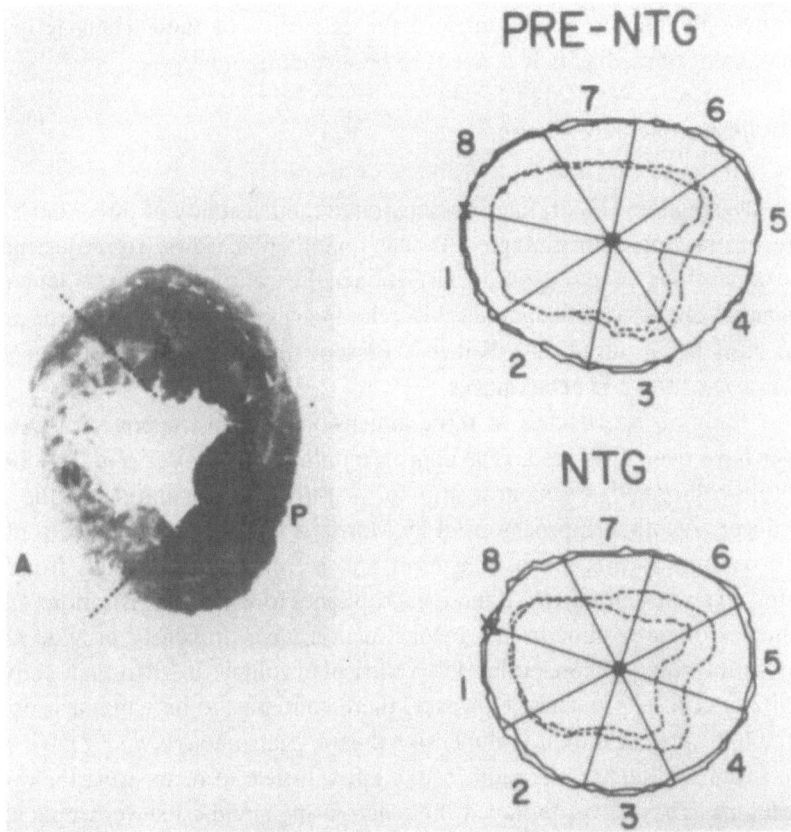

Figure 5. Triphenyltetrazolium chloride stained left ventricular slab equivalent to low papillary 2-D echocardiographic cross-section, along with superimposed 2-D echocardiographic endocardial and epicardial outlines obtained before and during nitroglycerin (NTG) testing 5 hr after left anterior descending artery occlusion. Note that the size of the nitroglycerin non-responsive region correlates well with the area of myocardial necrosis. (From reference 63, with permission of the author and the American Journal of Cardiology.) A = anterior; N = myocardial necrosis area; P = posterior; S = interventricular septum.

shape and geometry may sometimes be unjustified as assumptions regarding axisymmetric synergy and homogeneity of contraction may be unfounded even in the normal heart [37–40]. Heterogeneous contraction patterns can result from the anatomic variation in myocardial fiber mass and orientation in the wall of the heart [73–75]. Two-dimensional echocardiography, with its ability to provide circumferential, tomographic information, should provide further information regarding normal and abnormal shape and dynamic geometry of the beating heart [76]. Initial studies in man during physiologic maneuvers (Mueller maneuver [77]) and post myocardial infarction (infarct expansion [78]) have demonstrated the ability of 2-D echo to study acute and chronic alterations in left ventricular shape. Since it is presently unknown how changes in cardiac shape and structure contribute to alterations in function, the relevance of these changes to the development of cardiac failure needs to be further defined.

Three-dimensional reconstruction

Some investigators [79–81] have demonstrated the feasibility of three-dimensional reconstruction using multiple 2-D echo tomographic views. To reconstruct in three dimensions, precise spatial registration of the transducer in three-dimensional space is necessary. Sequential 2-D echo images gated to the electrocardiogram must be acquired and digitized. Present methods only involve manual digitization of the 2-D echo images.

Two common approaches to three-dimensional reconstruction of 2-D echo images have been described. One approach outlined by Geiser *et al.* [81] uses a precisely callibrated mechanical arm to measure the orientation of the 2-D transducer. Another approach used by Moritz *et al.* [80] uses spark-gap ultrasound emitters located on a transducer and measures transit times from the emitters to a reference array of three microphones for spatial registration. These techniques of three-dimensional reconstruction have proven to provide more accurate information concerning left ventricular volume in-vitro than conventional 2-D echo approaches. However, there continues to be a major problem related to display of the three-dimensional data. Matsumoto *et al.* [7] have used up to seven sagittal cross-sections of the left ventricle to reconstruct the three-dimensions. They have displayed their data using standard stereoscopic algorithms to orientate them in space and have used increasing shades of gray in order to denote depth. Moritz *et al.* [80] and Geiser *et al.* [81] have used an envelope corresponding to anatomical margin from multiple digitized outlines to indicate the left ventricle cavity (Figure 6). However, the problem of three-dimensional display is complex and not unique to echocardiography. Nevertheless, three-dimensional reconstruction of 2-D echo images should provide further opportunity to study left ventricular size and shape, and shape change. It may further enhance our ability to study complex congenital abnormalities.

Myocardial perfusion contrast echocardiography

Contrast echocardiography is based on the ability of ultrasound to visualize gaseous microbubbles in solution and has become an important clinical and research tool. An excellent monograph by Meltzer and Roelandt [82] provides a comprehensive review of its many applications in valvular and congenital heart disease.

More recently, there has been increasing interest in developing standardized echo contrast agents containing uniformly small and stable gaseous microbubbles

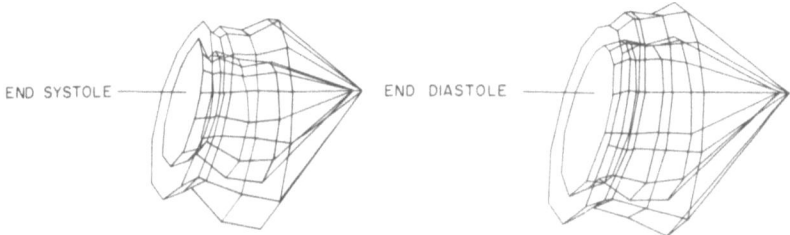

END SYSTOLE —

END DIASTOLE —

Figure 6. End-systolic and end-diastolic three-dimensional echocardiographic reconstruction. These are displayed in a 25-degree right anterior oblique position (From reference 81, with permission of the author and the American Heart Journal.)

for myocardial perfusion studies. A variety of contrast agents have been used in an attempt to develop a 2-D echo method for study of myocardial perfusion. These include: (1) commercially manufactured encapsulated microbubbles [83, 84], (2) carbon dioxide [84], (3) hydrogen peroxide [85], (4) agitated meglumine-saline mixture [86, 87], and (5) sonicated 70% sorbitol [88].

Several experimental studies [83, 85, 89] using a variety of contrast agents have demonstrated that 2-D echo with aortic root or intracoronary contrast injections may localize and accurately size the extent of a hypoperfused region of the myocardium. Armstrong *et al.* [83] used gelatin-encapsulated microbubbles as a contrast agent in an open chest model during circumflex coronary occlusion. Contrast enhancement as measured by commerical light meter correctly identified 48 of 51 octants (94%) with greater than 50% of normal coronary flow and 19 of 21 octants (90%) with reduced flow. Although regions of reduced perfusion were accurately detected, correlation between echo contrast enhancement and myocardial perfusion by the radioactive microsphere technique was poor. However, in their study, there was no attempt made to standardize injection volume, gain, depth, or gray scale settings which may have affected their correlations.

Kemper *et al.* [85] used a closed chest model with standardization of gain and depth settings by interactive use of an on-line color scale videodensitometer to study regional myocardial perfusion abnormalities. In their model, echo contrast defect was a considerably more accurate indicator of the state of regional myocardial perfusion and infarction than was wall motion (Figure 7). However, there were problems in using videodensitometry in that an unpredictable gradient in contrast enchancement was observed which made absolute quantification of regional flow by this technique difficult.

To further examine the dynamics of myocardial contrast, Tei *et al.* [86] digitized the video output of the 2-D echo left ventricular short axis image to analyze a myocardial echo contrast opacification disappearance rate index. They developed a computer algorithm which divided the left ventricle into 12 radial segments and determined the average echo contrast intensity within each segment. Myocardial contrast echo measurements in closed chest dogs with different degrees of plug-induced intracoronary stenosis indicated significant differences in the de-

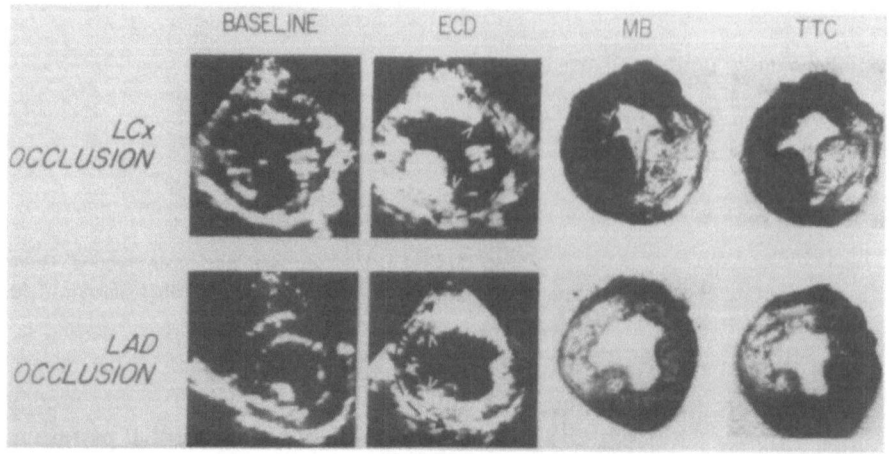

Figure 7. Examples of two-dimensional echocardiographic images and their corresponding left ventricle slices. (Top) After left circumflex (LCx) coronary artery ligation, a short-axis image of the midpapillary muscle level was obtained before injection of contrast agent (baseline). After injection of the H_2O_2/blood mixture, the myocardial area with normal perfusion lit up while the circumferential extent of ZD echo contrast defect (ECD) remained dark (white arrows). Abnormal wall motion was seen in real-time, which is designated by the black dashed line between black arrows. To determine the area at risk, monastral blue dye was injected in the left atriums of the dogs before they were killed. The area with abnormal myocardial perfusion was not impregnated with dye (light area). After incubating the slices in triphenyltetrazolium chloride (TTC) for 15 min at 37°C, the area of infarction remained unstained (light area). (Bottom) Similar sequence after left anterior descending (LAD) coronary ligation. Examples are from the middle to low papillary muscle levels. (From reference 85, with permission of the author and the American Heart Association, Inc.)

rived index. However, their methodology was unable to adequately describe the physiologic coronary flow rate within the contrast-perfused zone. It is possible that more standardized contrast agent agitation techniques with more reproducible and sufficiently small microbubble diameters may allow physiologic passage through the coronary microcirculation to allow for improved estimation of coronary flow. But, despite this, inherent limitations involved with regional texture differences in the video image, as discussed below, will continue to hamper efforts to accurately quantitate myocardial flow using this methodology.

Although the use of venous contrast agent injections during echocardiography appears to be safe in man [90], the safety of contrast agents for myocardial perfusion imaging in man remains to be proven. Further rigorous studies need to be performed in animal models before its application in man.

Tissue characterization

The clinical echocardiographer often notices inhomogeneity of echo intensities in the 2-D echo display often related to calcified structures within the heart. However, other inhomogeneities appear to be related to abnormalities of the structure or histology of myocardial tissue; for example, the peculiar texture of the septum in idiopathic hypertrophic subaortic stenosis, the 'ground glass' appearance of the myocardium in amyloidosis, and the intense echoes from areas of myocardium related to old myocardial infarction [91]. These observations have renewed interest in the area of tissue characterization using digital echocardiographic approaches.

Echocardiographic tissue characterization [92] can be defined as the assessment of the structure of tissue based on its acoustic properties. The implicit assumption is that acoustic properties of tissue is closely related to its histology so that abnormalities of acoustic properties may indicate alteration of normal histology or pathology.

Initial attempts at tissue characterization were performed using transmission techniques which measured acoustic impedance and attenuation [93–95]. These techniques involved having the source and the detector of the ultrasound on opposite sides of the specimen making them inapplicable for in-vivo work. Nevertheless, these initial investigations provided important data which demonstrated that acutely ischemic myocardial tissue could be detected by decreases in ultrasound attenuation [93, 94]. Similar decreases were noted in infarcted myocardium over an initial 24 hr period. However, as collagen content in infarcted tissue increased over the subsequent days, increased attenuation was noted at three days and at six weeks.

To be clinically useful, the use of reflected ultrasound in measurement of ultrasound backscatter is necessary. Subsequent investigations by Mimbs et al. [95–97] of tissue character therefore relied on measures of backscatter rather than abnormalities of acoustic impedance or attenuation. An increase in integrated backscatter was demonstrated within one hour of experimental coronary occlusion which persisted for weeks after infarction. This increase has been attributed to increases in edema during infarction [96]. In chronic infarction, the increase in collagen content in the healing process correlated with alterations in backscatter [95]. These same investigators identified myocardial doxorubicin toxicity by alterations in integrated backscatter measurements [91].

There have been recent attempts to perform tissue characterization using commercially available sector scanners. Skorton et al. [98] used regional average gray level as an analog of echo amplitude to investigate changes in tissue character during acute coronary occlusion in a closed chest canine model. Due to variability in gray level, the increase in gray level in the ischemic region could only be identified in comparison to a control echocardiogram. However, the shape of gray level frequency histograms proved to be a reliable discriminator of infarction.

These same investigators [99] studied quantitative texture measurements in an animal model after blunt left chest trauma producing myocardial contusion. They used four different algorithms as measures of texture: (1) gray level histogram statistics, (2) edges count, (3) gray level run-length statistics, and (4) gray level difference statistics. These texture measures were able to differentiate normal from abnormal myocardial tissue only when texture along the azimuthal direction was calculated.

Other investigators [100] performed 2-D echoes before and serially after coronary occlusion in four groups of dogs. The dogs were sacrificed at the following intervals: 24–48 hr, 1–2 weeks, 3 weeks, and 6–8 weeks. The 2-D echoes were digitized using a commercial video digitizer and the echo amplitudes were color encoded into eight regions of color. This color processing was performed to increase the dynamic range of echo information since the eye can distinguish considerably more colors than shades of gray. Using this color processing technique, they found that the progressive increase in echo amplitude paralleled the histopathologic evolution of myocardial infarction. Echo amplitude was greatest when hydroxyproline synthesis had increased and collagen deposition was at its fullest.

Although encouraging, these approaches to tissue characterization have significant limitations. Echo amplitude data vary significantly within the sector field of view as a function of range and azimuth within the scan [101, 102]. The causes of this variability include transducer geometry, changes in resolution, and the effect of signal detection and display processes. Current instrumentation can frequently make disease appear normal by way of typical TGC adjustments. In in-vitro experiments, this variability has been improved using line by line attenuation compensation (rational gain compensation) [103], as compared to the standard time-gain compensation which amplifies the entire azimuthal extent of the scan within each range interval.

Another approach has been the use of an empirical correction factor for attenuation based on measurements of excised chest wall specimens [104]. Using attenuation correction, measurements of integrated backscatter agreed closely with those obtained directly from the epicardial surface. However, regional alterations and image texture may not reflect actual pathology until methods are developed to correct for the significant regional differences in echo amplitude information.

Directly digitized RF data is necessary for significant tissue characterization using statistical analysis of the ultrasound signal. At present, the rapid sampling rate and large amount of digital data storage necessary to evaluate RF data have not permitted direct digitization of the entire 2-D echo field of view. However, Green et al. [105] digitized RF data from a single line of 2-D echo data and applied a stochastic approach [106] to the analysis of echo signals (Figure 8). Using this approach, the distribution of echo amplitudes within the received signal approximates the probability density function expected from on array of random, independent scatterers. These investigators used this stochastic approach to differentiate thrombus from artifact and myxoma.

The addition of two new parameters for quantitative display, frequency depen-

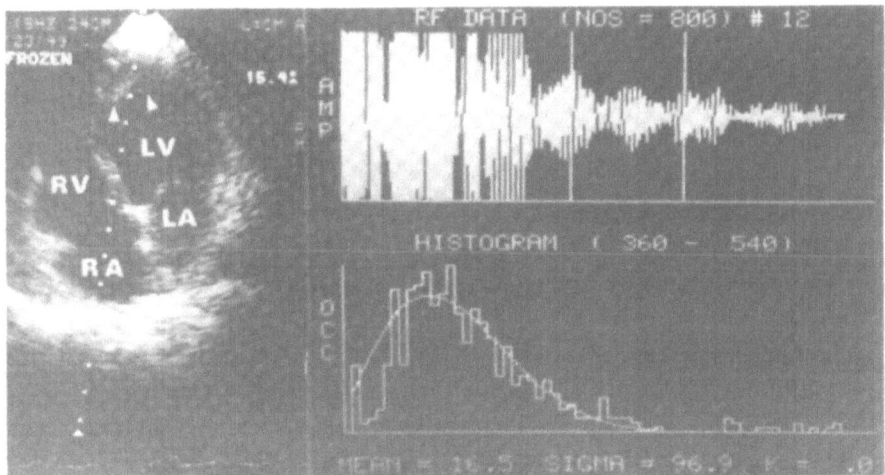

Figure 8. Composite of data obtained from a patient with an apical left ventricular thrombus confirmed at necropsy. The left panel shows a 2-dimensional echocardiographic image in the apical 4-chamber projection. The M-mode cursor passes through the thrombus (arrows), identifying the scan line from which the ultrasonic signal is sampled. The upper right panel is the 12th of 40 unprocessed signal samples and consists of 800 data points. Signal amplitude is represented on the ordinate and tissue depth on the abscissa. The operator-determined region of interest is enclosed by 2 vertical lines. The lower right panel depicts a histogram representing the number of occurences (ordinate) of the digitized component amplitudes (abscissa) of the signal from the region of interest. A theoretical probability density function, derived from the mean amplitude and variance of the signal, is superimposed on the histogram. The histogram is described by k = o, suggesting a random, independent collection of small scatterers. (From reference 105, with permission of the author and the American Journal of Cardiology.) AMP = amplitude; LA = left atrium; LV = left ventricle; OCC = number of occurrences of digitized component amplitude; RA = right atrium; RF = radiofrequency; RV = right ventricle.

dent backscattering and attenuation coefficient to clinical ultrasound imaging, as proposed by Meyer *et al.* [107], may allow differentiation of many of the current ambiguities and further improve the sensitivity and predictive value of ultrasound in tissue characterization.

Conclusion

Current 2-D echo instrumentation and technique are adequate for meaningful clinical diagnosis and investigation. However, further improvements in transducer design, and digital acquisition and processing techniques, will be necessary to allow for increased clinical use of quantitative measurements related to myocardial dynamics and tissue characterization. Only with further technologic advances will it be possible to perform frame by frame quantitative analysis of regional left ventricular function, three-dimensional reconstruction, myocardial

176

perfusion studies, and tissue characterization on a more routine clinical basis. The feasibility and importance of these techniques has now been demonstrated. The future development of digital 2-D echocardiography over the next decade should produce further advances in these areas.

Acknowledgements

This work was supported by grants from the American Heart Association of Michigan and Grant HL 29716 from the National Heart, Lung, and Blood Institute, National Institutes of Health, Bethesda, Maryland. The authors gratefully acknowledge the personnel in our Echocardiography, Computer, and Animal Research Laboratories for their continued enthusiasm and support of our efforts, and Mrs Sharon Haglund for preparing this manuscript.

References

1. Feigenbaum H: Echocardiography. Third edition. Lea & Febiger, Philadelphia, 1981.
2. Weyman AE: Cross-sectional echocardiography. Lea & Febiger, Philadelphia, 1982.
3. Wells PNT: Biomedical ultrasonics. Academic Press, New York, 1977.
4. Sahn DJ, Anderson F (eds): Two-dimensional anatomy of the heart: an atlas for echocardiographers. John Wiley & Sons, New York, 1982.
5. Hagan Ad, DiSeisa TG, Bloor CM, Calleja HB (eds): Two-dimensional echocardiography: clinical-pathological correlations in adult and congenital heart disease. Little, Brown & Co, Boston, 1984.
6. Skorton DJ, McNary CA, Child JS, Shah PM: Computerized image processing in cross-sectional echocardiography. Am J Cardiol 45: 403–486, 1980.
7. Matsumoto M, Matsuo H, Kitabalake A, Inoue M, Hamanka Y, Tamura A, Tanaka K, Hiroshi A: Three-dimensional echocardiograms and two-dimensional echocardiographic images at desired planes by a computerized system. Ultrasound Med Biol 3: 163–179, 1977.
8. Garrison JB, Weis JL, Manghan WL, Tuck ON, Guier WN, Fortuin NJ: Quantifying regional wall motion and thickening in two-dimensional echocardiography with a computer-aided contouring system. IEEE Computers in Cardiol 25–35, 1977.
9. Skolnick ML: A new approach to ultrasound image recording using a video disk recorder. Radiology 133: 530, 1979.
10. Garcia E, Gueret P, Bennett M, Corday E, Zwehl W, Meerbaum S, Corday S, Swan HJC, Berman D: Real-time computerization of two-dimensional echocardiography. Am Heart J 101: 763–792, 1981.
11. Jenkins JM, Qian G, Besozzi M, Delp EJ, Buda AJ: Computer processing of echocardiographic images for automated edge detection of left ventricular boundaries. IEEE Computers in Cardiol 391–394, 1981.
12. Wells PNT, Woodcock JP: Computers in ultrasonic diagnostics. Research Studies Press, Forest Grove, OR, 1977.
13. Robinson DE, Williams BG: Computer acquisition and processing of ultrasonic data. Ultrasonics in Medicine. Excerpta Medica, Amsterdam, 96–102, 1975.
14. Buda AJ, Delp EJ, Meyer CR, Jenkins JM, Smith DN, Bookstein FL, Pitt B: Automatic computer processing of digital two-dimensional echocardiograms. Am J Cardiol 52: 384–389, 1983.

15. Smith DN, Buda AJ, Delp EJ, Jenkins JM, Meyer CR, Splittgerber FH, Pitt B: Mitral valve tracking of directly digitized 2-D echocardiograms. IEEE Computers in Cardiol 329–332, 1982.

16. Delp EJ, Buda AJ, Swastek M, Smith DN, Jenkins JM, Meyer CR, Pitt B: The analysis of two-dimensional echocardiograms using a time-varying image approach. IEEE Computers in Cardiol 391–394, 1982.

17. Skorton DJ, McNary CA, Child JS, Newton FC, Shah PM: Digital image processing of two-dimensional echocardiograms: identification of the endocardium. Am J Cardiol 48: 479–486, 1981.

18. Zwehl W, Levy R, Garcia E, Haendchen RV, Childs W, Corday SR, Meerbaum S, Corday E: Validation of a computerized edge detection algorithm for quantitative two-dimensional echocardiography. Circulation 68 (5): 1127–1135, 1983.

19. Martin WN, Agfarwal JK: Dynamic scene analysis. Computers, Graphics, and Image Processing 14: 12–18, 1981.

20. Wyatt HL, Haendchen RV, Meerbaum S, Corday E: Assessment of quantitative methods for 2-dimensional echocardiography. Am J Cardiol 52: 396–402, 1983.

21. Wyatt HL, Heng MK, Meerbaum S, Hestenes JD, Cobo JM, Davison RM, Corday E: Cross-sectional echocardiography. I. Analysis of mathematic models for quantifying mass of the left ventricle in dogs. Circulation 60: 1104–1113, 1979.

22. Wyatt HL, Heng MK, Meerbaum S, Hestenes JD, Dula E, Corday E: Cross-sectional echocardiography. II. Analysis of mathematical models for quantifying volume of the formalin-fixed left ventricle. Circulation 61: 119–1125, 1980.

23. Wyatt HL, Meerbaum S, Heng MK, Gueret P, Corday E: Cross-sectional echocardiography. III. Analysis of mathematical models for quantifying volume of symmetric and asymmetric left ventricle. Am Heart J 100: 821–828, 1980.

24. Eaton LW, Maughan WL, Shoukas AA, Weiss JL: Accurate volume determination in the isolated ejecting canine left ventricle by two-dimensional echocardiography. Circulation 60: 320–326, 1979.

25. Schiller NB, Acquatella H, Ports TA, Drew D, Goerke J, Ringertz H, Silverman NH, Brundage B, Botvinick EH, Boswell R, Carlsson E, Parmley WW: Left ventricular volume from paired biplane two-dimensional echocardiography. Circulation 60: 547–555, 1979.

26. Folland ED, Parisi AF, Moynihan BS, Jones DR, Feldman CL, Tow DE: Assessment of left ventricular ejection fraction and volumes by real-time, two-dimensional echocardiography. Circulation 60: 760–766, 1979.

27. Helak JW, Reichek N: Quantitation of human left ventricular mass and volume by two-dimensional echocardiography; in vitro anatomic validation. Circulation 63: 1398–1407, 1981.

28. Stamm RB, Carabello BA, Mayers DL, Martin RP: Two-dimensional echocardiographic measurement of left ventricular ejection fraction: prospective analysis of what constitutes an adequate determination. Am Heart J 102: 136–144, 1982.

29. Schiller NB, Skiolderbrand CG, Schiller EJ, Mavroudis CC, Silverman NH, Rahimtoola SH, Lipton MJ: Canine left ventricular mass estimation by two-dimensional echocardiography. Circulation 68: 210–216, 1983.

30. Weiss JL, Eaton LW, Kallman CH, Maughan WL: Accuracy of volume determination by two-dimensional echocardiography: defining requirements under controlled conditions in the ejecting canine left ventricle. Circulation 67: 889–895, 1983.

31. Reichek N, Helak J, Plappert T, St John Sutton M, Weber KT: Anatomic validation of left ventricular mass estimates from clinical two-dimensional echocardiography: initial results. Circulation 67: 348–352, 1983.

32. Schnittger I, Fitzgerald PJ, Daughters GT, Ingels NB, Kantrowitz N, Schwartzkopf A, Meed CW, Popp RL: Limitations of comparing left ventricular volumes by two-dimensional echocardiography, myocardial markers and cineangiography. Am J Cardiol 50: 512–519, 1982.

33. Erbel R, Schweizer P, Lambertz H, Henh G, Meyer J, Krebs W, Effert S: Echoventriculogra-

178

phy – a simultaneous analysis of two-dimensional echocardiography and cineventriculography. Circulation 67: 205–215, 1983.

34. Moynihan PF, Parisi AF, Feldman CL: Quantitative detection of regional left ventricular contraction abnormalities by two-dimensional echocardiography. I. Analysis of methods. Circulation 63: 752–760, 1981.

35. Parisi AF, Moynihan PF, Folland ED, Feldman CL: Quantitative detection of regional left ventricular contraction abnormalities by two-dimensional echocardiography. II. Accuracy in coronary artery disease. Circulation 63: 761–767, 1981.

36. Sheehan FH, Mathey DG, Schofer J, Krebber H, Dodge HT: Effect of interventions in salvaging left ventricular function in acute myocardial infarction: a study of intracoronary streptokinase. Am J Cardiol 52: 431–443, 1983.

37. LeWinter MM, Kent RS, Kroener JM, Carew TE, Covell JW: Regional differences in myocardial performance in the left ventricle of the dog. Circ Res 37: 191–199, 1975.

38. Shapiro E, Marier DL, St John Sutton MG, Gibson DG: Regional non-uniformity of wall dynamics in normal left ventricle. Brit Heart J 45: 264–270, 1981.

39. Pandian NG, Skorton DJ, Collins SM, Falsetti HL, Burke ER, Kerber RE: Heterogeneity of left ventricular segmental wall thickening and excursion in 2-dimensional echocardiograms of normal human subjects. Am J Cardiol 51: 167–173, 1983.

40. Haendchen RV, Wyatt HL, Maurer G, Zwehl W, Bear M, Meerbaum S, Corday E: Quantitation of regional cardiac function by two-dimensional echocardiography. I. Patterns of contraction in the normal left ventricle. Circulation 67: 1234–1245, 1983.

41. Kerber RE, Marcus ML, Ehrhardt J, Wilson R, Abboud FM: Correlation between echocardiographically demonstrated segmental dyskinesis and regional myocardial perfusion. Circulation 52: 1097–1103, 1975.

42. Meltzer RS, Woythaler JN, Buda AJ, Griffin JC, Harrison WD, Martin RP, Harrison DC, Popp RL: Two-dimensional echocardiographic quantification of infarct size alteration by pharmacologic agents. Am J Cardiol 44: 257–262, 1979.

43. Meltzer RS, Woythaler JN, Buda AJ, Griffin JC, Kernoff R, Harrison DC, Popp RL, Martin RP: Non-invasive quantification of experimental canine myocardial infarct size using two-dimensional echocardiography. Eur J Cardiol 11: 215–225, 1980.

44. Wyatt HL, Meerbaum S, Heng MK, Rit H, Gueret P, Corday E: Experimental evaluation of the extent of myocardial dyssynergy and infarct size by two-dimensional echocardiography. Circulation 63: 607–614, 1981.

45. Lieberman AN, Weiss JL, Jugdutt BI, Becker LC, Bulkley BH, Garrison JG, Hutchins GM, Kallman CA, Weisfeldt ML: Two-dimensional echocardiography and infarct size: relationship of regional wall motion and thickening to the extent of myocardial infarction in the dog. Circulation 63: 739–746, 1981.

46. Nieminen M, Parisi AF, O'Boyle JE, Folland ED, Khuri S, Kloner RA: Serial evaluation of myocardial thickening and thinning in acute experimental infarction: identification and quantification using two-dimensional echocardiography Circulation 66: 174–180, 1982.

47. Henschke CI, Risser TA, Sandor T, Hanlon WB, Neumann A, Wynne J: Quantitative computer-assisted analysis of left ventricular wall thickening and motion by 2-dimensional echocardiography in acute myocardial infarction. Ann J Cardiol 52: 960–964, 1983.

48. O'Boyle JE, Parisi AF, Nieminen M, Kloner RA, Khuri S: Quantitative detection of regional left ventricular contraction abnormalities by 2-dimensional echocardiography. Am J Cardiol 51: 1732–1738, 1983.

49. Pandian NG, Koyanagi S, Skorton DJ, Collins SM, Eastham CL, Kieso RA, Marcus ML, Kerber RE: Relations between 2-dimensional echocardiographic wall thickening abnormalities, myocardial infarct size and coronary risk area in normal and hypertrophied myocardium in dogs. Am J Cardiol 52: 1318–1325, 1983.

50. Blumenthal DS, Becker LC, Bulkley BH, Hutchins GM, Weisfeldt ML, Weiss JL: Impaired

function of salvaged myocardium: two-dimensional echocardiographic quantification of regional wall thickening in the open-chest dog. Circulation 67: 225–233, 1983.

51. Ellis SG, Henschke CI, Sandor T, Wynne J, Braunwald E, Kloner RA: Time course of functional and biochemical recovery of myocardium salvaged by reperfusion. J Am Coll Cardiol 1: 1047–1055, 1983.

52. Pandian NG, Kerber RE: Two-dimensional echocardiography in experimental coronary stenosis. Circulation 66: 597–602, 1982.

53. Pandian NG, Kieso RA, Kerber RE: Two-dimensional echocardiography in experimental coronary stenosis. II. Relationship between systolic wall thinning and regional myocardial perfusion in severe coronary stenosis. Circulation 66: 603–611, 1982.

54. Theroux P, Franklin D, Ross J Jr, Kemper WS: Regional myocardial function during acute coronary occlusion and its modification by pharmacologic agents in the dog. Circ Res 35: 896–908, 1974.

55. Gallagher KP, Kumada T, Kaziol JA, McKown MD, Kemper WS, Ross J Jr: Significance of regional wall thickening abnormalities relative to transmural myocardial perfusion in anesthetized dogs. Circulation 62: 1266–1274, 1980.

56. Sasayama S, Gallagher KP, Kemper WS, Franklin D, Ross J Jr: Regional left ventricular wall thickness early and later after coronary occlusion in the dog. Am J Physiol 240: H293–H299, 1981.

57. Weiss RJ, Buda AJ, Pasyk S, O'Neill WW, Keyes JW Jr, Pitt B: Non-invasive quantification of jeopardized myocardial mass using two-dimensional echocardiography and thallium-201 tomography. Am J Cardiol 52: 1340–1344, 1983.

58. Buda AJ, Pasyk S, LeMire S, Smith DN, O'Neill WW, Keyes JW Jr, Pitt B: Immediate recovery of ischemic left ventricular regional function following coronary reperfusion: assessment by two-dimensional echocardiography. Clin Res (abstr) 31: 171A, 1983.

59. Buda AJ, Pasyk S, Keyes JW Jr, Pitt B: Interrelation of myocardial function and perfusion following coronary occlusion and reperfusion. Circulation (abstr) 68 (III): III–255, 1983.

60. Ellis SG, Wynne J, Braunwald E, Henschke CI, Sandor T, Kloner R: Response of reperfusion – salvaged, stunned myocardium to inotropic stimulation. Am Heart J 107: 13–19, 1984.

61. Theroux P, Ross J Jr, Franklin D, Kemper WS, Sasayama S: Coronary artery reperfusion. III. Early and late effects on regional myocardial function and dimensions in conscious dogs. Am J Cardiol 38: 599–606, 1976.

62. Gueret P, Meerbaum S, Corday E, Uchiyama T, Wyatt HL, Broffman J: Differential effects of nitroprusside on ischemic and non-ischemic myocardial segments demonstrated by computer-assisted two-dimensional echocardiography. Am J Cardiol 48: 59–68, 1981.

63. Shimoura K, Meerbaum S, Sakamaki T, Kondo S, Fishbein MC, Y-Rit J, Tei C, Shah PM, Corday E: Relation between functional response to nitroglycerin and extent of myocardial necrosis in dogs: mapping of the left ventricle by 2-dimensional echocardiography. Am J Cardiol 52: 177–183, 1983.

64. Uchiyama T, Corday E, Meerbaum S, Lang T, Gueret P, Povzhitkov M, Peter T: Characterization of left ventricular mechanical function during arrhythmias with two-dimensional echocardiography. I. Premature ventricular contractions. Am J Cardiol 48: 679–689, 1981.

65. Torres MAR, Corday E, Meerbaum S, Sakamaki T, Peter T, Uchiyama T: Characterization of left ventricular mechanical function during arrhythmias by two-dimensional echocardiography. II. Location of the site of onset of premature ventricular systoles. J Am Coll Cardiol 1: 819–829, 1983.

66. Clayton PD, Jeppson GM, Klausner SC: Should a fixed external reference system be used to analyze left ventricular wall motion? Circulation 65: 1518–1521, 1982.

67. Bookstein FL, Buda AJ: Mean tensor analysis of cardiac wall motion: a quantitative, coordinate-free approach to regional left ventricular function. Clin Res (abstr) 31: 169A, 1983.

68. Bookstein FL: The measurement of biological shape and shape change. Lecture Notes in Biomathematics, Vol 24. Springer-Verlag, New York, 1978.

69. Rankin JS, McHale PAS, Arentzen CE, Ling D, Greenfield JC, Anderson RW: The three-dimensional geometry of the left ventricle in the conscious dog. Circulation 39: 304–313, 1976.

70. Weber KT, Hawthorne EW: Descriptor and determinants of cardiac shape: an overview. Federation Proc 40: 2005–2010, 1981.

71. Janicki JS, Weber KT, Shroff S: Regional and global shape and size of the intact myocardium. Federation Proc 40: 2017–2022, 1981.

72. Olsen CO, Van Tright P, Rankin JS: Dynamic geometry of the intact left ventricle. Federation Proc 40: 2023–2030, 1981.

73. Streeter DD, Spotnitz MN, Patel DJ, Ross J, Sonnenblick EH: Fiber orientation in the canine left ventricle during diastole and systole. Circ Res 24: 339–347, 1969.

74. Streeter DD, Hanna WI: Engineering mechanics for successive states in canine left ventricular myocardium. I. Cavity and wall geometry. Circ Res 33: 639–655, 1973.

75. Streeter DD, Hanna WI: Engineering mechanics for successive stages in canine left ventricular myocardium. II. Fiber angle and sarcomere length. Circ Res 33: 656–664, 1973.

76. Weiss JL, Eaton LW, Manghan WL, Brinker JA, Bulkey B, Guzman P, Yiu FCP: Ventricular size and shape by two-dimensional echocardiography. Federation Proc 40: 2031–2036, 1981.

77. Brinker JA, Weiss JL, Lappe DL, Robson JL, Summer WK, Permutt S, Weisfeldt ML: Leftward septal displacement during right ventricular loading in man. Circulation 61: 626–633, 1980.

78. Eaton LW, Weiss JL, Bulkley BH, Garrison JB, Weisfeldt ML: Regional cardiac dilatation after acute myocardial infarction: recognition by two-dimensional echocardiography. N Engl J Med 300: 57–62, 1979.

79. Geiser EA, Lupkiewicz SM, Chirstie LG, Ariet M, Conetta DA, Conti CR: A framework for three-dimensional time-varying reconstruction of the human left ventricle: sources of error and estimation of their magnitude. Computers and Biomed Res 13: 225–241, 1980.

80. Moritz WE, Medema DK, McCabe D, Pearlman AS: Three-dimensional imaging and volume determination using a series of two-dimensional ultrasonic scans. Echocardiology. Martinus Nijhoff, The Hague, 1981, p 449.

81. Geiser EA, Ariet M, Conetta DA, Lupkiewicz SM, Christie LG Jr, Conti CR: Dynamic three-dimensional echocardiographic reconstruction of the intact human left ventricles: technique and initial observations in patients. Am Heart J 103: 1056–1065, 1982.

82. Meltzer RS, Roelandt J (eds): Contrast echocardiography. Martinus Nijhoff, The Hague, 1982.

83. Armstrong WF, Mueller TM, Kinney EL, Tickner EG, Dillon JC, Feigenbaum H: Assessment of myocardial perfusion abnormalities with contrast-enhanced two-dimensional echocardiography. Circulation 66: 166–173, 1982.

84. DeMaria AN, Bommer WJ, Riggs K et al.: Echocardiographic visualization of myocardial perfusion by left heart and intracoronary injections of echo contrast agents. Circulation (abstr) 60 (II): II–143, 1980.

85. Kemper AJ, O'Boyle JE, Sharma S, Cohen CA, Kloner RA, Khuri SF, Parisi AF: Hydrogen peroxide contrast-enhanced two-dimensional echocardiography: real-time in vivo delineation of regional myocardial perfusion. Circulation 68: 603–611, 1983.

86. Tei C, Kondo S, Meerbaum S, Ong K, Maurer G, Wood F, Sakamaki T, Shimoura K, Corday E, Shah PM: Correlation of myocardial echo contrast disappearance rate ('washout') and severity of experimental coronary stenosis. J Am Coll Cardiol 3: 39–46, 1984.

87. Maurer G, Ong K, Haendchen R, Torres M, Tei C, Wood F, Meerbaum S, Shah P, Corday E: Myocardial contrast two-dimensional echocardiography: comparison of contrast disappearance rates in normal and underperfused myocardium. Circulation 69: 418–429, 1984.

88. Feinstein SB, Ten Cate FJ, Zwehl W, Ong K, Maurer G, Tei C, Shah PM, Meerbaum S, Corday E: Two-dimensional contrast echocardiography. I. In vitro development and quantitative analysis of echo contrast agents. J Am Coll Cardiol 3: 14–20, 1984.

89. Sakamaki T, Tei C, Meerbaum S, Shimoura K, Kondo S, Fishbein MC, Y-Rit J, Shah PM,

Corday E: Verification of myocardial contrast two-dimensional echocardiographic assessment of perfusion defects in ischemic myocardium. J Am Coll Cardiol 3: 34–38, 1984.

90. Bommer WJ, Shah PM, Allen H, Meltzer R, Kisslo J: The safety of contrast echocardiography: report of the committee on contrast echocardiography for the American Society of Echocardiography. J Am Coll Cardiol 3: 6–13, 1984.

91. Bhandari AK, Nanda NC: Myocardial texture characterization by two-dimensional echocardiography. Am J Cardiol 51: 817–825, 1983.

92. Chivers RC: Tissue characterization. Ultrasound Med Biol 7: 1–20, 1980.

93. Mimbs JW, Yuhas DE, Miller JG, Weiss AN, Sobel BE: Detection of myocardial infarction based on altered attenuation of ultrasound. Circ Res 41: 192–198, 1977.

94. Mimbs JW, O'Donnell M, Miller JG, Sobel BE: Changes in ultrasonic attenuation indicative of early myocardial ischemic injury. Am J Physiol 236: H340–H344, 1979.

95. Mimbs JW, O'Donnel M, Bauwens D, Miller JG, Sobel BE: The dependence of ultrasonic attenuation and backscatter on collagen content in dog and rabbit hearts. Circ Res 47: 49–58, 1980.

96. Mimbs JW, Bauwens D, Cohen RD, O'Donnell M, Miller JG, Sobel BE: Effects of myocardial ischemia on quantitative ultrasonic backscatter and identification of responsible determinants. Circ Res 49: 89–96, 1981.

97. Mimbs JW, O'Donnel M, Miller JG, Sobel BE: Detection of cardiomyopathic changes induced by doxorubicin based on quantitative analysis of ultrasonic backscatter. Am J Cardiol 47: 1056–1060, 1981.

98. Skorton DJ, Melton HE Jr, Pandian NG, Nichols J, Koyanagi NS, Marcus ML, Collins SM, Kerber RE: Detection of acute myocardial infarction in closed-chest dogs by analysis of regional two-dimensional echocardiographic gray-level distributions. Circ Res 52: 36–44, 1983.

99. Skorton DJ, Collins SM, Nichols J, Pandian NG, Bean JA, Kerber RE: Quantitative texture analysis in two-dimensional echocardiography: application to the diagnosis of experimental myocardial contusion. Circulation 68: 217–223, 1983.

100. Parisi AF, Nieminen M, O'Boyle JE, Moynhan PF, Khuri SF, Kloner RA, Folland ED, Schoen FJ: Enhanced detection of the evolution of tissue changes after acute myocardial infarction using color-encoded two-dimensional echocardiography. Circulation 66: 764–770, 1982.

101. Flax SW, Glover GH, Pelc NJ: Textural variations in B-mode ultrasonography; a stochastic model. Ultrasonic Imaging 3: 235–257, 1981.

102. Skorton DJ, Collins SM, Woskoff SD, Bean JA, Melton HE: Range- and azimuth-dependent variability of image texture in two-dimensional echocardiograms. Circulation 68: 834–840, 1983.

103. Melton HE Jr, Skorton DJ: Rational gain compensation for attenuation: a step toward quantitative two-dimensional echocardiography. Am J Cardiol (abstr) 49: 931, 1982.

104. Cohen RD, Mottley JG, Miller JG, Kurnik PB, Sobel BE: Detection of ischemic myocardium in vivo through the chest wall by quantitative ultrasonic tissue characterization. Am J Cardiol 50: 838–843, 1982.

105. Green SE, Joynt LF, Fitzgerald PJ, Rubenson DS, Popp RL: In vivo ultrasonic tissue characterization of human intracardiac masses. Am J Cardiol 51: 231–236, 1983.

106. Joynt LF: A stochastic approach to ultrasonic tissue characterization. Technical report G557-4, Integrated Circuits Laboratory, Stanford Electronics Laboratories, Stanford University, Stanford, CA, 1979.

107. Meyer CR: Preliminary results on a system for wideband, reflectionmode, ultrasonic attenuation imaging. IEEE Trans Sonics and Ultrasonics 29: 12–17, 1982.

12. Doppler echocardiography: Basic principles and clinical applications

A. REBECCA SNIDER

In recent years, Doppler ultrasound has been used extensively to evaluate blood flow patterns within the heart and peripheral vessels. This technology can be used qualitatively to diagnose valvular and congenital heart disease; and, because it is a safe and non-invasive technique, Doppler ultrasound can be used for the serial assessment of the defect. In addition, recent studies have shown that the severity of the flow abnormality can be accurately quantitated from the Doppler examination in many cases. The purposes of this chapter are: (1) to examine the basic physical principles of Doppler ultrasound, and (2) to review the clinical applications of this technique.

Physical principles of Doppler ultrasound

The Doppler effect

If a person is moving toward a sound source, he will hear a tone with higher frequency or pitch than when he is at rest. Conversely, if he is moving away from the sound source, he will hear a tone with lower frequency (Figure 1). The same effect occurs when the sound source is moving and the receiver is stationary. The change in frequency is called the Doppler shift in frequency or the Doppler frequency and was first described by the Austrian physicist Christian Johann Doppler (1803–1853) [1].

The Doppler effect applies to all types of waves where the source and the receiver are moving relative to one another (i.e. light from a moving star, radar waves, etc.). In medical applications, an emitted ultrasound pulse strikes a moving red blood cell and the reflected pulses are shifted in frequency compared to the emitted pulse. The change in frequency is related to the velocity and direction of red blood cell flow as well as to other factors such as the angle between the Doppler ultrasound beam and the blood flow and the speed of sound in tissue. The mathematical relationship of these factors is described by the

STATIONARY RECEIVER

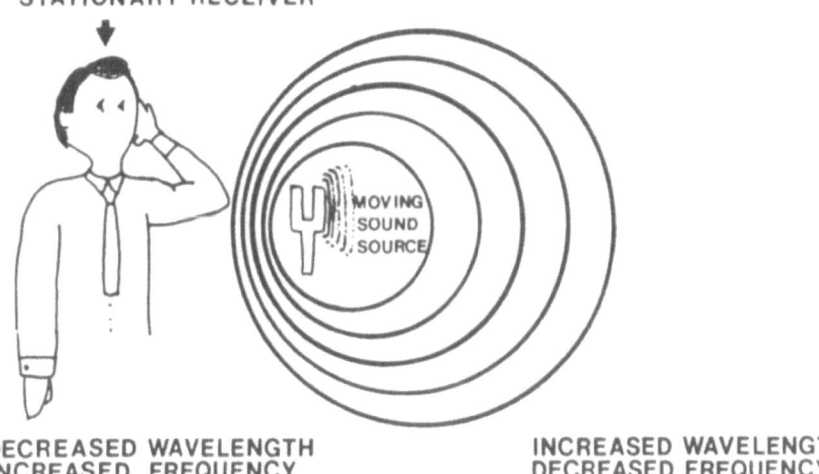

DECREASED WAVELENGTH
INCREASED FREQUENCY

INCREASED WAVELENGTH
DECREASED FREQUENCY

Figure 1. Schematic illustration of the Doppler effect. (The figure was redrawn with permission from Hatle & Angelsen [1], page 2.)

Doppler Equation:

$$f_d = \frac{2\,f_o}{c}\, v \cos \theta$$

where
f_d = observed Doppler frequency shift
f_o = the transmitted frequency
c = velocity of sound in human tissue at 37° C
(approximately 1560 m/s)
v = blood flow velocity
θ = angle between the ultrasound beam and the blood flow.

In the remainder of this section, we will examine each of the variables of this relationship in more detail.

For medical diagnostic work, transmitted frequencies in the range of 1 to 10 MHz (one million cycles per second) are used depending upon the clinical application. From the Doppler equation, velocity is inversely proportional to the transmitted frequency; therefore, the maximum velocity that can be measured at a given depth with a 5 MHz transducer is less than the maximum velocity that can be detected at the same depth with a 3 MHz transducer. On the other hand, the resolution is reduced as the transmitted frequency is reduced. Thus, one should use a Doppler transducer which gives the best resolution possible but not at the expense of missing higher frequency shifts or velocities [2].

The observed Doppler frequency shift is usually in the order of several kilohertz (kHz = 1000 cycles/s) and produces, therefore, an audible signal (audible range = 20–20 000 Hz). There are several methods by which the audible signal can be electronically processed and displayed graphically, thereby providing two outputs (audio signal and graphical display) from the Doppler examination. Most commonly, the Doppler spectrum undergoes a fast Fourier transform (FFT) analysis. The FFT process transforms the original complex Doppler waveform into its frequency components and corresponding amplitudes. The Doppler spectral tracing produced by the FFT device is graphically displayed with frequency shift or velocity on the vertical axis, time on the horizontal axis, and amplitude or power as shades of gray. Doppler signals from blood flow toward the transducer are displayed above the baseline and Doppler signals from blood flow away from the transducer are displayed below the baseline.

The Doppler signal contains a spectrum of frequencies rather than just one single frequency. In normal blood flow, the variation in frequency distribution is related to factors such as: (1) unequal distribution of flow velocity over the cross-sectional area of the vessel due to viscous friction (flow velocity is lower near the vessel walls); (2) variations in red blood cell interspaces; and (3) divergence and non-uniformity of sound beams [3]. In spite of these variations, when the blood flow through a cardiac chamber or peripheral vessel is laminar, the red blood cells are generally moving in a parallel fashion and with similar velocities. In this situation, the Doppler frequency shifts are uniform and produce a tonal or 'music-like' sound as an audio output and a narrow frequency bandwidth on the graphic display. When blood flow is disturbed (as in turbulent flow), the red blood cells are moving in random directions and with varying velocities. In the situation of disturbed flow, the Doppler spectrum is composed of multiple, widely varying frequencies. The audio output is harsh or 'scratchy' and the graphic display has a wide frequency bandwidth [4].

Both echocardiographic imaging and Doppler flowmetry rely on backscattered ultrasound that results from the interaction of the transmitted wave and the tissue. For ultrasonic imaging, the scatterers are relatively large (i.e. cardiac walls, valves, etc.) and the strongest reflections occur when the scatterer is perpendicular to the transmitted beam. For Doppler flowmetry, the scatterers (red blood cells) are relatively small, and it is the component of the flow velocity parallel to the ultrasound beam that produces the Doppler frequency shifts. For a right angle triangle, this component of the velocity vector, known as the radial velocity, is v cos θ (Figure 2). This is the origin of the term v cos θ in the Doppler equation [1].

Rearranging the Doppler equation in order to solve for velocity, we find that:

$$V = \frac{c f_d}{2 f_o \cos \theta} .$$

The Doppler frequency shift f_d is the only measured physical parameter. The velocity is a mathematically derived value and is, therefore, subject to error. One source of error is in the measurement of the angle θ between the ultrasound beam

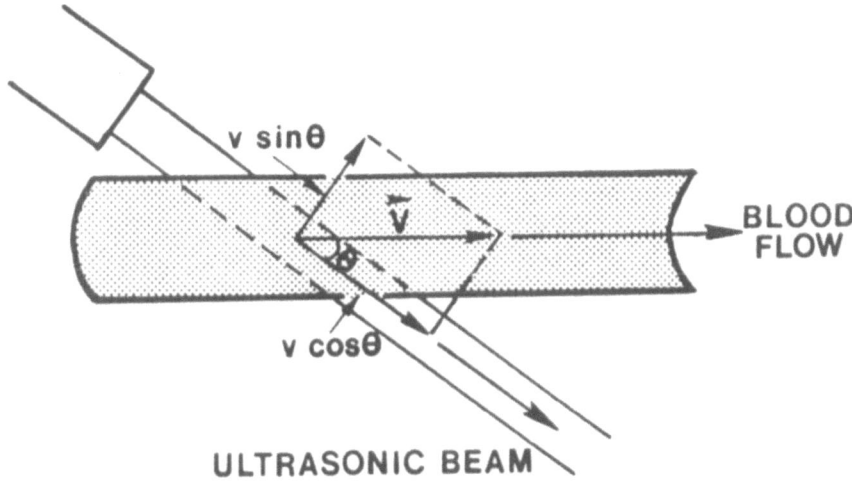

Figure 2. The component of the velocity vector (v) which is parallel to the ultrasound beam gives rise to the Doppler shift in frequency. For a right angle triangle, this component (called the radial velocity) is equal to v cos θ where θ is the angle between the ultrasound beam and the direction of blood flow in the vessel. (The figure was redrawn with permission from Hatle & Angelsen [1], page 15.)

and the red blood cell flow. For angles of less than 20°, the cos θ is so close to 1 that it can be neglected in the equation without introducing significant error. For example, by neglecting the angle in the calculation, the underestimation of the velocity is 6% at an angle of 20° [1]. For angles greater than 20°, the angle must be measured and cos θ included in the Doppler equation in order to minimize errors in the calculation of the velocity. Several problems can arise in measuring θ and cos θ:

1. Even with the use of a two-dimensional echocardiographic display, it is difficult to measure θ with certainty. From the two-dimensional echocardiographic image, θ can be estimated in the x and y planes; however, one is never sure where the beam lies relative to the blood flow in the z or azimuthal (elevational) plane [5];

2. The angle θ calculated from the two-dimensional image is the angle between the ultrasound beam and the vessel walls. The direction of blood flow in the vessel may not be parallel to the vessel wall. For example, with an eccentric, stenotic aortic valve, the jet flow through the valve is usually directed toward the right border of the ascending aorta (from angiographic studies) rather than parallel to the walls of the ascending aorta;

3. Because the cosine is a circular function, for angles on the curve of the circle (30° to 60°), v cos θ is a less accurate estimator of the radial velocity [1].

Instrumentation

Two types of Doppler equipment have been developed for interrogating flow in

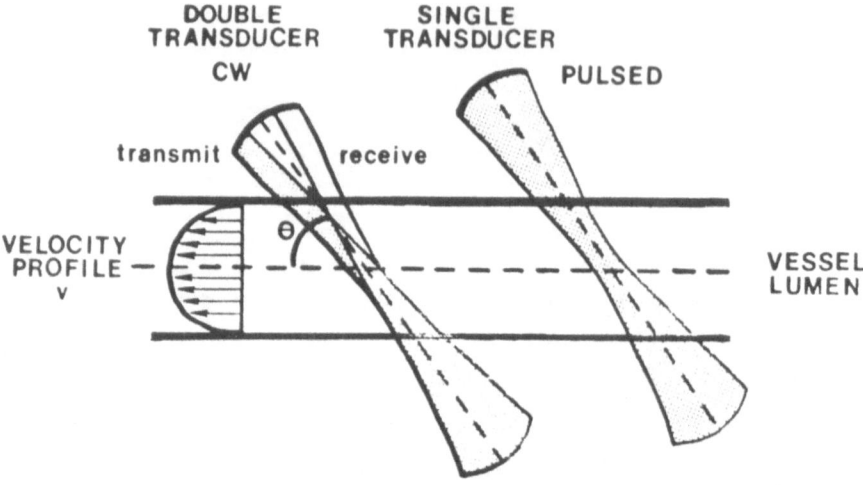

Figure 3. For cardiac applications, there are two basic types of Doppler ultrasound equipment – continuous wave Doppler (CW) and pulsed Doppler. With CW Doppler, there are two transducers – one is continuously transmitting the ultrasound beam and the other is continuously receiving the ultrasound beam. With pulsed Doppler, a single transducer alternately transmits and receives short bursts of ultrasound. (This figure was redrawn with permission from Hatle & Angelsen [1], page 35.)

the cardiac chambers and peripheral vessels. Historically, the first type of Doppler ultrasound system used was the continuous wave (CW) Doppler. This system was used initially to examine blood flow in peripheral vessels. In CW Doppler systems (Figure 3), there are two transducers – one is continuously transmitting an ultrasound beam while the other is continuously receiving backscattered pulses. Thus, Doppler signals from all blood flow along the path of the ultrasound beam are received and summated. There is no range resolution – one cannot interrogate flow in a specific chamber of the heart. Examination of intracardiac flow with CW Doppler can be thought of as aiming a flashlight beam at the heart. A major advantage of CW Doppler is that there is no limit on the maximum velocity that can be measured. Sampling theory states that in order to detect or display a wave of a certain frequency, one must be sampling at (at least) that frequency. In CW Doppler, sampling is continuous, the sampling rate is infinite, and there is no limit to the ability to display very high frequency shifts [1].

In the range-gated pulsed Doppler system (Figure 3), there is one transducer which alternately transmits and receives the ultrasound signal. Thus, a short burst of ultrasound is transmitted to a selected depth at a rate called the pulse repetition frequency (PRF). The backscattered signal is received with the same transducer. Using a time delay or range-gating control, the operator can selectively sample signals arising from red blood cell flow at a given depth in a range cell called the sample volume. For example, with the two-dimensional (2-D) range-gated pulsed Doppler system, the vessel to be interrogated is imaged directly on the 2-D

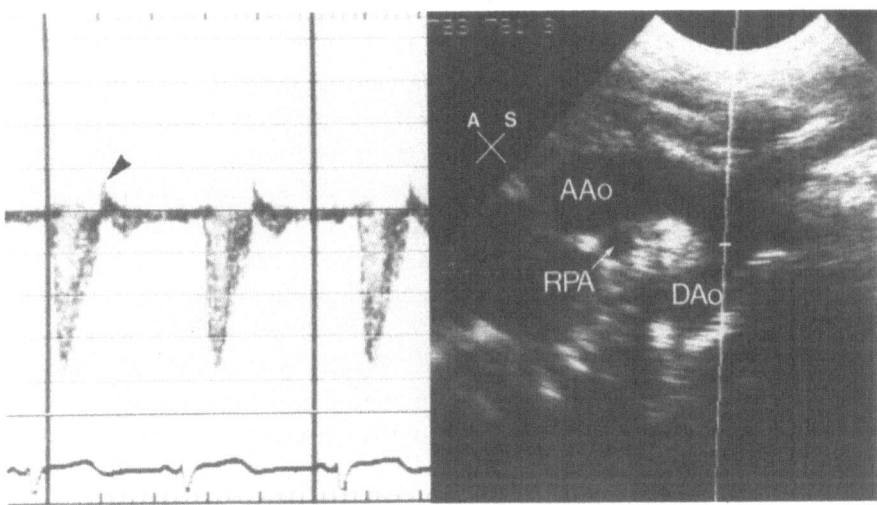

Figure 4. Doppler spectral recording from the descending aorta (DAo) of a normal infant. The freeze-frame image (right) from the suprasternal notch long axis view shows the position of the sample volume (cross-bar on the cursor line) when the Doppler recording was made. The Doppler recording on the left shows a large deflection in systole below the baseline indicating normal systolic forward flow down the DAo and away from the transducer. In diastole, there is no significant flow. The small Doppler signal in early diastole above the baseline (black arrow) is the normal small amount of retrograde flow that occurs in the aorta associated with aortic valve closure. A = anterior; AAo = ascending aorta; RPA = right pulmonary artery; S = superior.

echo system (Figure 4). The Doppler cursor line which indicates the direction of the Doppler ultrasound beam is placed in the vessel to be examined. The position of the range cell or sample volume along the cursor line is operator controlled and indicated on the display by a cross bar on the Doppler line. Range-gating means that the receiver only analyzes signals that return to the transducer at a pre-selected time period which is proportional to the distance of the sample volume from the transducer. The sample volume has a finite size – its width is the beam width and its length is the pulse duration [5].

Pulsed Doppler has a major advantage of range resolution – one can sample blood flow in a specific small area whose location and depth can be varied. However, a disadvantage of pulsed Doppler is that there are limits to the maximum frequency shifts that can be detected at each depth. The limit on the maximum detectable frequency shift is explained by the sampling theorem. To avoid range ambiguity, the ultrasound pulse must travel down to the selected depth and back before the next pulse can enter the heart. Therefore, the pulse repetition frequency (PRF) or sampling rate is limited at each depth. At shallower depths, the PRF and, therefore, the maximum detectable frequency is higher than at deeper depths. The maximum detectable frequency is called the Nyquist limit and, if the display is divided into forward and reverse channels, is equivalent to ± PRF/2. For example, if the Doppler system has a PRF of 12 800 bursts per second at a depth of 5 cm, then the Nyquist limit at 5 cm is ± 6 400 cps (12 800/2) or ± 6.4 kHz. If the depth setting is increased to 11 cm, then the emitted pulse must travel twice as far before the next pulse can enter the heart; therefore, the PRF is approximately halved. If at 11 cm, the PRF is 6 400 bursts per second, then the Nyquist limit at 11 cm is ± 3 200 cps (6 400/2) or ± 3.2 kHz [1].

In the pulsed Doppler system, if a frequency shift occurs which exceeds the Nyquist limit, then the equipment cuts off the true signal, electronically folds or wraps the signal around, and displays it ambiguously in the opposite channel or direction (Figure 5). This phenomenon is called wraparound or frequency aliasing. With very high velocity jets in pulsed Doppler systems, the signal may be wrapped on itself several times creating the appearance of a dispersed signal with a wide bandwidth and equal amounts of positive and negative velocities. This has caused some confusion between Doppler signals arising from turbulent flow and Doppler signals with severe aliasing (high velocity jets). Recently, two newer technical modalities have been used to increase the Nyquist limit on pulsed Doppler instruments: (1) adaptive Doppler or extended range Doppler – the PRF is increased so that several pulses are in the heart at the same time; this system introduces some range ambiguity in order to increase the Nyquist limit; (2) zero shift method – this system examines only one sign or channel of the Doppler shift; therefore, the system can display (in one direction) frequency shifts from zero up to PRF (instead of ± PRF/2) [1, 6].

Clinical applications of Doppler ultrasound

Velocity profiles: normal and turbulent flow

The viscous frictional forces between the moving red blood cells and the vessel wall and between the adjacent layers of moving red blood cells lead to different velocities across the vessel lumen. The velocity depicted as a function of position in the vessel cross section is called the velocity profile. Acceleration of the blood when the heart contracts also effects the velocity distribution in the vessel by flattening the velocity profile. Thus, both viscosity and acceleration are determinants of the velocity profile [1].

In the normal circulation, because of the viscosity of the blood and the low velocities, blood flows in a regular fashion called laminar flow. At the inlet of a circular blood vessel or orifice, the velocity profile is flattened (i.e. fairly uniform velocities occur across the vessel lumen). At a far distance from the inlet, viscous resistance to flow in the vessel causes the velocity profile to become parabolic. Acceleration of the blood flattens the velocity profile. Less acceleration of the blood is required to flatten the velocity profile in the aorta than in a smaller vessel where the viscous resistance to flow is higher [1].

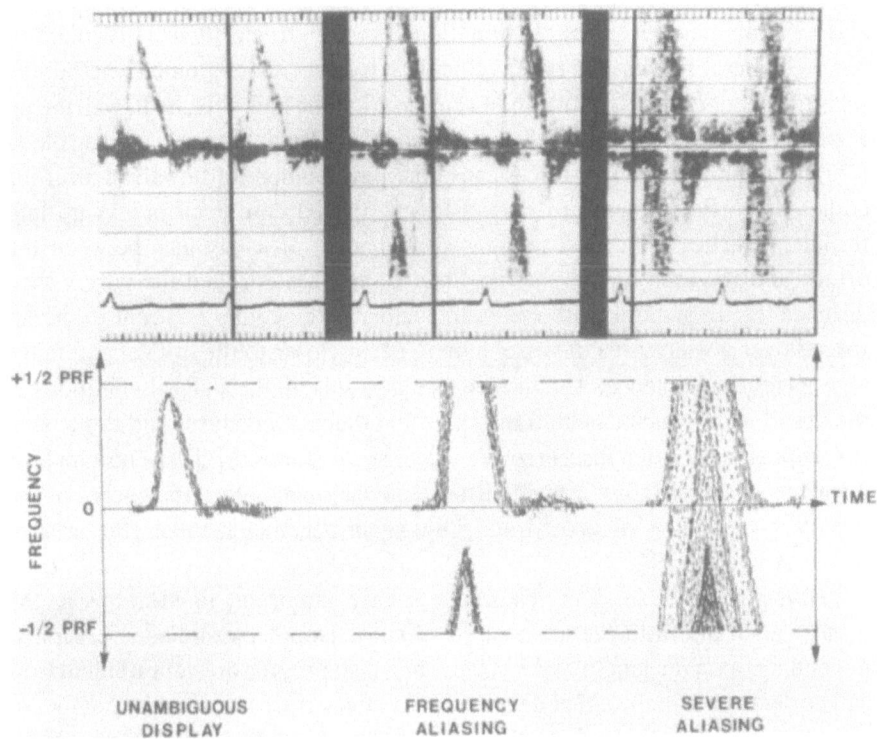

Figure 5. Examples of frequency aliasing. These Doppler recordings were all taken from the ascending aorta (suprasternal notch view) of the same patient but at different depth settings. In the left hand panel, the depth setting is 5 cm, the pulse repetition frequency (PRF) for this particular Doppler instrument at 5 cm is 12 800 bursts per second, and the Nyquist limit for this depth is ± 6.4 kHz. Notice that at this depth setting the maximum frequency shift recorded in the ascending aorta does not exceed the Nyquist limit and the Doppler tracing can be displayed fully or unambiguously. In the middle panel, the depth setting is 9 cm, the PRF is 7 600 bursts per second, and the Nyquist limit is 3.8 kHz. The maximum frequency shift in the ascending aorta exceeds the Nyquist limit so that the Doppler signal cannot be fully displayed. The portion of the Doppler recording exceeding the Nyquist limit is cut-off and folded over into the opposite channel or direction. This is called frequency aliasing or wraparound. In the right hand panel, the depth setting is 17 cm, the PRF is 4 200 bursts per second and the Nyquist limit is 2.1 kHz. The maximum frequency shift in the ascending aorta greatly exceeds the Nyquist limit; therefore, the Doppler signal is folded over onto itself several times. Notice that this form of severe aliasing can mimic turbulent flow, which we know is not present in this patient when the depth setting is appropriate.

As the velocity increases, regular laminar flow changes to turbulent flow. In turbulent flow, red blood cells are moving at random velocities and in random directions. In turbulent flow, a component of the velocity vector is transverse to the vessel axis causing additional resistance to flow. The velocity at which laminar flow decomposes into turbulent flow is difficult to determine precisely and is related to rheologic factors such as fluid density, vessel diameter, and fluid viscosity [1, 7]. In the circulation, high velocity jets can occur with septal defects and with valvular stenosis or regurgitation. These high velocity jets stream into a region of blood flowing at a lower velocity. It is as yet undetermined whether the jet is turbulent or not. In vitro studies suggest that the high velocity flow in the jet is laminar [1]. At the boundary layer between the jet and the slowly moving blood (parajet region), frictional forces cause the development of turbulent, whirling eddies or vortices (Figure 6). Downstream, the jet core itself breaks up into turbulent vortices (the post jet flow disturbance). The distance between the orifice and the area of the post jet flow disturbance is called the vortex shed distance [8]. In general, with increasing velocity, the eddies adjacent to the jet spread over a wider area of vessel lumen, occur closer to the orifice, and move with increasing violence. The disturbance also sets up mechanical vibrations in the vessel walls which can be transmitted to adjacent structures and to the skin (i.e. suprasternal notch thrill in severe valvar aortic stenosis) [7]. The post jet flow disturbance persists for a certain distance downstream before the energy of the turbulent vortices is dissipated and flow again becomes laminar (the area of relaminarization) [8].

These physics of jet flow disturbances have important implications in the performance and interpretation of the clinical Doppler examination. Firstly, depending upon the length of the vortex shed distance, the area of turbulent flow can be detected initially either near the obstructive orifice or even one chamber or great vessel downstream from the origin of the jet. Secondly, because of the length of the post jet flow disturbance, flow disturbances can be detected in cardiac chambers or great vessels located downstream from the primary site of the defect. This persistence of disturbed flow for some distance downstream in contiguous cardiac chambers or great vessels is called the series effect. For example, on the Doppler examination, disturbed flow in systole in the main pulmonary artery could be caused by either valvar pulmonic stenosis or a ventricular septal defect. As a result of the series effect, the downstream persistence of the post jet flow disturbance from one obstructive site can mask a flow disturbance from a second nearby obstructive site. For example, in a patient with subaortic stenosis and valvar aortic stenosis, the turbulent flow produced by the subaortic narrowing may persist into the ascending aorta and mask an additional flow disturbance at the level of the aortic valve [8]. Finally, a severe flow disturbance can cause mechanical vibrations in the vessel walls which are transmitted to the walls of an adjacent vessel causing the flow in the adjacent vessel to become disturbed. This effect is known as induction. For example, in patients with severe pulmonic stenosis, a flow disturbance can often be detected in the aorta as well as in the main pulmonary artery. Induction also explains the presence of a palpable suprasternal notch thrill in patients with valvar pulmonic stenosis [9].

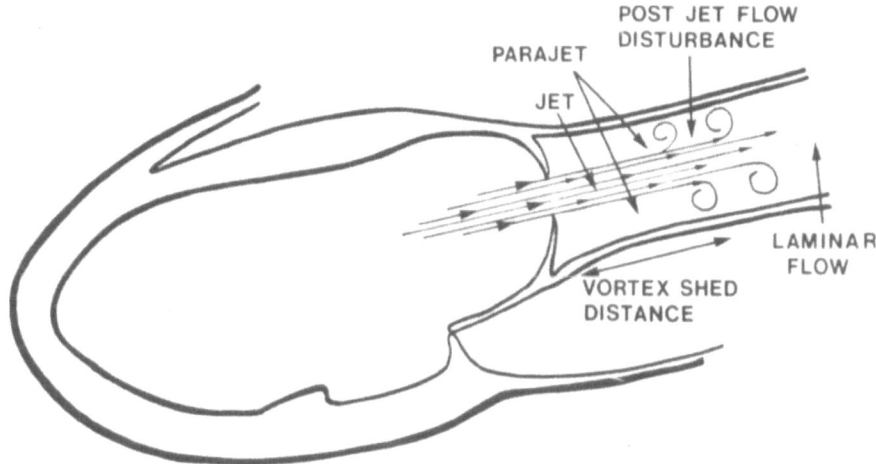

Figure 6. Diagrammatic representation of the anatomy of a jet. Flow in the jet is regular or laminar. In the parajet regions adjacent to the vessel wall, the blood flow velocity is reduced. At a distance from the obstructive orifice, the jet dissipates into whirling eddies. This distance is called the vortex shed distance. Further downstream from the post jet flow disturbance, flow again becomes laminar.

Quantitation of the pressure drop across an obstruction

For fluid flowing in a rigid tube, the volumetric flow is equal to the fluid velocity times the cross-sectional area of the tube. Figure 7 depicts fluid flow in a tube with an area of constriction (A_2). If there is no loss of fluid volume from the tube, then the volumetric flow at area 1 must be the same as the volumetric flow at area 2 ($v_1 A_1 = v_2 A_2$). In other words, to move the same volume of fluid through a restricted area, a higher velocity must be generated. This acceleration of fluid to a higher velocity is called convective acceleration and is achieved by a pressure drop across the area of flow obstruction. The Bernoulli equation shows the relation between the pressure drop and the velocity:

$$P1 - P2 = \frac{1}{2}\varrho \, (v_2^2 - v_1^2) + \varrho \int_1^2 \frac{dv}{dt} \, ds + R \, (v)$$

where subscript 1 indicates pressure (p) or velocity (v) proximal to the obstruction and subscript 2 indicates pressure or velocity in the jet; ϱ = mass density of blood; v = velocity vector of the blood along the flow path; ds = path element; and R = viscous resistance. The first term in the equation is due to convective acceleration, the middle term represents acceleration caused by velocity changes with time (inertial forces), and the third term is caused by viscous frictional losses. Since the velocity (v_1) proximal to the jet is much smaller than the velocity (v_2) in the jet, v_1 can be neglected for practical purposes. In addition, since the velocity profile in the inlet of the obstructive orifice is flat, viscous friction in the center of the lumen can be neglected. Also, in clinical applications, the pressure drop

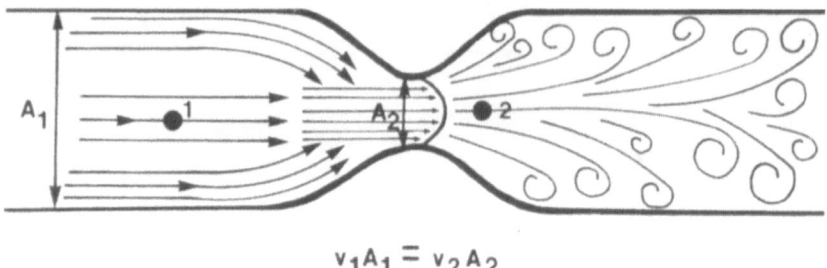

$$v_1 A_1 \doteq v_2 A_2$$

A = vessel cross-sectional area
v = velocity

Figure 7. Diagrammatic illustration of a flow obstruction. Flow is equal to the blood velocity (v) times the vessel cross-sectional area (A). Therefore, in order to get the same amount of blood through an obstructed area (A_2), an increase in velocity (v_2) must occur.

required to overcome inertial forces is negligible and a simplified Bernoulli equation is used to calculate the pressure drop across the obstruction to flow:

$$P1 - P2 = 4v_2{}^2$$

For v_2 expressed in m/s, the calculated pressure drop is in mm Hg [1, 10, 11].

The equation $P1 - P2 = 4v_2{}^2$ can be used to estimate the pressure gradient across a stenotic valve or across a septal defect. Likewise, the maximum velocity in the jet of a regurgitant atrioventricular valve can be used to estimate ventricular systolic pressure. Clinical studies using the above formula have shown excellent correlation between the pressure gradient predicted by Doppler ultrasound and the pressure gradient measured at cardiac catheterization in patients with mitral stenosis [10–12], pulmonic stenosis [13], aortic stenosis [14–16], and prosthetic valves [17, 18].

There are several errors or limitations that can occur when using the maximum jet velocity to predict the pressure drop across an obstruction. Firstly, from Poiseuille's Law, the viscous resistance,

$$R = \frac{8\mu\,l}{\pi\,a^4}$$

where μ = blood viscosity
l = length of the vessel
a = radius of the vessel lumen

Therefore, viscous resistance increases as vessel size decreases. In vitro studies [19] have shown that for an orifice diameter of 8 mm or greater viscous forces are negligible, and the pressure gradient can be accurately predicted from convective forces alone. At an orifice diameter of 3.5 mm, $4v^2$ underestimates the actual pressure drop, especially for smaller velocities (<3 m/s). For a 1.5 mm orifice diameter, the pressure drop predicted from the modified Bernoulli equation is approximately $1/2$ the actual pressure drop [1]. Secondly, the pressure drop associated with flow acceleration can be significant in certain clinical situations (i.e. when estimating the pressure drop across a severely stenotic aortic valve).

Quantitation of volumetric flow

The blood flow in l/min can be calculated by the following equation:

$$\text{Blood flow (l/min)} = \frac{\text{mean flow velocity} \times A \times 60\,\text{s/min}}{1000\,\text{cc/l}}$$

where A = vessel cross-sectional area in cm^2.

The temporal mean flow velocity throughout the cardiac cycle is determined by digitizing and integrating the area under the Doppler waveform over several complete cardiac cycles (this area is the velocity time integral) and dividing the velocity time integral by the total duration of the traced beats (beat duration). In digitizing and integrating the area under the Doppler curve, the densest portion of the tracing (the modal velocity shift) should be used. If the Doppler was recorded at an angle θ of greater than 20° from the blood flow direction, then the mean flow velocity should be divided by $\cos \theta$ in order to correct for the angle [20].

Using the above Doppler technique for calculation of blood flow, several investigators have shown excellent correlation between Doppler measurements of flow and invasive measurements of flows in experimental animals (i.e., using electromagnetic flowmeters, thermodilution techniques, etc.) [21, 22]. Additionally, other investigators have shown excellent correlation between Doppler measurements of flow and invasive measurements of flow in humans [23, 24]. In experimental animals and in humans, the Doppler technique has been used successfully to determine the magnitude of the left-to-right shunt using Doppler recordings from the aorta and main pulmonary artery [20, 25–28]. In addition, a method using the mitral valve inflow Doppler to reflect systemic flow in patients with no left-to-right shunt or to reflect pulmonary blood flow in patients with a left-to-right shunt and intact atrial septum has been described and validated [29]. In all of these studies, the major source of error in calculating volumetric flow from the Doppler ultrasound examination has been in the estimation of the vessel cross-sectional area.

Doppler findings in various cardiac defects

Obstructive lesions

In calculating the severity of an obstructive lesion from the Doppler examination,

194

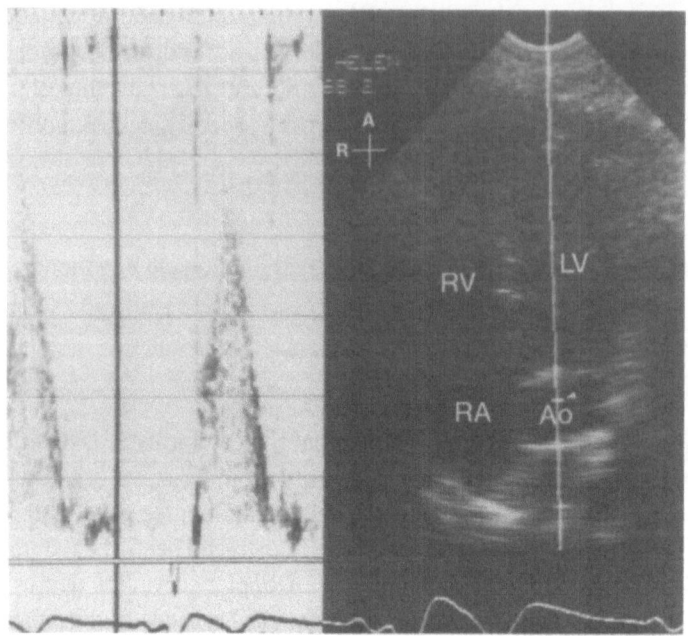

Figure 8. Doppler recording from the ascending aorta (Ao) of a patient with aortic valve stenosis. The freeze-frame image on the right shows the position (arrow) of the sample volume above the aortic valve in the apical four-chamber view. The Doppler spectral recording on the left shows a high velocity jet in systole. In order to display the jet unambiguously, the Doppler baseline has been shifted to the bottom of the recording (zero-shift). Each calibration line represents a 2 kHz frequency shift; therefore, the cardiac cycle on the far left shows a peak systolic frequency shift of 10 kHz. For a 3 mHz transducer, this is a velocity of 2.6 m/s and predicts a pressure drop across the aortic valve of 27 mm Hg. A = apex; LV = left ventricle; R = right; RA = right atrium; RV = right ventricle.

one must angle the ultrasound beam until the highest-pitched (clear and tone-like) audio signal is found. Use of a wall filter setting in the range of 200–800 Hz will eliminate the high amplitude, low frequency wall noises, making it easier to evaluate the audio signal from the jet. In patients with aortic valve stenosis, the jet can be detected from the suprasternal notch, apex, or right parasternal regions. Figure 8 shows a high velocity jet recorded from the ascending aorta from the cardiac apex. In this example, the peak systolic frequency is nearly 10 kHz (in the first beat), which is a velocity of 2.6 m/s for an angle of 0° and a 3 MHz carrier frequency. The predicted pressure drop is $4 \times (2.6)^2$ or 27 mmHg. Also, in aortic valve stenosis, the time from aortic valve opening to the peak velocity is delayed. When normalized for heart rate, the ratio of time to peak velocity divided by the left ventricular ejection time is less than 0.5 in mild obstruction and greater than 0.55 in severe obstruction [1, 14, 30].

In pulmonary stenosis, the jet velocities are usually best recorded from the parasternal short axis view; however, in small infants, the subcostal view of the

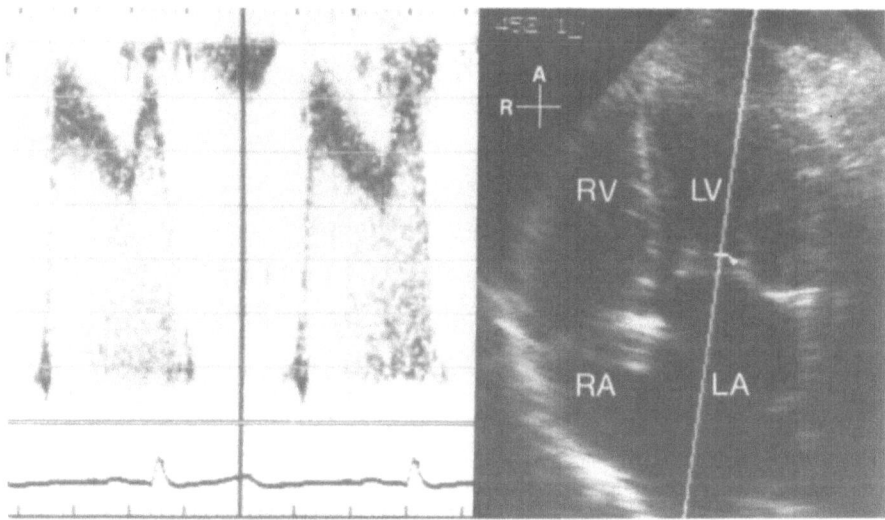

Figure 9. Doppler recording from a patient with mitral stenosis. The freeze-frame image (right) is an apical four-chamber view showing the position of the sample volume (arrow) in the left ventricle (LV) just distal to the mitral valve when the Doppler recording was made. The Doppler spectral tracing on the left shows a high velocity jet which peaks in early diastole and is followed by a slow rate of decrease in the peak velocity. In order to display the Doppler frequency shifts unambiguously, the baseline has been shifted to the bottom (zero-shift). Each Doppler calibration line represents a 1 kHz frequency shift. A = apex; LA = left atrium; R = right; RA = right atrium; RV = right ventricle.

right ventricle may be very useful. An increased velocity in the main pulmonary artery can indicate either pulmonic stenosis or increased flow (i.e. left-to-right shunt, pulmonary regurgitation). If the increased velocity is due to increased flow, then both the right ventricular and pulmonary artery Doppler recordings will have a high velocity; whereas, if the increased velocity is due to pulmonic stenosis, the right ventricular Doppler recording will have a normal velocity [1, 13].

In mitral stenosis, the jet velocity is best recorded from the apical four-chamber view. In the normal patient, the mitral valve Doppler tracing shows a maximum velocity in early diastole followed by a rapid decrease in velocity and a second increase in velocity associated with atrial contraction. In patients with mitral stenosis (Figure 9), the maximum velocity is increased followed by a slower rate of fall of the velocity prior to atrial contraction. Several studies have shown a good correlation between mean diastolic pressure drop calculated from the Doppler tracing and pressure drop at catheterization [10, 11]. The velocity across the mitral valve is increased with obstruction or with increased flow across the valve; however, the rate of decline of the velocity from the early peak velocity is altered by obstruction rather than flow. Several investigators have used the slope of the decline in the maximum velocity to estimate the pressure half-time (the time it takes until the initial pressure drop is halved). The pressure half-time is

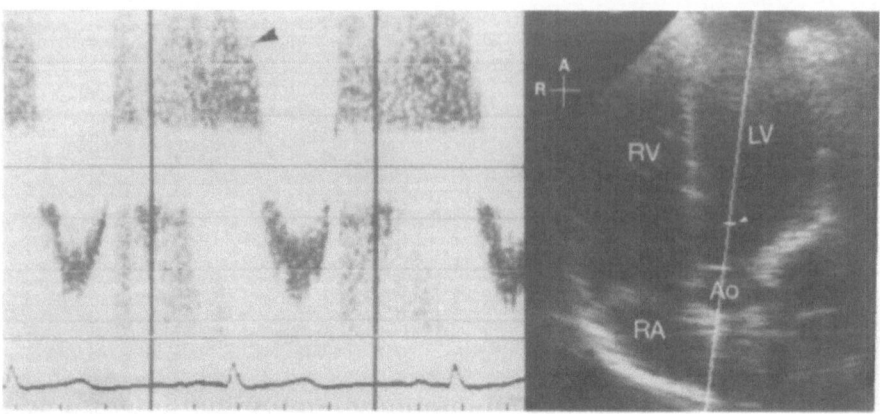

Figure 10. Doppler spectral tracing from a patient with aortic insufficiency. The freeze-frame image of the apical four-chamber view on the right shows the position of the sample volume (arrow) in the left ventricular outflow tract just beneath the aortic valve when the Doppler tracing was recorded. The Doppler spectral tracing on the left shows normal forward flow away from the transducer and, therefore, below the baseline in systole. In diastole, there is a high velocity jet above the baseline indicating regurgitant flow through the aortic valve and toward the transducer. The regurgitant flow signals exceed the Nyquist limit of the equipment and are displayed ambiguously (frequency aliasing). A = apex; Ao = aorta; LV = left ventricle; R = right; RA = right atrium; RV = right ventricle.

calculated by dividing the peak velocity by 1.4 and measuring the time from peak velocity to where the velocity is decreased to peak velocity/1.4. Pressure half-time, which is independent of flow across the valve, is less than 60 ms in normal patients, 100 to 400 ms in patients with mitral stenosis, and associated with a valve area of less than $1.0 \, cm^2$ when greater than 220 ms. Pressure half-time can be used to estimate mitral valve area from the following equation:

$$MVA \ (cm^2) = \frac{220}{Pressure \ half\text{-}time} \tag{1}$$

Regurgitant lesions

Aortic insufficiency can be detected in the left ventricular outflow tract from the apical four-chamber view as flow signals toward the transducer in diastole (Figures 10, 11). Aortic insufficiency is apparent from the suprasternal notch view as reverse diastolic flow. In the apical four-chamber view, care must be taken not to mistake Doppler signals from mitral valve inflow for a regurgitant aortic valve. The position of the sample volume, the timing of the signals (aortic regurgitation starts before mitral valve opening), and the peak velocity of the signal may help distinguish aortic regurgitation from mitral valve inflow. The amount of aortic regurgitation may be evaluated by comparing the areas of the reverse and forward flow on the aortic Doppler tracing or by determing how far toward the left ventricular apex the regurgitant signals can be detected [31].

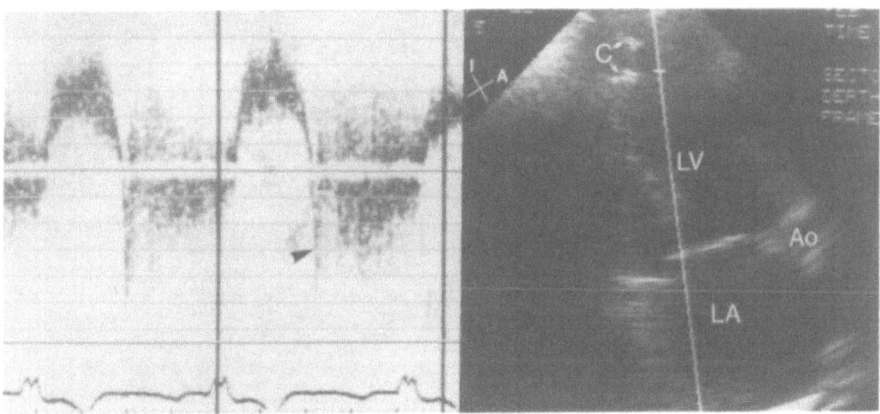

Figure 11. Doppler recording taken from the apical long axis view of a patient with severe aortic stenosis, a left ventricular-to-descending aorta apical conduit, and conduit insufficiency. The freeze-frame image on the right shows the position of the sample volume (cross-bar on the cursor line) in the left ventricular apex adjacent to the conduit orifice (C). The Doppler spectral tracing on the left shows a laminar signal above the baseline throughout systole indicating forward flow toward the transducer from the left ventricle (LV) to the conduit. In diastole (black arrow), there are signals below the baseline indicating blood flow away from the transducer. These signals represent a regurgitant jet from the conduit. A = anterior; Ao = aorta; I = inferior; LA = left atrium.

Mitral insufficiency can be detected on the Doppler examination by recording the flow signals proximal to the mitral valve in the left atrium from the apical four-chamber view (Figure 12). In this view, the regurgitant signals occur throughout systole and are displayed below the baseline indicating blood flow away from the transducer. The amount of mitral insufficiency can be roughly assessed by noting how far back in the left atrium the regurgitant jet can be detected [32–36]. Also, the maximum velocity of the regurgitant jet can be used to estimate the pressure drop from the left ventricle to the left atrium in systole.

Tricuspid regurgitation can be detected by recording the flow signals in the right atrium proximal to the tricuspid valve from either the apical four chamber or parasternal short axis view (Figure 13). As with mitral insufficiency, reverse flow signals are seen throughout systole. Usually, respiratory variation of the Doppler signals is evident. The maximum velocity in the regurgitant jet can be used to estimate the pressure drop in systole from the right ventricle to the right atrium. The extension of the regurgitant jet into the right atrium correlates well with the angiographic assessment of the severity of the lesion [37, 38].

Pulmonary regurgitation can be detected on the Doppler examination by recording diastolic flow signals toward the transducer in the right ventricular outflow tract in the parasternal short axis view (Figure 14). The regurgitant flow signals can also be recorded in the main pulmonary artery (Figure 15). Respiratory variation of the Doppler flow signals is usually evident. As with the other regurgitant lesions, the amount of regurgitation can be evaluated by noting the

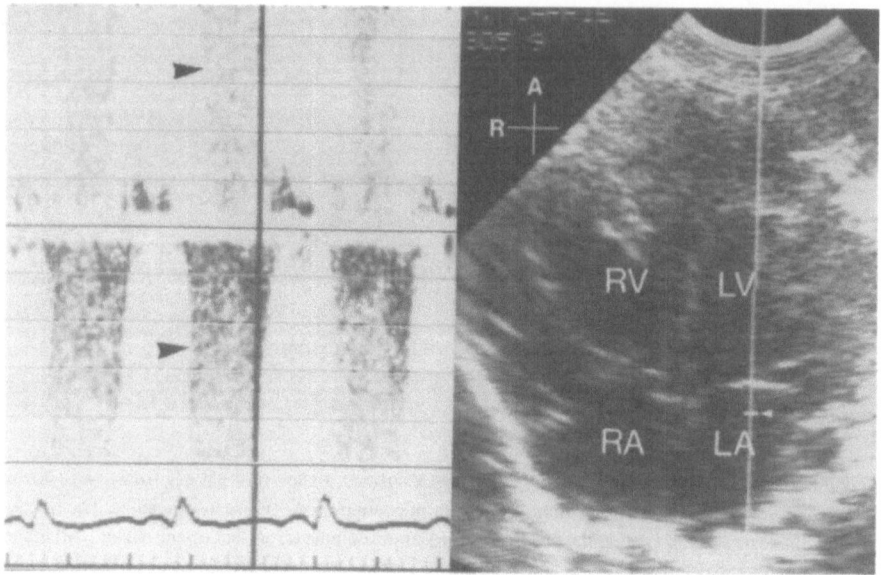

Figure 12. Doppler recording from an infant with asphyxia and mitral insufficiency. The freeze-frame image of the apical four-chamber view on the right shows the position of the sample volume (arrow) in the left atrium (LA) at the time of the Doppler recording. The Doppler spectral tracing on the left shows signals above the baseline in diastole representing normal forward flow through the mitral valve. In systole, there is a high velocity jet displayed below the baseline with wraparound (aliasing) which represents regurgitant flow away from the transducer through the mitral valve. A = apex; LV = left ventricle; R = right; RA = right atrium; RV = right ventricle.

extension of the regurgitant flow into the right ventricle. In patients with pulmonary regurgitation and a low pulmonary artery diastolic pressure, the velocity of the regurgitant Doppler flow decreases rapidly throughout diastole and ends before systole (see Figure 14). In patients with pulmonary hypertension and pulmonary regurgitation, the velocity of the regurgitant flow remains high throughout diastole because a pressure drop is still present at end-diastole between the right ventricle and pulmonary artery [1, 32].

Left-to-right shunts

With an atrial septal defect, disturbed flow can be recorded in the right atrium from the apical four-chamber or parasternal short axis view (Figure 16). The disturbed flow, which is directed toward the transducer, starts in mid-systole and increases at end-systole. A second increase in flow velocity occurs with atrial contraction. In patients with an atrial septal defect, the subcostal four-chamber view can be used to position the sample volume parallel to the flow through the defect in order to detect the maximum velocity in the shunt flow and estimate the pressure drop across the atrial septal defect. Doppler tracings from the main

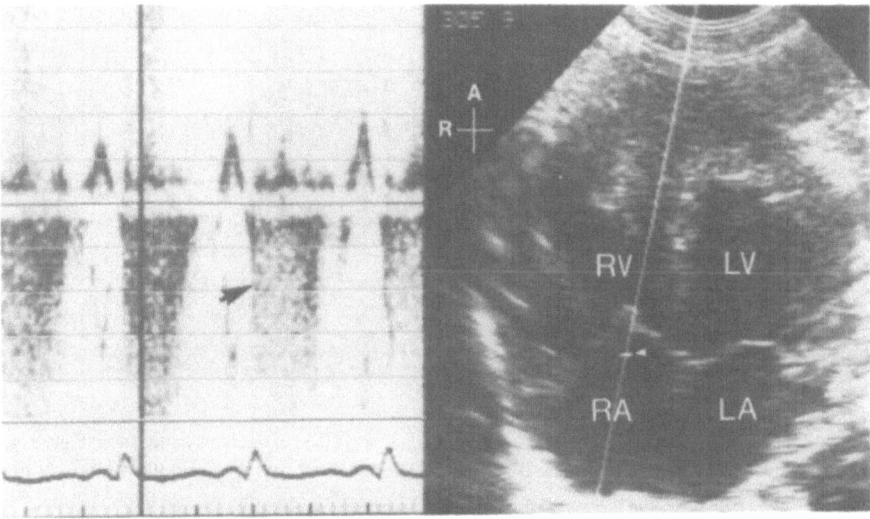

Figure 13. Doppler recording from the same infant as in Figure 12 showing tricuspid insufficiency. The freeze-frame image of the apical four-chamber view on the right shows the position of the sample volume (arrow) in the right atrium (RA) when the Doppler recording was made. The Doppler spectral tracing on the left shows signals above the baseline in diastole representing normal forward flow toward the transducer through the tricuspid valve. In systole, a high velocity jet (black arrow) is displayed below the baseline indicating regurgitant flow through the tricuspid valve and away from the transducer. A = apex; LA = left atrium; LV = left ventricle; R = right; RV = right ventricle.

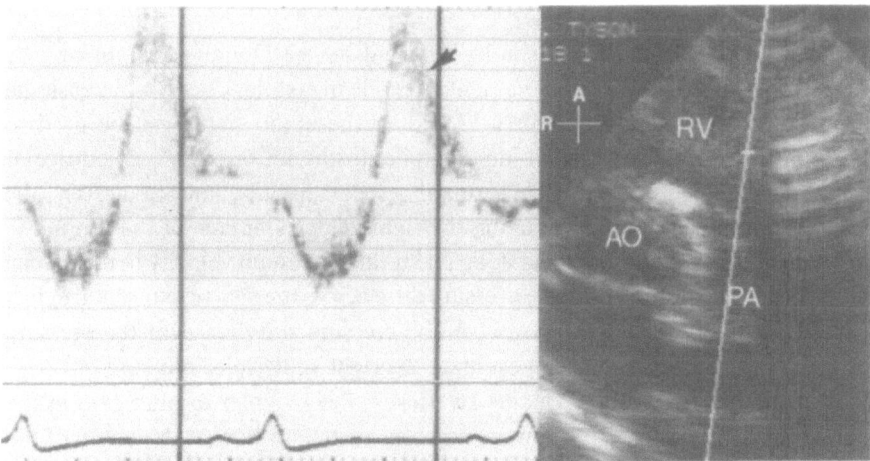

Figure 14. Doppler spectral tracing from a patient with pulmonary insufficiency following repair of tetralogy of Fallot. The freeze-frame image (right) from the parasternal short axis view shows the position of the sample volume in the right ventricle (RV) proximal to the pulmonary valve. The Doppler spectral tracing on the left shows a signal throughout systole below the baseline indicating forward flow from the RV to the pulmonary artery (PA) away from the transducer. In diastole, there is a large deflection above the baseline (black arrow) indicating regurgitant flow through the pulmonary valve toward the transducer. This signal does not persist until the end of diastole, indicating a low pulmonary artery diastolic pressure. A = anterior; Ao = aorta; R = right.

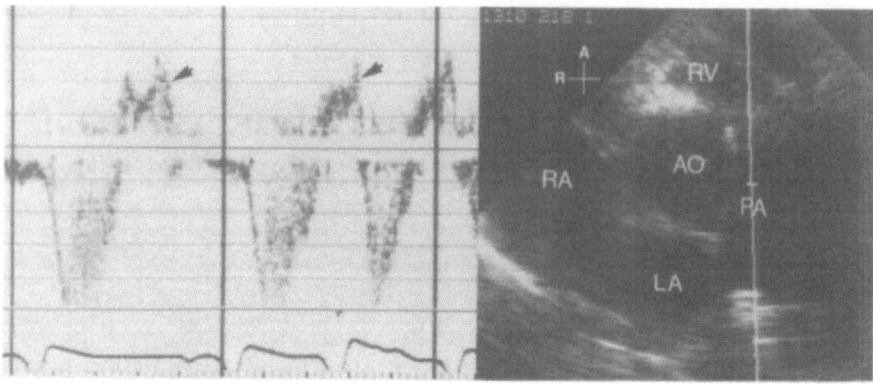

Figure 15. Doppler spectral tracing from the pulmonary artery (PA) of the same patient as in Figure 14. The freeze-frame image on the right shows the parasternal short axis view and the position of the sample volume in the PA at the time of the Doppler recording. On the left, the Doppler spectral tracing shows signals below the baseline in systole indicating normal forward flow away from the transducer from the right ventricle (RV) to the PA. In diastole, there is a large deflection above the baseline (black arrows) indicating reverse flow in the PA toward the transducer. This reverse flow is caused by pulmonary insufficiency. A = anterior; AO = aorta; LA = left atrium; R = right; RA = right atrium.

pulmonary artery and ascending aorta combined with a two-dimensional echocardiographic measurement of the diameters of the great vessels can be used to calculate the pulmonary blood flow, the systemic blood flow, and the magnitude of the left-to-right shunt [27, 39].

A ventricular septal defect can be detected on the Doppler examination by recording a high velocity jet in the right ventricle in systole. The two-dimensional echocardiographic image (Figures 17, 18) or the audio signal can be used to position the Doppler sample volume parallel to the jet through the ventricular septal defect; or, if the ventricular septal defect cannot be imaged directly, the sample volume can be moved along the right ventricular side of the septum in order to detect a high velocity systolic jet. If the maximum velocity in the jet can be recorded accurately, then the pressure drop across the ventricular septal defect can be calculated. Using the systolic blood pressure and the calculated pressure drop across the defect, one can estimate the right ventricular pressure [40–42].

In patients with a patent ductus arteriosus, the Doppler examination in the parasternal short axis view shows continuous turbulent flow at the origin of the left pulmonary artery (Figure 19). Closer to the pulmonary valve, the Doppler recording usually shows laminar systolic forward flow through the pulmonary valve and disturbed diastolic flow directed toward the transducer from the patent ductus arteriosus. Usually, the disturbed flow persists until the end of diastole; however, in patients with elevated pulmonary vascular resistance, the diastolic flow is of shorter duration. In addition, the Doppler recording from the descending aorta of patients with a patent ductus arteriosus shows evidence of retrograde

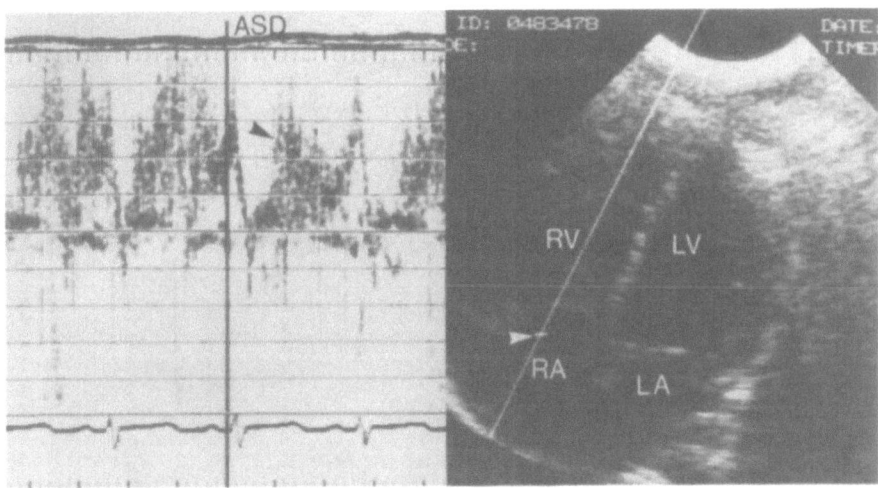

Figure 16. Doppler spectral tracing from an infant with a secundum atrial septal defect. The freeze-frame image (right) of the apical four-chamber view shows the position of the sample volume (white arrow) in the right atrium (RA) at the time of the Doppler recording. The Doppler spectral tracing on the left shows disturbed flow toward the transducer which begins in mid-systole and peaks at the end of systole. This flow pattern represents a left-to-right shunt at the atrial level. LA = left atrium; LV = left ventricle; RV = right ventricle.

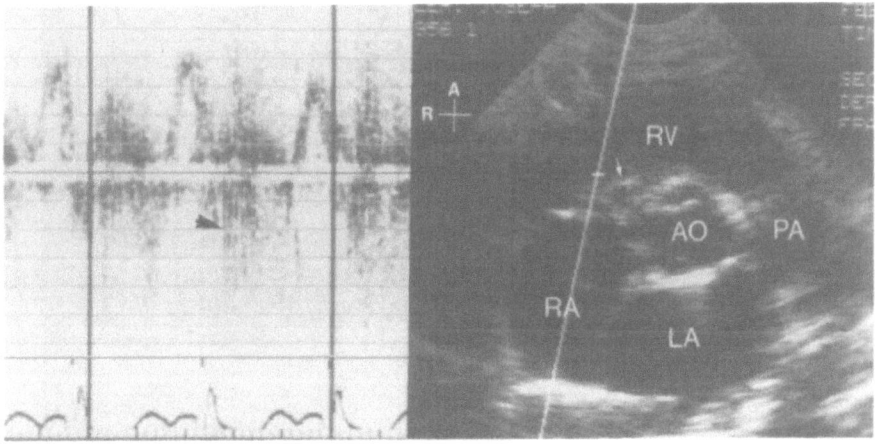

Figure 17. Doppler spectral recording from a child with a membranous ventricular septal defect and a ventricular septal aneurysm. The freeze-frame image on the right from the parasternal short axis view shows the position of the sample volume adjacent to the ventricular septal aneurysm (white arrow) when the Doppler recording was made. The Doppler spectral tracing on the left shows laminar signals above the baseline in diastole indicating forward flow through the tricuspid valve from the right atrium (RA) to the right ventricle (RV). There is disturbed flow throughout systole (black arrow) caused by a jet of blood passing through the ventricular septal defect. A = anterior; AO = aorta; LA = left atrium; PA = pulmonary artery; R = right.

202

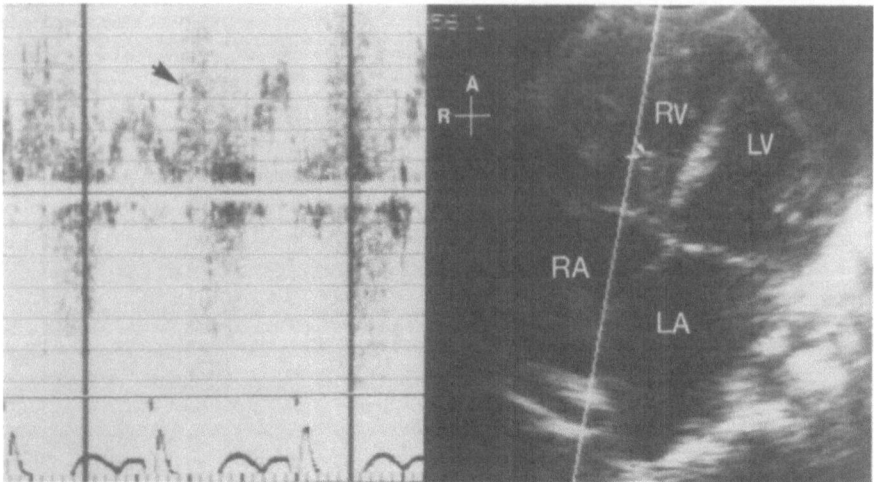

Figure 18. Doppler spectral tracing from the same patient as in Figure 17. The freeze-frame image from the apical four-chamber view on the right shows the position of the sample volume adjacent to the ventricular septal aneurysm (white arrow) at the time of the Doppler recording. The Doppler spectral tracing on the left shows a laminar signal throughout diastole above the baseline indicating forward flow toward the transducer from the right atrium (RA) to the right ventricle (RV). In systole, there is a high velocity jet displayed above the baseline with wraparound (black arrow). This jet is caused by the left-to-right shunt through the ventricular septal defect and toward the transducer. A = apex; LA = left atrium; LV = left ventricle; R = right.

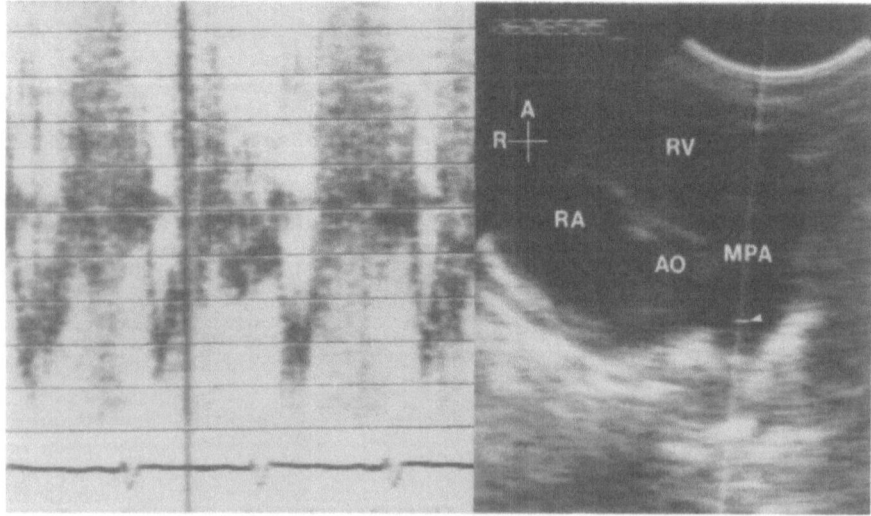

Figure 19. Doppler spectral recording from a newborn infant with a patent ductus arteriosus. The freeze-frame image of the parasternal short axis view on the right shows the position of the sample volume (arrow) in the main pulmonary artery (MPA) toward the origin of the left pulmonary artery. The Doppler spectral tracing on the left shows laminar flow signals throughout systole below the baseline indicating forward flow from the right ventricle (RV) to the MPA. In diastole, there is a high velocity jet displayed above the baseline indicating forward flow toward the transducer through the ductus arteriosus. A = anterior; AO = aorta; R = right RA = right atrium.

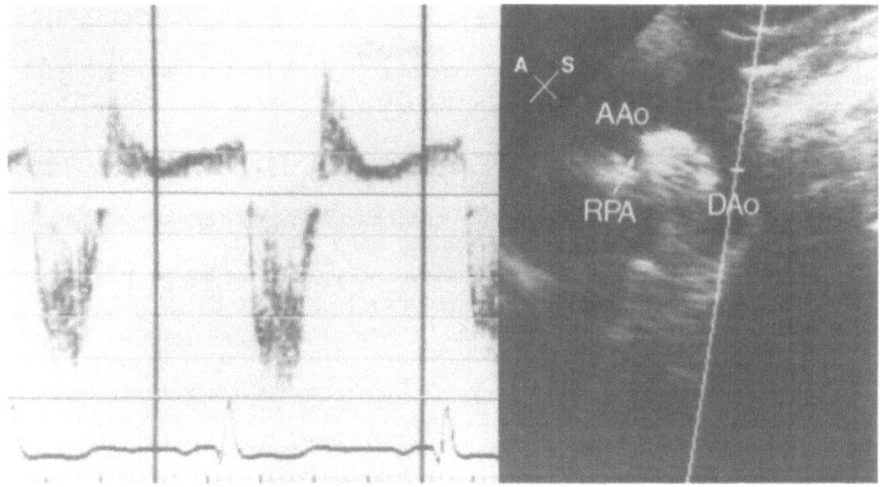

Figure 20. Doppler recording from an infant with a large patent ductus arteriosus. The freeze-frame image of the suprasternal notch view on the right shows the position of the sample volume in the descending aorta (DAo) at the time the Doppler recording was made. The Doppler spectral tracing on the left shows a laminar signal below the baseline indicating forward flow in the DAo away from the transducer in systole. In diastole, there is a large deflection above the baseline indicating retrograde flow in the DAo toward the transducer. This retrograde flow is due to the diastolic shunting of blood from the descending aorta through the ductus arteriosus to the main pulmonary artery. A = anterior; AAo = ascending aorta; RPA = right pulmonary artery; S = superior.

diastolic flow from the descending aorta to the pulmonary arteries (Figure 20). The amount of reverse diastolic flow gives a rough approximation of the size of the left-to-right shunt [43–46].

Conclusion

Doppler ultrasound provides a safe, non-invasive technique for detecting and localizing flow disturbances in the heart and peripheral vessels. This technique has added significant quantitative information (pressure drop across obstructions and volumetric flow rates) to the anatomic information obtained from the two-dimensional echocardiographic examination. Doppler ultrasound has proven to be invaluable in the initial diagnosis and in the serial assessment of valvular and congenital heart disease.

Acknowledgements

The author wishes to thank Mrs Margaret Young for assistance in preparation of the manuscript and Ms Jane Gretka for technical assistance.

204

References

1. Hatle L, Angelsen B: Doppler ultrasound in cardiology. Lea & Febiger, Philadelphia, 1982.
2. Strandness DE Jr: The use of ultrasound in the evaluation of peripheral vascular disease. Prog CV Dis 20: 403–422, 1978.
3. Reid JM, Baker DW: Physics and electronics of the ultrasonic Doppler method. In: Egermann H (ed.), Ultrasonographia Medica. (Publisher), Wien, 1971, p 109.
4. Pearlman AS, Stevenson JG, Baker DW: Doppler echocardiography: applications, limitations and future directions. Am J Cardiol 46: 1256–1262, 1980.
5. Valdes-Cruz LM, Sahn DJ: Two-dimensional echo Doppler for non-invasive quantitation of cardiac flow: a status report. Modern Concepts of Cardiovasc Dis 51: 123–128, 1982.
6. Baker DW, Rubenstein SA, Lorch GS: Pulsed Doppler echocardiography: principles and applications. Am J Med 63: 69–80, 1977.
7. Johnson SL, Baker DW, Lute RA, Dodge HT: Doppler echocardiography: the localization of cardiac murmurs. Circulation 48: 810–822, 1973.
8. Kececioglu-Draelos Z, Goldberg SJ, Areias J, Sahn DJ: Verification and clinical demonstration of the echo Doppler series effect and vortex shed distance. Circulation 63: 1422–1428, 1981.
9. Goldberg SJ, Areias J, Feldman L, Sahn DJ, Allen HD: Lesions that cause aortic flow disturbance. Circulation 60: 1539–1547, 1979.
10. Holen J, Aaslid R, Landmark K, Simonsen S: Determination of pressure gradient in mitral stenosis with a non-invasive ultrasound Doppler technique. Acta Med Scand 199: 455–460, 1976.
11. Hatle L, Brubakk A, Tromsdal A, Angelsen B: Non-invasive assessment of pressure drop in mitral stenosis by Doppler ultrasound. Brit Heart J 40: 131–140, 1978.
12. Holen J, Hoie J, Froysaker T: Determination of pre- and postoperative flow obstruction in patients undergoing closed mitral commissurotomy from non-invasive ultrasound Doppler data and cardiac output. Am Heart J 97: 499–504, 1979.
13. Lima CO, Sahn DJ, Valdes-Cruz LM, Goldberg SJ, Barron JV, Allen HD, Grenadier E: Non-invasive prediction of transvalvular pressure gradient in patients with pulmonary stenosis by quantitative two-dimensional echocardiographic Doppler studies. Circulation 67: 866–871, 1983.
14. Hatle L, Angelsen BA, Tromsdal A: Non-invasive assessment of aortic stenosis by Doppler ultrasound. Brit Heart J 43: 284–292, 1980.
15. Hatle L: Non-invasive assessment and differentiation of left ventricular outflow obstruction by Doppler ultrasound. Circulation 64: 381–387, 1981.
16. Cannon SR, Richards KL, Rollwitz WT: Digital Fourier techniques in the diagnosis and quantification of aortic stenosis with pulsed-Doppler echocardiography. JCU 10: 101–107, 1982.
17. Holen J, Hoie J, Semb B: Obstructive characteristics of Bjork-Shiley, Hancock, and Lillehei-Kaster prosthetic mitral valves in the immediate postoperative period. Acta Med Scand 204:5–11, 1978.
18. Holen J, Simonsen S, Froysaker T: An ultrasound Doppler technique for the non-invasive determination of the pressure gradient in the Bjork-Shiley mitral valve. Circulation 59: 436–442, 1979.
19. Holen J, Aaslid R, Landmark K, Simonsen S, Ostrem T: Determination of effective orifice area in mitral stenosis from non-invasive ultrasound Doppler data and mitral flow rate. Acta Med Scand 201: 83–88, 1977.
20. Valdes-Cruz LM, Horowitz S, Mesel E, Sahn DJ, Fisher DC, Larson D, Goldberg SJ, Allen HD: A pulsed Doppler echocardiographic method for calculation of pulmonary and systemic flow: accuracy in a canine model with ventricular septal defect. Circulation 68: 597–602, 1983.
21. Colocousis JS, Huntsman LL, Curreri PW: Estimation of stroke volume changes by ultrasonic Doppler. Circulation 56: 914–924, 1977.
22. Friedman MJ, Sahn DJ, Larson D, Flint A: 2D echo-range gated Doppler measurements of cardiac output and stroke volume in open chest dogs. Circulation (abstr) 62: 101, 1980.

23. Huntsman LL, Stewart DK, Barnes SR, Franklin SB, Colocousis JS, Hessel EA: Non-invasive Doppler determination of cardiac output in man. Clinical validation. Circulation 67: 593–602, 1983.

24. Alverson DC, Eldridge M, Dillon T, Yabek SM, Berman W Jr: Non-invasive pulsed Doppler determination of cardiac output in neonates and children. J Pediatr 101: 46–50, 1982.

25. Goldberg SJ, Sahn DJ, Allen HD, Valdes-Cruz LM, Hoenecke H, Carnahan Y: Evaluation of pulmonary and systemic blood flow by 2-dimensional Doppler echocardiography using fast Fourier transform spectral analysis. Am J Cardiol 50: 1394–1400, 1982.

26. Sanders SP, Yeager S, Williams RG: Measurement of systemic and pulmonary blood flow and QP/QS ratio using Doppler and two-dimensional echocardiography. Am J Cardiol 51: 952–956, 1983.

27. Valdes-Cruz LM, Horowitz S, Mesel E, Sahn DJ, Fisher DC, Larson D: A pulsed Doppler echocardiographic method for calculating pulmonary and systemic blood flow in atrial level shunts: validation studies in animals and initial human experience. Circulation 69: 80–86, 1984.

28. Meijboom EJ, Valdes-Cruz LM, Horowitz S, Sahn DJ, Larson DF, Young KA, Lima CO, Goldberg SJ, Allen HD: A two-dimensional Doppler echocardiographic method for calculation of pulmonary and systemic blood flow in a canine model with a variable-sized left-to-right extracardiac shunt. Circulation 68: 437–445, 1983.

29. Fisher DC, Sahn DJ, Friedman MJ, Larson D, Valdes-Cruz LM, Horowitz S, Goldberg SJ, Allen HD: The mitral valve orifice method for non-invasive two-dimensional echo Doppler determinations of cardiac output. Circulation 67: 872–877, 1983.

30. Lima CO, Sahn DJ, Valdes-Cruz LM, Allen HD, Goldberg SJ, Grenadier E, Barron JV: Prediction of the severity of left ventricular outflow tract obstruction by quantitative two-dimensional echocardiographic Doppler studies. Circulation 68: 348–354, 1983.

31. Jenni R, Hubscher W, Casty M, Anliker M, Krayenbuehl HP: Quantitation of aortic regurgitation by a percutaneous 128-channel digital ultrasound Doppler instrument. In: Lancee CT (ed.), Echocardiology. Martinus Nijhoff, The Hague, 1979, pp 241–243.

32. Brubakk AO, Angelsen BAJ, Hatle L: Diagnosis of valvular heart disease using transcutaneous Doppler ultrasound. Cardiovasc Res 11: 461–469, 1977.

33. Stevenson JG, Kawabori I, Guntheroth WG: Differentiation of ventricular septal defects from mitral regurgitation by pulsed Doppler echocardiography. Circulation 56: 14–18, 1977.

34. Miyatake K, Kinoshita N, Nagata S, Beppu S, Park Y, Sakakibara H, Nimura Y: Intracardiac flow pattern in mitral regurgitation studied with combined use of the ultrasonic pulsed Doppler technique and cross-sectional echocardiography. Am J Cardiol 45: 155–162, 1980.

35. Nichol PM, Boughner DR, Persaud JA: Non-invasive assessment of mitral regurgitation by transcutaneous Doppler ultrasound. Circulation 54: 656–661, 1976.

36. Abbasi AS, Allen MW, De Christofaro D, Ungar J: Detection and estimation of the degree of mitral regurgitation by range-gated pulsed Doppler echocardiography. Circulation 61: 143–147, 1980.

37. Skiaerpe T, Hatle L: Diagnosis and assessment of tricuspid regurgitation with Doppler ultrasound. In: Rijsterborgh H (ed.), Echocardiology. Martinus Nijhoff, The Hague, 1981, pp 299–304.

38. Fantini F, Magherini A: Detection of tricuspid regurgitation with pulsed Doppler echocardiography. In: Lancee CT (ed.), Echocardiology. Martinus Nijhoff, The Hague, 1979, pp 233–235.

39. Goldberg SJ, Areias JC, Spitaels SEC, De Villeneuve VH: Use of time interval histographic output from echo-Doppler to detect left-to-right atrial shunts. Circulation 58: 147–152, 1978.

40. Hatle L, Rokseth R: Non-invasive diagnosis and assessment of ventricular septal defect by Doppler ultrasound. Acta Med Scand Suppl 645: 47–56, 1981.

41. Stevenson JG, Kawabori I, Dooley T, Guntheroth WG: Diagnosis of ventricular septal defect by pulsed Doppler echocardiography – sensitivity, specificity and limitations. Circulation 58: 322–326, 1978.

42. Magherini A, Azzolina G, Wiechmann V, Fantini F: Pulsed Doppler echocardiography for diagnosis of ventricular septal defects. Brit Heart J 43: 143–147, 1980.

43. Stevenson JG, Kawabori I, Guntheroth WG: Non-invasive detection of pulmonary hypertension in patent ductus arteriosus by pulsed Doppler echocardiography. Circulation 60: 355–359, 1979.

44. Stevenson JG, Kawabori I, Guntheroth WG: Pulsed Doppler echocardiographic diagnosis of patent ductus arteriosus: sensitivity, specificity, limitations and technical features. Cathet Cardiovasc Diagn 6: 255–263, 1980.

45. Gentile R, Stevenson G, Dooley T, Franklin D, Kawabori I, Pearlman A: Pulsed Doppler echocardiographic determination of time of ductal closure in normal newborn infants. J Pediatr 98: 443–448, 1981.

46. Serwer GA, Armstrong BE, Anderson PAW: Non-invasive detection of retrograde descending aortic flow in infants using continuous wave Doppler ultrasonography. J Pediatr 97: 394–400, 1980.

13. Radionuclide imaging of the heart

JACK E. JUNI and ANDREW J. BUDA

Introduction

One on the first fields to make widespread use of the digital computer in cardiac imaging was nuclear medicine. Dedicated minicomputers designed specifically for acquisition and manipulation of digital radionuclide images have been available commercially for almost fourteen years.

The field of nuclear cardiology has continued to expand both in depth and breadth and has, in fact, become almost a subspeciality in itself. In this chapter, we will attempt to review the field of nuclear cardiac imaging with a special emphasis on techniques relevant to other digital imaging modalities. Of necessity, this can be but an overall description. The interested reader is strongly urged to investigate the reference bibliography for further details.

Essentially all nuclear medicine imaging of the heart, with the exception of positron emission tomography (PET scanning) which is described in chapter 14, is done by means of the Anger or 'gamma' camera [1, 2]. This device (see Figure 1) consists of a 10–20 inch diameter single crystal of sodium iodide (NaI) which is between $1/4$ and $1/2$ inch in thickness. A collimator is fastened to one side of this crystal and consists of a thick lead plate with several thousand small parallel (usually) holes drilled through it (Figure 2). This permits only those gamma particles traveling *directly towards* the crystal to pass through and interact with the crystal itself. In this manner, the collimator functions in roughly the same capacity as a photographic lens. The reverse side of the NaI crystal is covered by an array of photomultiplier tubes, each of which has its own pre-amplifier and is connected directly to analog position computing circuitry (Figure 3). When a gamma particle successfully passes through the collimator and strikes the sodium iodide crystal, it interacts, producing a small flash of light or scintillation. This light spreads for some distance through the crystal and is detected by several of the photo-multiplier tubes on the rear of the crystal. The relative intensity of the light detected by each photomultiplier tube is dependent on the position in the crystal of the original light flash. By analyzing the relative strength of the various

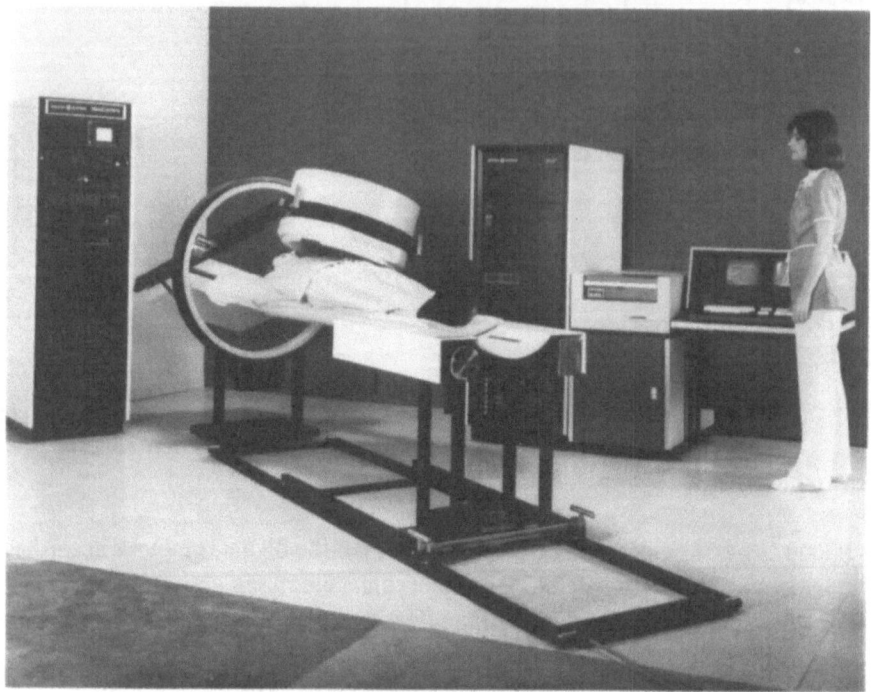

Figure 1. Typical state-of-the-art gamma camera with associated computer. (Photograph provided through the courtesy of General Electric Corporation.)

photomultiplier output signals, the analog computing circuitry is able to calculate the position in the crystal at which the scintillation must have occurred. This information, in the form of an X, Y coordinate pair is sent, along with other information regarding the energy of the detected particle, in analog form to a mini- or microcomputer with an analog-to-digital converter which converts the X, Y coordinate pairs to digital form and stores the information on a two-dimensional image matrix [3]. In routine clinical use, this matrix is 64 × 64 or 128 × 128 pixels. The final image, represents the sum of hundreds of thousands of individual X, Y coordinate pairs, each representing a single gamma particle-NaI crystal interaction and its resulting scintillation.

Other imaging devices such as the rectilinear scanner [4], and multiwire proportional counting chambers [5] have been used for cardiac imaging. These devices have only minimal impact on the current practice of nuclear cardiology.

Equilibrium gated blood pool imaging

Gated blood pool imaging is, arguably, the most commonly performed radionuclide imaging study of the heart at the present time [6–8]. In actual fact, the

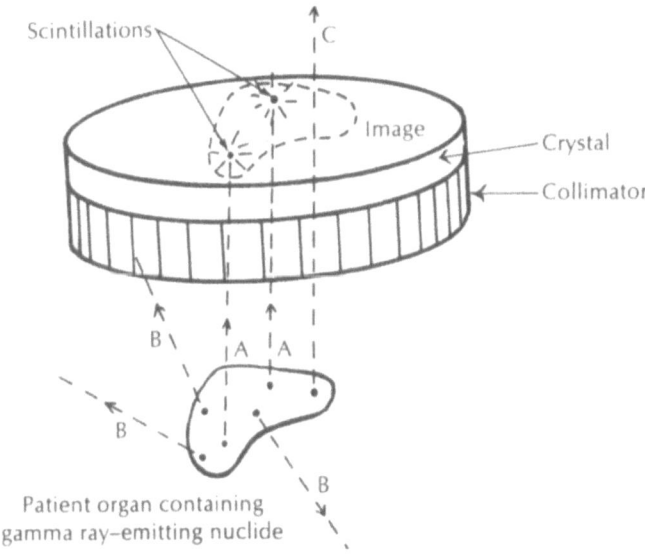

Figure 2. Parallel hole collimator used to 'focus' radionuclide image onto face of the gamma camera. A = gamma rays used to construct image; B = gamma rays that do not reach crystal; C = gamma ray that passes through crystal without being absorbed.

heart itself is not directly imaged. The patient's red blood cells are labeled with a tracer [9, 10], typically technetium-99 m with a half-life of 6 hr, and it is this pool of labeled red blood cells that is actually imaged. When the gamma camera is aimed at a patient's chest, the largest collection of red blood cells are in the chambers of the heart and in the great blood vessels. The heart itself is surrounded by the airfilled lungs which have a relatively low concentration of red blood cells. Thus, the most visible structures in the chest are the pools of blood in the cardiac chambers, in particular the ventricles, and it is these pools of blood rather than the myocardium itself which are imaged. The resulting images have a ventricular blood pool-to-lung or target-to-background ratio of approximately 3:2 [11]. With sufficient image enhancement, this is suitable for imaging. the structure and function of the myocardium itself, is inferred from the shape, indentations, and movement of the ventricular blood pools [12, 13].

The amount of radioactivity that one may safely administer to a patient is relatively small. Since, in gated blood pool imaging, only a relatively small portion of the total labeled blood volume (about 5%) is in the heart at any given point in time, the amount of radioactivity in the region of interest and thus the number of counts coming from that region in any given period of time is quite small. In fact, far too few counts are given off by the cardiac structures over the duration of a single cardiac cycle to form a meaningful image. Since the heart is constantly moving, one would ideally wish to acquire a series of images representing the heart at each portion of the cardiac cycle, unblurred by movement of the heart during image acquisition. This is accomplished by a process called gating [3,

210

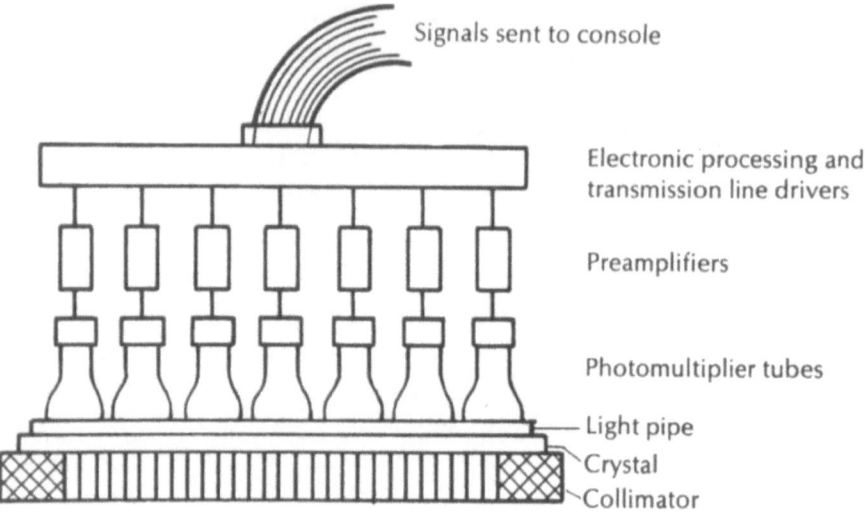

Signals sent to console

Electronic processing and transmission line drivers

Preamplifiers

Photomultiplier tubes

Light pipe
Crystal
Collimator

Figure 3. Schematic diagram of the 'head' of a typical gamma camera showing the collimator, crystal, and multiple photomultiplier tubes, each with associated preamplifier and analog positioning circuitry.

14, 15]. Each cardiac contraction is preceeded by a QRS complex on the electrocardiogram. The patient's ECG is monitored continuously during the image procedure and each QRS complex is detected by a 'trigger sensor' which then sends a pulse to the image acquisition computer. The time period of each cardiac cycle, the R-R interval, is broken down into a series of typically 16–32 time segments (Figure 4). Data acquired during each of these segments of the cardiac cycle is accumulated over the course of 200–400 cardiac cycles. The gamma camera produces an almost continuous stream of X, Y coordinate signals. Using the QRS trigger as a guide, the computer then sorts this image data into the appropriate bin or frame according to the time interval which has passed since the last received QRS trigger signal. Thus, after 200–400 cycles, a series of 16–32 images will have been created. These images are analogous to the frames of a movie and represent the summed data of all the cardiac cycles in the acquisition. These images may be displayed in rapid sequence in an 'endless loop' fashion to provide a cinematic display of the beating heart. Visual analysis of these images provides valuable information as to qualitative wall motion and cardiac function.

By defining a region-of-interest around, for example, the left ventricle, and determining these counts in each frame through the cycle, a time-activity curve may be generated [16, 17, 22]. The shape of this curve directly represents the changes in left ventricular volume occurring through a given cardiac cycle plus a relatively constant amount of radioactivity contributed by scatter from adjacent structures such as liver and spleen and 'background' activity from overlying and underlying lung and soft tissues. The amount of background activity can be approximately determined by measuring the activity per pixel in an area immedi-

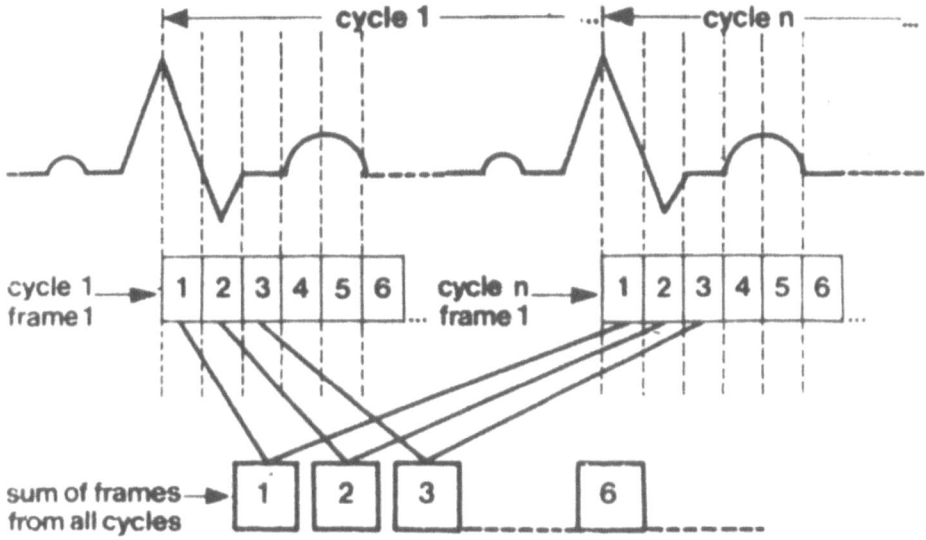

Figure 4. Each cardiac cycle is broken down into a series of 16–64 time intervals. Data acquired during each of these intervals is accumulated in a separate image frame. A total of 200–400 cardiac cycles are accumulated to build up a image series.

ately adjacent to the heart. This background activity is then subtracted as a constant from the ventricular time-activity curve to give a curve representing actual ventricular volume changes. Analysis of this ventricular volume curve has proven to be an extremely productive area of research.

One of the first aspects of cardiac function to be evaluated by this means was the ejection fraction (Figure 5). By looking at the number of counts of the background corrected left ventricular time-activity curve at end-diastole and subtracting this from the number of counts at end-systole, the relative stroke volume can be determined. Dividing the stroke volume by the end-diastolic counts gives the cardiac ejection fraction. This is has been found to correlate quite closely with ejection fraction as determined by contrast angiographic techniques [17]. Gated blood pool images is performed almost as easily during exercise as when the patient is at rest [18]. The comparison of exercise to resting ejection fraction in the individual patient has proven to be a sensitive indicator of coronary artery disease. Normal volunteers will show a significant increase in ejection fraction with exercise while most persons with significant coronary artery disease show a fall, or at least no increase in ejection fraction with exercise [19–21, 25–27].

A number of other parameters have been measured from these 'global' left ventricular time-activity curves. Analysis of the fraction of blood ejected during the first one-third of systole (first-third ejection fraction) [23, 24, 28, 29] and the peak ejection rate during systole have been advocated as indicators of coronary artery disease. Recently, evaluation of the diastolic portion of the time-activity curve has generated great interest [30–34]. By determining the slope of an appropriately filtered or smoothed time-activity curve at any point along its length, the rate of blood flow into or out of the ventricle at that point in time can be measured. Thus, the first derivative of the time-activity curve represents a plot of the rates of ventricular filling and ejection.

Bonow and his colleagues at the National Institutes of Health have used this technique to measure the peak filling rate (PFR) and the time from end-systole to the occurrence of the peak filling rate (TPFR) in a wide variety of patients (Figure 6) [30]. They have found that these parameters, while not specific for coronary artery disease, are abnormal in virtually all patients with coronary artery disease even when measured at rest. Reduto *et al.* [31] have examined these parameters as well as a third measurement, the percent of overall filling occurring in the first third of diastole, both at rest and at exercise using a first-pass technique (to be discussed below). They found that diastolic function was even more abnormal in coronary artery disease patients when evaluated with exercise.

An interesting technique for evaluation of the intrinsic shape of the left ventricular volume curve, the cardiac flow-volume loop [35, 38] has recently been proposed (Figure 7). This approach is designed to demonstrate the dynamic relationship between instantaneous ventricular volume and the simultaneous rate of blood flow. A plot is derived, as demonstrated in the figure, by plotting left ventricular flow (the derivative of ventricular volume) against the simultaneous ventricular volume. This results in a mapping of the entire cardiac cycle into a closed loop. The construction of the loop may be best appreciated by comparing the time-activity curve to its corresponding flow-volume loop. Corresponding points on the two curves are labeled. The flow-volume loop is normalized so that the horizontal or volume axis ranges from 0–100% of the individual's stroke volume while the vertical axis represents flow either into (negative) or out of (positive) the ventricle. This axis is normalized so that the greatest flow, either positive or negative, represents 100 units. The NIH group has found the flow-volume loop to be capable of differentiating and identifying patients with coronary artery disease when derived from resting left ventricular time-activity curves [37, 38]. This finding is particularly remarkable in view of the fact that the methods of construction and normalization of the flow-volume loop eliminate any ability to measure absolute rates of ventricular filling or ejection and by virtue of normalization of the volume axis, eliminate measurement of ejection fraction.

Cardiac function is frequently not uniform. Many diseases, in particular coronary artery disease, affect some segments of the ventricle more than others. A number of groups have investigated approaches to the regional analysis of ventricular function [39–41]. In particular, measurements of regional ejection fraction have proven useful in many hands. While details of technique vary, in most, the ventricle is subdivided into three to thirty segments or pie shaped wedges. These wedge shaped regions are applied to each of the frames in the

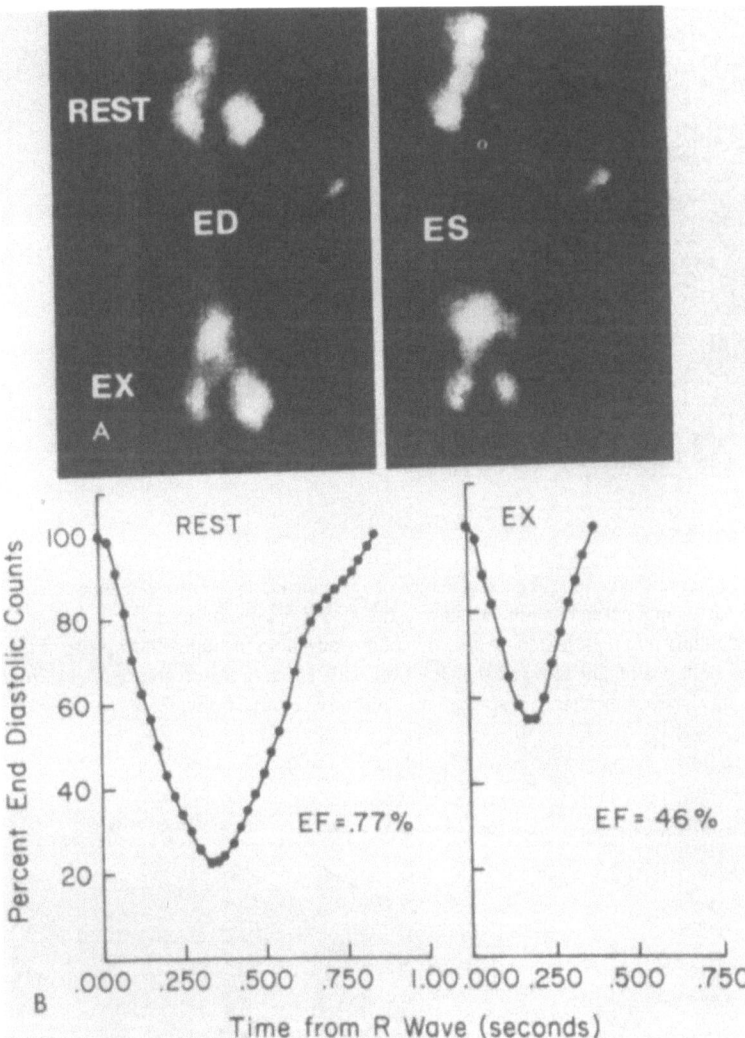

Figure 5. Typical gated radionuclide image is taken at end-diastole and end-systole with associated left ventricular volume curve derived by plotting left ventricular counts at each frame in the image series.

image series yielding an individual time-activity or volume curve for each region. Normal limits for regional ejection fraction of each part of the heart have been developed and applied prospectively to many groups of patients [40]. While some controversy still exists as to the degree of advantage this sort of analysis provides over visual analysis of wall motion by highly trained observers, there is no doubt that it provides an objective way of quantifying regional myocardial function.

214

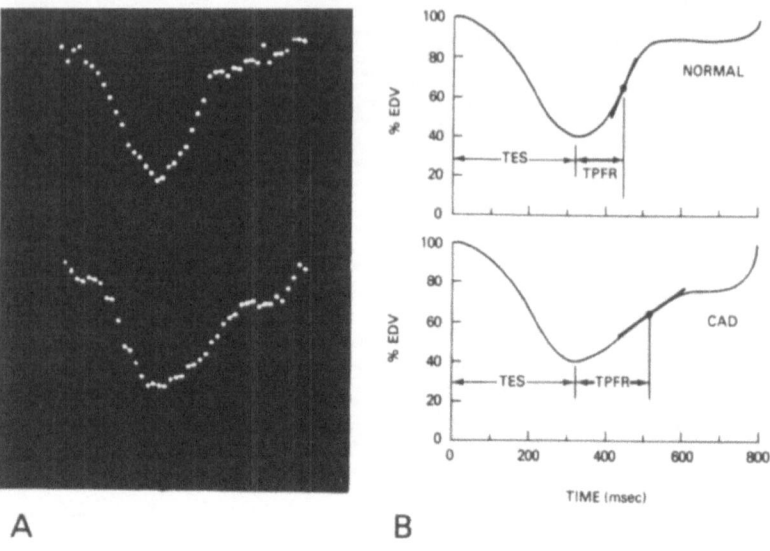

A   B

Figure 6. Unprocessed and schematic versions of radionuclide left ventricular time-activity (time-volume) curves in a normal volunteer (above) and a patient with coronary artery disease (below). Note peak filling rate represented by the slope of the tangent to the rapid filling phase of the curve. Note how both peak filling rate and the time from end-systole to the occurence of peak filling rate (TPFR) are significantly altered in the patient with coronary artery disease.

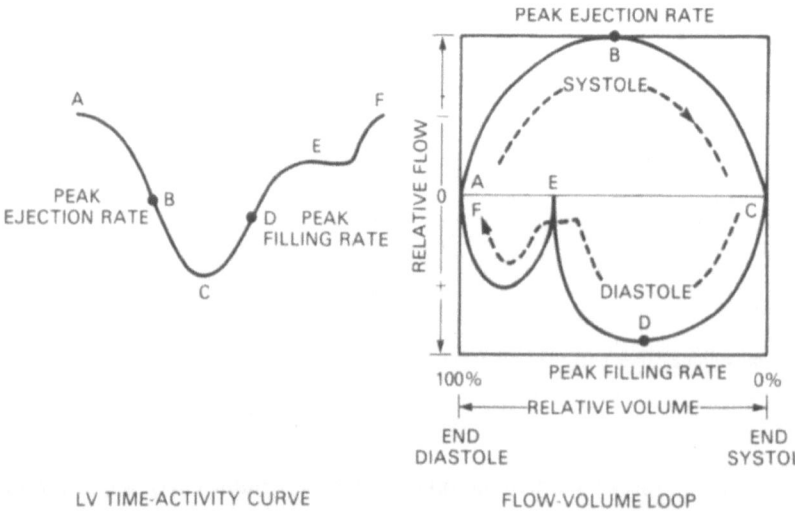

LV TIME-ACTIVITY CURVE   FLOW-VOLUME LOOP

Figure 7. Cardiac flow-volume loop derived by plotting the left ventricular volume against the simultaneous rate of blood flow at each point through the cardiac cycle. This approach has proved useful in appreciating the subtle relationship of left ventricular filling and emptying to the associated ventricular volume.

Phase analysis

A new and intriguing approach to analysis of regional volume curves has been proposed by Vitale and the group from NIH [42]. Each regional volume curve is fitted to a cosine curve with a frequency of exactly one cycle per cardiac cycle length. The amplitude of this fitted curve reflects the regional stroke volume while the phase shift of the fitted curve reflects both the timing of contraction and of relaxation of that ventricular region. Their group has found this technique to be quite reliable in detection of coronary artery disease. Mahac *et al.* [43], have found this approach to quantifying the regional timing of contraction to be useful in evaluation of interventricular conduction abnormalities.

Fitting time-activity curves from small regions of the ventricular image series has been applied widely in the form now generically referred to as 'phase analysis' or 'Fourier analysis'. This technique, first described by Adams *et al.* [44] in 1979 as well as others involves creation of a time-activity curve for each pixel of the image series throughout the recorded cardiac cycle. These individual pixel curves are each fitted with a single cosine function curve with a frequency corresponding to that of the cardiac cycle. Two *parametric* images are obtained by this technique. One, the amplitude image, is a single image in which the intensity or color of each pixel represents the amplitude of the cosine curve fitted to that particular pixel over the time span of the original image series. Thus, those areas with a large cyclic variation in counts, e.g. pixels within the region of the ventricles, will have a large amplitude of the fitted curve and will appear as intense or brightly colored regions of the amplitude image. Those images with little cyclic fluctuation at the primary frequency of cardiac contraction, e.g. those areas representing background or lung activity, will have a low amplitude of the fitted curve and will thus have a low intensity or different color on the parametric amplitude image. Such images are of particular interest in defining the limits of the cardiac structures. The relative 'amplitude' of the left ventricular region as obtained by summing the amplitudes of all pixels within this region has been compared to the relative overall 'amplitude' of the right ventricle for measurement of intracardiac shunting and valvular regurgitation with encouraging results.

The second parametric image generated by this technique, *the phase* image, has attracted the greatest attention and discussion. In this parametric image, the intensity or color of each pixel represents the timing of phase shift of a single cosine function fitted to the time-activity curve of that pixel. Thus, a pixel in the region of the left ventricle would have a fitted cosine wave approximately 180° out-of-phase with the curve fitted to a pixel representing the left atrium. On the parametric phase display, these pixels would be represented with different colors and/or intensities reflecting the difference in timing of overall contraction and relaxation. The uniformity of phase between the right and left ventricles in a normal individual is quite remarkable. Likewise the atria, while 180° out-of-phase from the ventricles, are relatively uniform in phase between themselves. In the

216

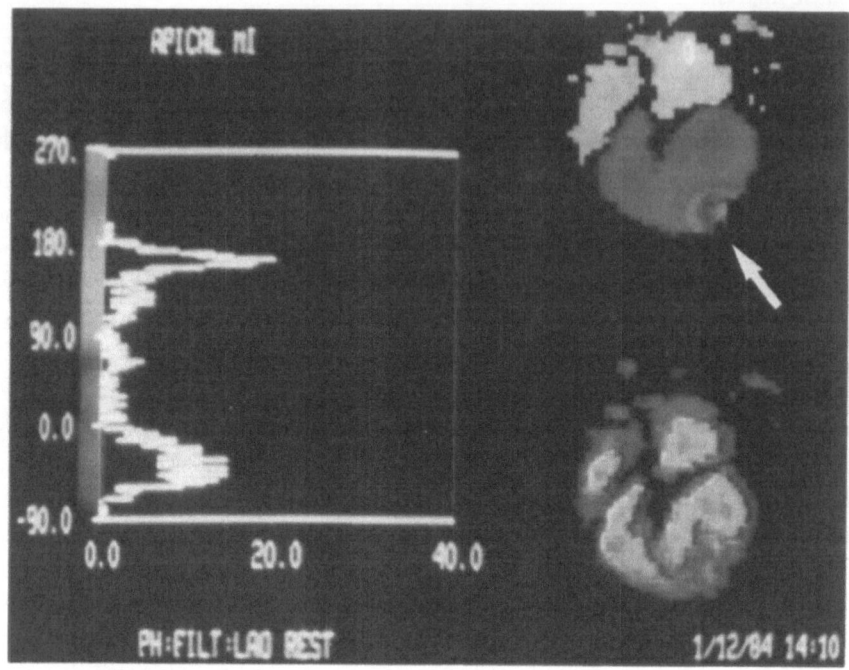

Figure 8. Typical 'phase' parametric images of a normal heart (on the left) and a heart with an apical aneurysm (on the right). Note the marked phase delay in the region of the aneurysm represented by a difference in color relative to the remainder of the ventricle.

presence of inter- or intraventricular conduction delays or in regional wall motion abnormalities, this uniformity of cyclic variation is destroyed (Figure 8). While the phase image is derived from the original series of intensity images and thus provides no information not intrinsically available in the original sequence, these parametric images do provide detailed information about the timing of blood volume changes across the entire image at a single glance [44–55]. Many groups now use phase images routinely in evaluation of patients for coronary artery disease regional wall motion abnormalities, and intraventricular conduction delays [45, 47, 48, 52, 55]. Phase images have also been successfully used to localize abnormal ventricular activation pathways in patients with Wolff-Parkinson-White (WPW) syndrome [49, 50, 59], electronic pacemakers [50, 51], and even ventricular tachycardia [53]. Some recent work has indicated that phase images may be capable of detecting subtle intraventricular conduction delays which may not be evident on resting electrocardiogram [54].

Quantitative phase analysis

By totaling and plotting the number of pixels demonstrating each possible overall phase shift, a *phase angle histogram* can be generated (see Figure 9). In the

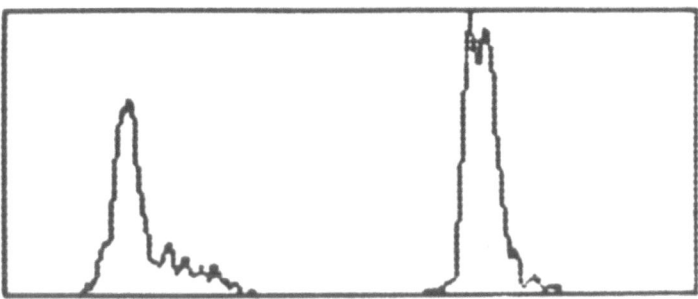

Figure 9. Phase angle histogram demonstrating the large ventricular peak and smaller atrial peak. The size of each peak represents the number of image pixels varying in intensity at each phase angle.

normal heart, this histogram will consist of two main peaks approximately 180° out-of-phase from each other. The smaller peak represents the contraction of the atria while the larger peak represents the contraction of both ventricles. Cases with complete left or right bundle branch block may demonstrate dual ventricular histogram peaks representing the difference in timing between the two ventricles (Figure 10). More subtle cases of regional abnormalities of timing may simply produce a widening or shift of the phase histogram without resulting in an additonal detectable peak. The width of the phase histogram at one-half maximum, the standard deviation and skewness of ventricular phase histogram have all proven useful in identifying such abnormalities and have been advocated in the routine evaluation of patients for wall motion abnormalities of coronary artery disease [50, 52, 56]. The actual sensitivity of such techniques and their application in routine clinical practice remains to be determined definitively. A recently presented technique for accentuating phase abnormalities by variable weighting of pixels with unusual phase shifts according to their spatial clustersing or lack thereof [57] represents an exciting concept which has yet to reach clinical application.

The eventual clinical role of phase imaging is an area on ongoing controversy. Other forms of parametric imaging have been described as alternatives and adjuncts to phase imaging as described above [58]. These techniques generally all work by producing an image in which the intensity or color of each pixel reflects some characteristic of that pixel's individual time-activity curve. Since the overall phase shift of a time-activity curve reflects both contraction and relaxation phases of the cycle equally, some groups have generated parametric images in which color or intensity reflect only the time to occurrence of end-systole with other images reflecting only the time to occurrence of the peak diastolic filling rate in an attempt to separate the systolic and diastolic components of the cycle. Parametric images showing the peak filling rate and peak ejection rate have also been produced. Software for production of these images is routinely available on most presently available commercial systems.

218

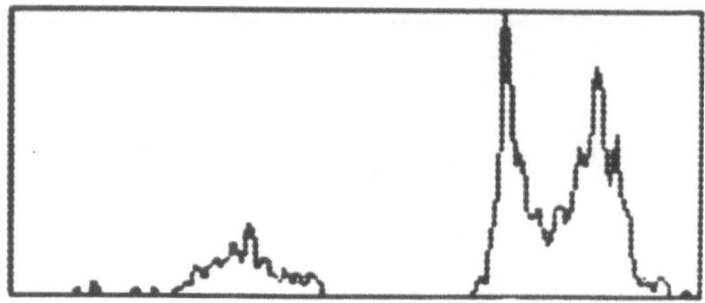

Figure 10. Phase angle histogram on patient with right bundle branch block. Note that a separate peak is visible for the right and the left ventricle.

Multi-harmonic analysis

Fitting a single frequency co-sine function to the left ventricular time-activity curve or to individual pixel time-activity curves obviously results in an over-simplification of the shape of these curves [60, 61]. In attempts to overcome this, some investigators have looked into the use of 'multiple harmonic curves' [61, 62]. Such curves, represent a time-activity curve reconstructed by adding together either the first, second, third, etc., frequency harmonics of the Fourier transform view of the original curve. By reconstructing this curve for more than one harmonic, a closer approximation to the original curve can be obtained while still removing some of the random noise which is especially evident in single pixel time-activity curves. The optimal number of harmonics to be used in such curve regeneration or smoothing has generally been found to be between 2–3 harmonics for single pixel curves [62, 63]. While this work is still relatively new, it is the opinion of these authors that optimal reproduction of single pixel time-activity or time-volume curves with removal of as much noise as possible will require application of a more sophicated digital filter which includes weighted amounts of many harmonics. Future work will hopefully clarify this controversy.

Arrythmia filtration

The method of image acquisition may have profound effects on the quality and physiologic significance of the resulting images. As described earlier, most gated blood pool images are acquired directly onto a computer. The data is sorted into the appropriate bin or image frame by measurement of the time elapsed since the most recently received QRS trigger pulse. This method assumes that all cardiac cycles are exactly identical in timing. In actual patients, this is rarely the case. Small amounts of cycle length variability are present in all individuals and are frequently as much as 10–15% of the mean cardiac cycle length. This variability is considered normal and is generally reflective of parasympathetic nervous system tone and its response to normal respiration. These variations cause some cycles to be shorter than others. If, during image acquisition, the computer receives a new QRS trigger impulse, it goes back to the beginning of the image sequence, adding the incoming camera data to the first frame again. If the QRS trigger impulse comes relatively early due to a relatively short preceeding cycle, the computer will still reset back to the first frame and start a new cycle over. This results in relatively less data being placed in the latter frames of the study as compared to the earlier ones. If a large number of 'short' beats are present, this process results in a significant reduction in count and information density in the latter frames [3]. This is commonly seen in routine gated blood pool studies and can be seen as a flicker at the end of the image sequence or as an abrupt drop-off in counts on the global left ventricular time-activity curve over the last few frames (Figure 11). This drop-off obviously does not represent an actual fall in cardiac volume and in fact is artifactual. Data has been presented indicating that the artifact induced by even normal cycle length variability is enough to significantly alter measurements of diastolic filling parameters [64].

Several acquistion methods are available to combat this problem. The most widely available is known as serial-mode or list-mode acquisition [3] (Figure 12). Using this technique, the incoming camera and QRS trigger data streams are not used to sort out image data as it is received by the computer. Rather, all X, Y coordinate pairs from the camera are stored on a high capacity disk along with the QRS trigger impulses and a rapid (1–10 ms) clock timing marker. No attempt is made to format the data into images as it is being acquired. Rather, after acquisition is complete, the stored data is read from the disk in the order of acquisition. Each cardiac cycle is evaluated for cycle length and checked to see if it falls within preset operator determined limits. If it does, the data is then

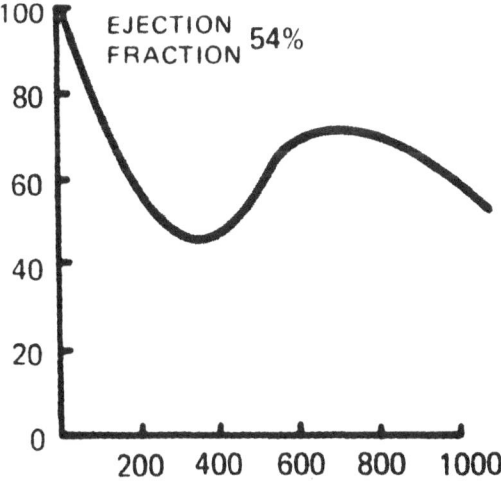

Figure 11. Left ventricular time-activity curve showing abrupt dropoff in the last portion of the study. This is an artifact generated by variation in heart rate during acquisition.

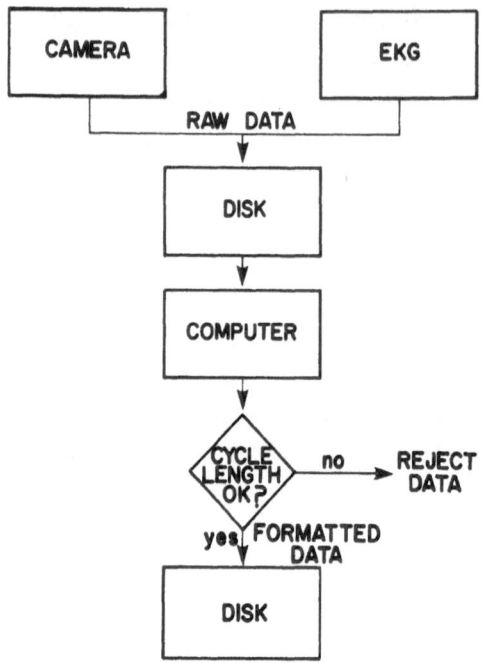

Figure 12. Schematic diagram of 'list mode' acquisition technique. All image, EKG, and timing data is stored on high capacity magnetic disks for future formatting.

formatted into multiple image frames as described previously. If the data does not fit within operator determined cycle length limits, it is discarded. This technique permits one to set very narrow limits of acceptable cardiac cycle length and to process the data in any way desired or in multiple ways after acquisition is complete. By limiting variability of accepted cycles, the problems of count drop-off in the terminal frames of the study can be eliminated.

More recently, several commercial vendors have made available systems which permit 'on-the-fly' arrythmia filtration [65] (Figure 13). These systems use an intermediate buffer consisting of either of a high speed Winchester magnetic disk or a large amount of peripheral random access memory to store the data stream, or small sections of it, as it comes in from the camera. The computer, working several beats behind the actual input data stream, then evaluates the cycle length of each beat residing in this buffer and decides whether or not the beat falls within acceptable limits. If it does not, it is discarded. The net result of these on-the-fly techniques and serial mode techniques is quite similar. The on-the-fly or dynamic techniques have the advantage of requiring less high speed disk storage and requiring less operator time in reformatting the studies after-the-fact. They suffer from the disadvantage of being unable to retrospectively alter the limits of acceptability and reformat the study. With the dynamic systems, once a study has been acquired, the individual cycles making up that study cannot be reanalyzed.

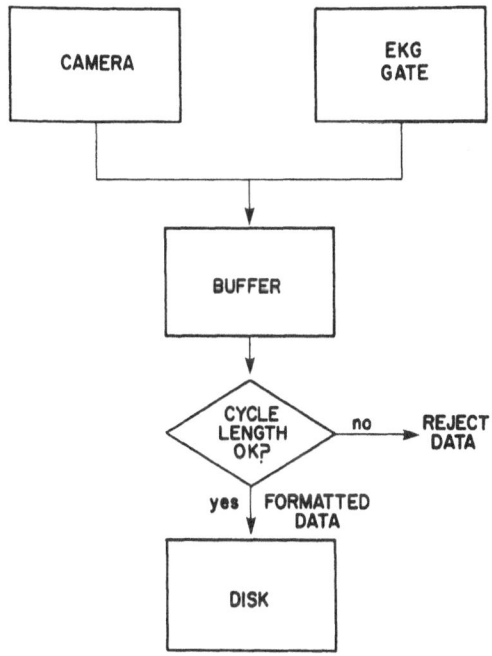

Figure 13. Schematic diagram of 'dynamic arrhythmia filtration'. Incoming image, EKG, and timing data are buffered temporarily and evaluated for appropriateness of cycle length. Cycles falling within a preset cycle length acceptance window are incorporated into the gated study while all other cycles are rejected.

First-pass radionuclide ventriculography

First-pass techniques are used in many centers as an alternative or an adjunct to gated equilibrium blood pool imaging. The technique is, in essence, quite simple. The gamma camera is positioned over the patients chest prior to injection of radiotracer. The tracer is then injected as a single rapid bolus directly into the most proximal vein available or, in many institutions, into a central venous catheter. The gamma camera output is sent directly to a computer which is instructed to format the data into sequential images at a very rapid rate, typically 25 or more frames per second [3]. Image acquisition usually continues until the majority of the first pass of tracer has gone beyond the left ventricle. Examination of the individual frames of the study will reveal detail of the various cardiac structures (Figure 14). Because the entire bolus is present within the heart at essentially the same time, very good counting statistics may be obtained, thus permitting such rapid framing rates. The high counting rates required, is far beyond the ability of most standard single crystal gamma cameras [66, 67]. Most work with first-pass ventriculography has been done using 'multicrystal' cameras [68]. These cameras consist of a number, usually approximately 64, of single sodium iodide crystals arranged in a rectangular array. Each crystal is provided

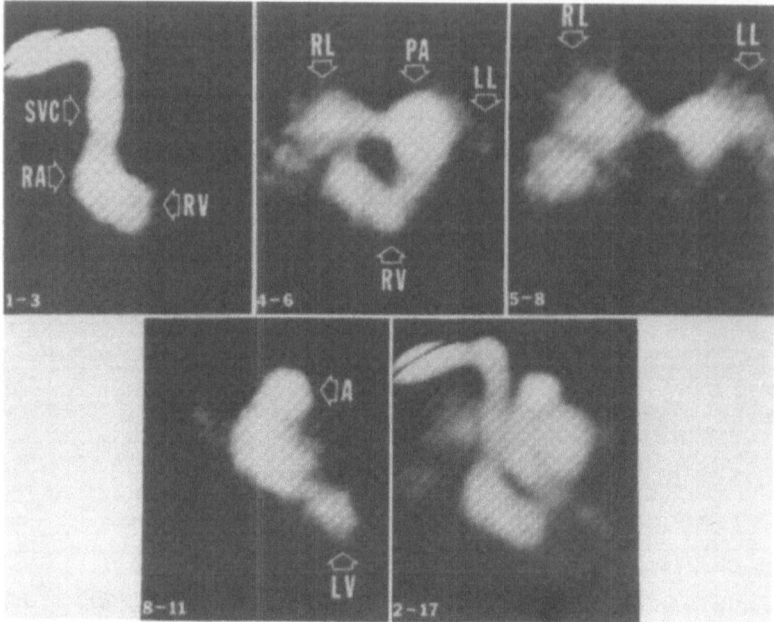

Figure 14. Selected images from a first-pass radionuclide study. Note initial passage of the tracer through the superior vena cava (SVC), into the right atrium (RA), and right ventricle (RV). The tracer then passes through the lungs, the left atrium and left ventricles and is eventually expelled through the ascending and decending aorta (A). LL = left lung; RL = right lung.

with its own photomultiplier tube. No position detecting circuitry is necessary, thus permitting the very high count rate capabilities of this type of camera. Unfortunately, the spatial resolution of the images is limited to the width of each crystal and thus is quite low relative to single-crystal gamma cameras. For most users, the trade-off between high spatial resolution and high count rate sensitivity must be considered when choosing equipment and deciding whether to acquire cardiac studies via the first-pass or gated equilibrium approach. Recently, some single-crystal gamma cameras with digital position sensing circuitry have been introduced which offer count rate capabilities sufficient for performance of first-pass ventriculography. When these cameras operate in high count rate mode, however, spatial resolution is usually significantly impared and is not greatly different from that of the multicrystal camera.

Gated equilibrium vs. first-pass

The first-pass ventriculogram has several advantages over the gated equilibrium study. The right and left ventricle may be easily evaluated in isolation without concern for overlap. Thus, the right ventricular ejection fraction can be easily determined without interferance from adjacent structures. In addition, the study is over in approximately one minute as compared to the 3–4 min required for each gated equilibrium acquisition. There are a number of disadvantages inherent in the first-pass technique which are partially responsible for its limited use and the apparently rising popularity of the gated equilibrium technique. As mentioned above, the spatial resolution of the first-pass technique is poor. It is generally only possible to obtain a single view of the heart with each injection. With equilibrium techniques, it is routine procedure to obtain 3–4 views of the heart at each study. This is felt to permit better evaluation of regional wall motion than a single view. It is difficult to do multiple sequential first-pass studies in order to evaluate the effects of an intervention such as exercise. It is possible to inject the patient once with a tracer which is rapidly cleared by the kidneys or liver and then give a second injection at peak exercise. This approach, however, does not allow multiple views at each level and does not permit any imaging to be done between rest and maximal exercise. Thus, the gated equilibrium approach is generally felt to be most useful when serial images are to be obtained through exercise or other situations where multiple images are to be obtained pre- and post-intervention.

Ventricular volume determination

Measurement of absolute left ventricular volume has wide-spread clinical importance as an indicator of cardiac function. Changes in end-diastolic and end-systolic volume reflect the ventricle's overall ability to respond to the preload and afterload demands placed on it. Knowledge of left ventricular stroke volume and heart rate permits calculation of cardiac output. Invasive measurement of these parameters is routinely performed in acutely ill patients but requires left heart catheterization and typically, injection of relatively large volumes of contrast material with subsequent hemodynamic effects [100], as well as, the possibility of transient renal dysfunction or allergic reaction.

Many authors have described non-invasive methods of determining left ventricular volumes by radionuclide techniques [101–115]. Radionuclide approaches to volume determination tend to fall in two categories – geometric and count-based.

Geometric approaches have been applied to both first-pass [101, 102] and gated equilibrium blood pool studies [102]. In essence, these techniques are direct decendents of the geometric volume calculations described for contrast angiography by Sandler and Dodge [104, 105]. A number of measurements of the length and width of the ventricle are made from one or more views. The ventricle is assumed to have a given geometric shape, typically a prolate ellipsoid [106]. The ventricular volume is determined by fitting this shape to the various measurements. If the physical dimensions represented by one image pixel are known, these calculations may be made from radionuclide images of the heart with an excellent correlation to measurements made by contrast angiography. Correlation co-efficients are typically better than 0.90 [103].

These geometric techniques all assume a predetermined ventricular shape which may not apply to all patients. And, probably do not apply to patients with severe congestive heart failure or with extremely small ventricles. To avoid these shape assumptions, a number of investigators have proposed count-based methods of volume measurement [107–111]. Rather than directly measuring the physical dimensions of the ventricle, these techniques involve determination of the count rate from the left ventricle, typically during a single frame of an equilibrium gated blood pool study. Since ventricular counts are proportional to ventricular blood volume, if a blood sample is drawn and counted to determine the count rate per minute per cc of blood, the total ventricular volume during that part of the cycle can be calculated.

This approach gives volume measurements which correlate highly with those determined by contrast angiography, but consistently underestimate contrast volumes. This underestimation is due to the absorption or attenuation of gamma photons emitted from within the ventricle by overlying thoracic tissues. This results in a reduction in the number of photons reaching the gamma camera detector. Some workers have corrected for this by determining a regression equation of count-based volumes to geometric contrast volumes and applying this regression equation to all radionuclide measurements [107, 108]. Others have attempted to measure the attenuation factor directly by determining cardiac depth from multiple views [109–111] and using an assumed standard attenuation factor for thoracic tissue or by use of transmission measurements [112]. These techniques provide an excellent correlation with contrast volumes and, while somewhat more complicated than simple geometric techniques, are simple enough for routine application. Attenuation correction clearly improves the accuracy of measurement and is likely to be reliable in patients with a wider variation in body habitus than regression techniques [111].

Recently, some preliminary work has been performed in measurements of chamber volume by gated single photon emission computed tomography of gated equilibrium blood pool images [113, 114]. A description of single photon emission tomography is given later in this chapter. By measuring the ventricle from the resulting three-dimensional images, volumes may be determined without prior assumptions as to the three-dimensional shape of the ventricle. The preliminary studies have shown excellent correlation with contrast volumes but the technique is, at present, expensive and time-consuming. Recent advances in tomographic techniques [115] may make this a practical approach in the future.

Myocardial perfusion imaging

The myocardial perfusion agent of choice, first proposed fourteen years ago [69], is thallium-201 chloride. Thallium is an analog of potassium and is taken up by essentially all muscle cells via the sodium-potassium ATP-ase pump [70]. Its initial uptake into the myocardium on the first-pass has been shown to be directly and linearly proportional to myocardial blood flow over an extremely wide range [71–73]. Approximately 90% of thallium presented to the myocardium is extracted in the first-pass. Thus, the amount of tracer concentrated in the myocardium immediately after administration reflects the relative blood flow to that region. As time passes after injection, thallium gradually washes out of the myocardial tissue. Its rate of washout is approximately inversely proportional to the rate of regional blood flow, that is, those areas with diminished blood flow and thus diminished uptake, will demonstrate the slowest washout of thallium over time [74–76]. This interesting pattern of tracer kinetics, in which areas with good perfusion have high initial uptake but then wash out very rapidly, while those areas with poor perfusion have low initial uptake but markedly delayed washout has been capitalized on in routine thallium imaging. If a sufficient time has been allowed following injection for the normal areas to have undergone significant washout and the heart is then reimaged, what appeared as perfusion defects or areas of reduced tracer uptake on initial imaging may appear to have 'filled in'. This phenomenon which has been termed 'redistribution' of thallium is due to the delayed washout of thallium in the relatively hypoperfused zone [77]. Thus, with time, thallium has either failed to washout or may, in fact, have continued to accumulate thallium from the blood stream while the more normally perfused tissue has undergone continuous washout. Thus, at later periods of time, the hypoperfused and the normally perfused areas may appear to show approximately equal tracer content. The redistribution pattern, that is, an initial defect which is no longer evident on delayed imaging, identifies tissue which is hypoperfused but remains viable. Areas of myocardial infarction, will have minimal or no thallium uptake initially and will not take up thallium with time. Thus, those areas will have a persistent defect in the delayed images. The filling in or persistence of a perfusion defect permits one to differentiate between hypoperfused but viable myocardium and that which is non-functional or scar tissue (Figure 15).

Since its introduction, thallium imaging has proved highly useful in identification and diagnosis of coronary artery disease. Typical reported sensitivities are 80–90% with 85–95% specificity for detection coronary artery disease [78]. The typical imaging procedure is performed by stressing the patient on an upright treadmill using a standard exercise protocol. When the patient's maximum workload is achieved or symptoms and/or ECG findings typical of ischemia occur, he or she is injected with 2–3 mCi of thallium-201 chloride. Exercise continues for approximately 1 more minute. The patient is then placed under the gamma camera with image acquisition beginning immediately. After an initial set of images from multiple views have been obtained, the patient then rests and returns in approximately 3 hr for repeat imaging.

Thallium imaging may be performed with the standard single crystal gamma camera. Due to the low photon energy (81 keV) and the relatively poor dosimetric factors of thallium [79] which limit the administered dose, the presence of

226

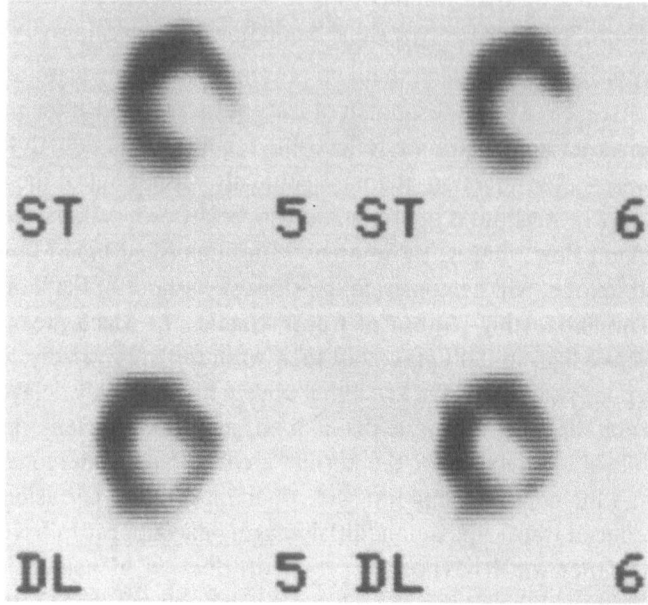

Figure 15. Typical thallium-201 perfusion image in a patient with hypoperfused but viable myocardium. Note that the initial image (ST) reveals an area of myocardium which appears not to take up thallium. On delayed (DL) images, this 'defect' has filled in. This represents gradual accumulation of thallium in the hypoperfused area with simultaneous washout of thallium initially accumulated in the well-perfused myocardium.

noise, background activity, and tissue cross-talk are particularly important. Statistical noise in thallium images have been handled by a variety of low pass filtering techniques which are discussed in Chapter 2. Correction for background activity is considerably more complex than in gated blood pool imaging. Since thallium is taken up by all muscle tissue, there is significant activity in the chest wall musculature as well as the paraspinous musculature. This results in a non-uniform background and foreground activity which is superimposition upon the myocardial activity. This irregular superimposition makes it difficult to judge areas of significant alterations in myocardial tracer uptake. One of the most interesting and most widely applied background correction techniques has been the interpolative method originally developed by Goris *et al.* [80]. Many variations and modifications of the original concept have been devised and are marketed commercially. The underlying principle is similar in all. The operator defines a border zone, typically a rectangle or ellipse surrounding the myocardium (Figure 16). The computer algorithm measures activity along the edges of this region and uses this to predict background activity on a pixel-by-pixel basis within the region of interest. This assumes a fairly continuous distribution of background activity from that outside the region to that within the region. Since one edge of the region

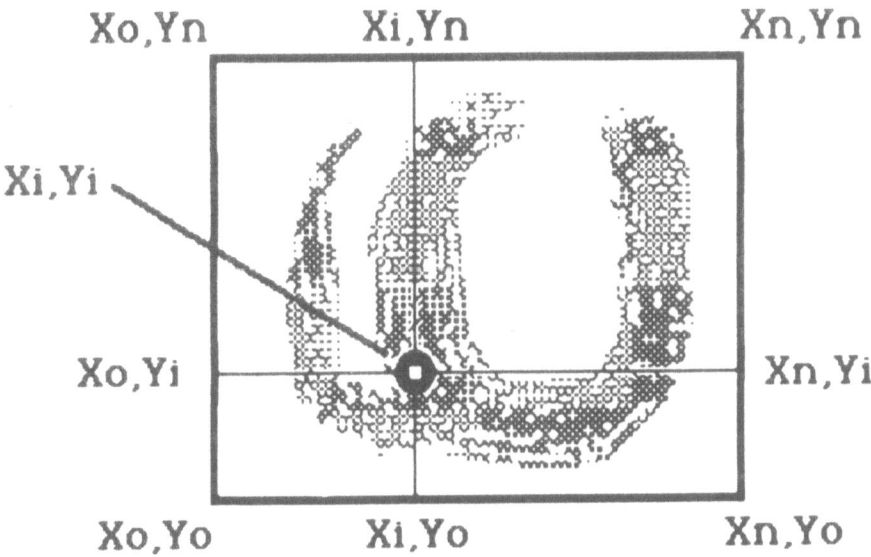

Figure 16. Interpolative background subtraction. The operator defines a border region (typically rectangular or elliptical) enclosing the myocardium. 'Background' activity to be subtracted from each pixel within is determined by that pixel's distance from pixels at the edge of the region and the relative intensity of those edge pixels. Thus, for any pixel (X_i, Y_i) within the region, a value interpolated from activity in the boundary pixels along both horizontal and vertical axes is subtracted. In this manner, the value subtracted from X_i, Y_i is a smooth function of the distance of that pixel from the boundary pixels and the relative intensity of these boundary pixels.

of interest may show significantly more background activity than another the interpolative technique will subtract the most 'background' activity from those pixels within the region closest to the 'hot' edge and will substract less and less background as it moves towards the 'cooler' opposite side of the region. Various modification of the technique have allowed for linear or non-linear interpolation of background from one edge to the next [81]. Some techniques have compared edges across only one axis usually the horizontal axis of the region of interest while other techniques interpolate in both the horizontal and the vertical directions simultaneously. This technique has gained wide acceptance and, while it is unlikely to represent perfection in background subtraction, is generally felt to provide reasonable results with introduction of a minimum of artifact.

Quantitative analysis

Since it is the relative intensity of tracer uptake by the myocardium, rather than its exact spatial distribution which is of most interest in evaluating thallium myocardial perfusion images, quantitative techniques for analysis of tracer uptake have been widely proposed and applied [86]. One technique, proposed by Beller, Watson *et al.* [82] and widely used, has been that of drawing horizontal profiles

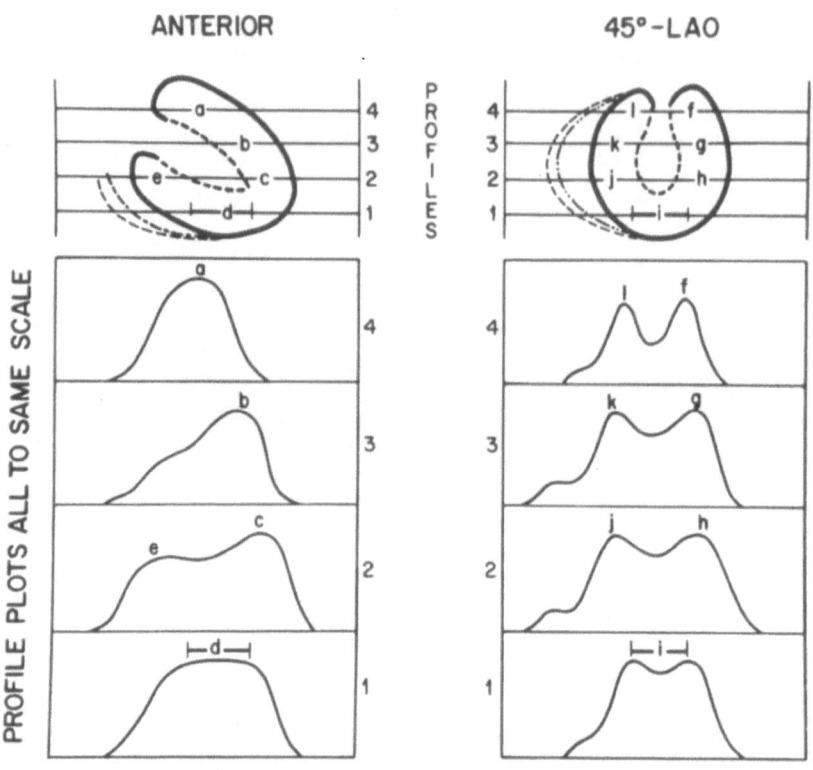

Figure 17. Horizontal profiles drawn through thallium images. This technique may be useful in detecting subtle asymmetry of uptake between opposing walls of the heart.

(Figure 17). A series of horizontal lines or profiles are drawn through the computer image such that they cross opposite myocardial walls. The relative intensity of activity along this profile is plotted on a two-dimensional graph. This simplifies comparison of activity at various levels along a myocardial wall and, especially, comparison of activity in opposite walls. It does not, however, provide absolute quantitation and the relative normal patterns for horizontal profiles through multiple views must at the present time be memorized by the observer and applied subjectively.

An interesting and widely used technique is that of the circumferential profile [83, 84]. This approach is basically a radial transformation of the image data. The operator defines the center of the left ventricle and some arbitrary limits enclosing the heart. The computer algorithm then proceeds to search outward from the center along a series of rays, typically at 6–10° angles. The region of greatest image intensity or tracer activity along each ray is noted. When a full 360° of radii have been constructed, the computer plots the activity on a horizontal display as shown in Figure 18. The horizontal axis of such a display represents the angle of each

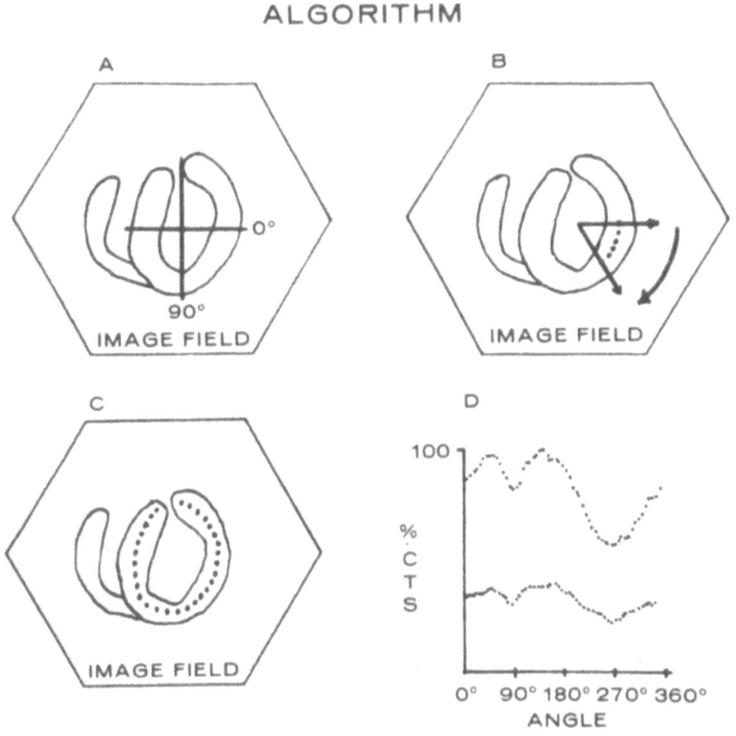

ALGORITHM

Figure 18. The circumferential profile approach to quantitation of thallium activity. The computer calculates maximum activity along a number of radii extending 360° around an operator defined central point. The maximum activity along each ray is then plotted.

radius in degrees such that by moving along this horizontal plot, one may see the maximum activity at each radius along the full 360° circumference of the image. The vertical axis of such a plot represents the intensity or activity of that particular radius. This technique is appealing in that it provides an objective approach to interpretation which is almost completely automated. Several groups have defined normal limits for maximum and minimum uptake at each point along the circumference [85]. By overlaying the circumferential curve with a plot of the previously defined normal limits, it may be readily seen whether uptake in any region of the heart falls outside of limits for that view. This technique has won some general acceptance and has been shown to provide a significant improvement in sensitivity and specificity for the detection of coronary artery disease when compared to subjective visual interpretation [87]. The circumferential profile technique is often combined with interpolative background subtraction. Many centers, perform circumferential activity calculations on both initial and delayed images and display these side-by-side or in a superimposed fashion [87]. This allows determination of the relative rate of washout at each region along the circumference of myocardium and may thus give a feel for the presence of 'redistribution' or delayed washout in any region or regions.

While it is quite conceivable that the circumferential profile technique will become the quantitative technique of choice in the near future, many centers at present have had difficulty in implementing the technique, frequently due to failure of various commercial algorithms to adequately track the myocardial circumference.

Tomographic thallium imaging

The preceeding discussion has brought out a number of the problems associated with planar imaging of the heart. One of the most severe such limitations is that of foreground and background activity. Another limitation is the superimposition of cardiac structures in any given view. To help alleviate both of these problems, single photon emission tomography has been applied to thallium perfusion imaging. A number of techniques have been proposed, most notably the 7-pinhole technique of Vogel *et al.* and the rotating slant hole collimator technique [88–90]. At the present time, the standard method of choice is generally felt to be the rotating gamma camera technique [91–93]. This technique involves a gamma camera similar to those described previously. The camera is, however, mounted on a stand which permits it to rotate around the patient under exact computer guidance and to stop at predetermined positions to acquire images. Images of the heart are obtained from multiple views, typically 64 or 128 views over 180° of arc. These views provide a number of two-dimensional projections of the three-dimensional structure of the heart. Using computer algorithms similar to those used in transmission computed tomography, a three-dimensional matrix containing the reconstructed three-dimensional districution of thallium activity in the chest is formed. Two-dimensional 'slices' of this three-dimensional matrix may be viewed to given effects similar to that of X-ray computed tomography. In this case, however, the image is composed of virtually only myocardial activity. Background activity is eliminated and all overlying or underlying structures have been removed. Most groups have reported tomography yielding much greater accuracy than planar imaging [93, 94].

Tomography may be further enhanced by use of so-called 'oblique angle reconstruction' techniques. Using these techniques, the data in the three-dimensional matrix of reconstructed activity is re-sorted in such a manner as to effectively realign the slices relative to the heart [95]. This process allows one to view 'slices' through the heart at any angle desired. Most typically, short axis cuts of the left ventricle are obtained similar to those used in two-dimensional echocardiography (Figures 19 and 20). Additional views are often obtained with orientation along the axis of the individual patient's heart, typically horizontal and vertical long axis views. This technique offers the very real advantage of giving comparible views for each patient's heart, regardless of the angulation of the

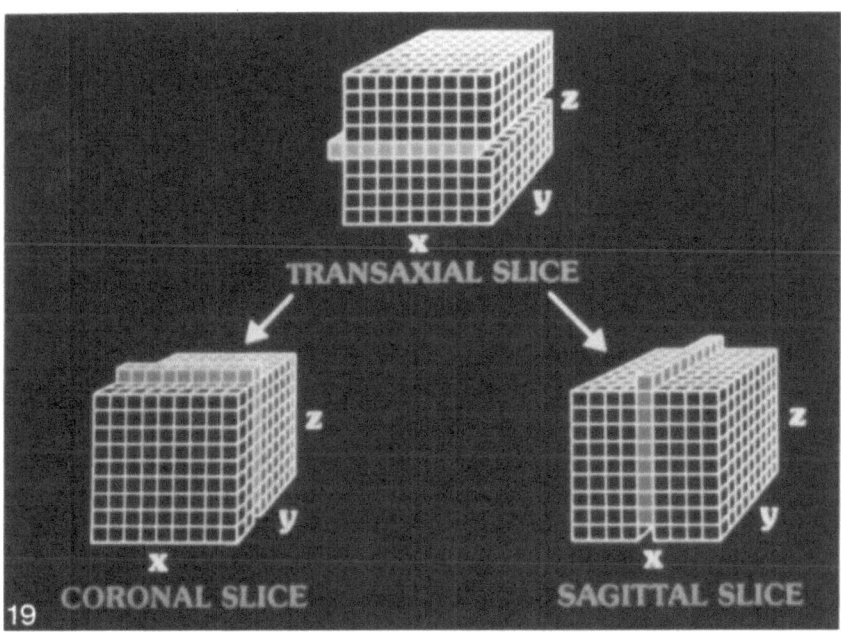

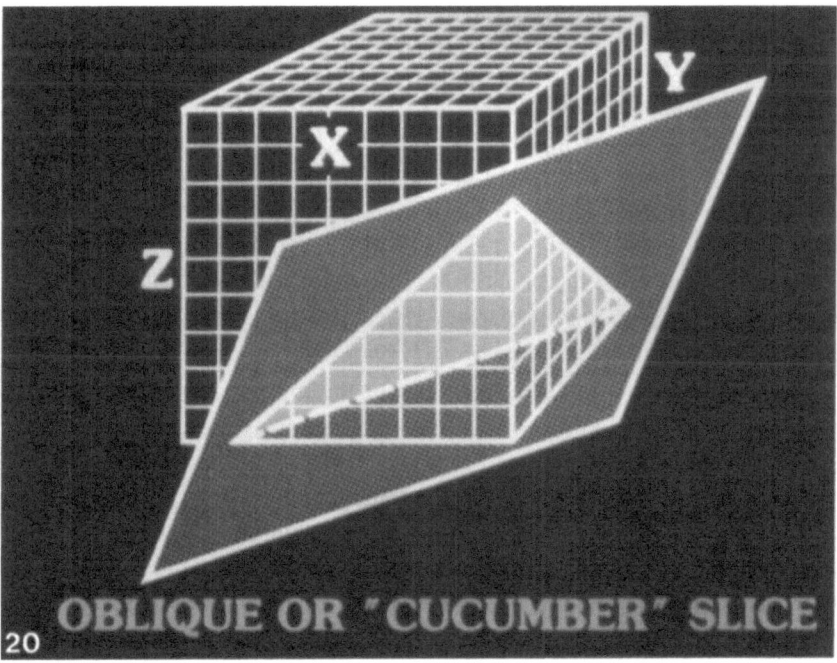

Figures 19 and 20. By resorting three-dimensional image matrix data, oblique angle 'slices' may be obtained through any axis of the heart.

heart in a given patient's chest. Thus, oblique angle reconstruction permits images of the heart from every patient in equivalent views and thus permits more accurate comparisons of identical regions of the heart from patient to patient and from a given patient to collected sets of normals.

The circumferential profile technique of quantitation has been applied to short axis tomographic slices with some success. The exact role of quantification in tomographic thallium imaging remains to be fully determined. Due to the intrinsic capability of tomography to remove foreground and background structure, no background subtraction, interprolative or otherwise, is required.

Tomographic thallium images have been combined with other image modalities to give even further information. For example, following acquisition of thallium tomographic images, a patient may have their red cells labeled with technetium-99 m and a tomographic gated blood pool image may be obtained demonstrating the full three-dimensional structure of the cardiac chambers both in diastole and systole [96]. These images may be then superimposed on the equivalent tomographic thallium slices to give a simultaneous feel for sectional anatomy, perfusion and contraction. Tomographic thallium images have also been performed in conjunction with technetium pyrophosphate images [97]. Technetium pyrophosphate is a tracer which is accumulated in areas of myocardial infarction. There is no accumulation in normal myocardium. By combining tomographic images of thallium which will show a cold defect in the region of an infarct with the 'hot spot' imaging of technetium pyrophosphate, it is possible to both delineate the zone of hypoperfusion surrounding an infarct as well as identify and measure the area of infarction.

Keyes and others [98, 99] have demonstrated that it is possible to accurately quantitate the area and mass of infarction and a presumably, ischemia, by computerized planimetry of multiple tomographic thallium sections. By determining the total volume of perfused functional myocardium from a thallium image and using two-dimensional echo techniques to determine the total mass of myocardium (both viable and non-viable) and then subtracting the volume determined by thallium tomography from that determined by echocardiography, accurate measurements of hypoperfused volume have been obtained in animals [99]. Such techniques hold great promise for the future both in terms of quantification of infarction size but also in terms of quantifying regions of myocardium at risk and defining a mass of myocardium which is potentially salvagable by revascularization techniques such as coronary artery bypass grafting or percutaneous transluminal coronary angioplasty. In addition, such techniques offer promise of quantitating the results of these interventions.

Perfusion imaging has been attempted using a number of other agents besides thallium. The ideal agent would have a higher imaging energy and better dosimetric calculations permitting one to give greater amounts of activity and thus obtain images of greater statistical accuracy. A number of technetium labeled alternatives have been proposed in recent years. Perhaps the best well-known of these is technetium-99m-DMPE. This agent showed dramatic myocardial uptake in certain animals which was shown to be linearly related to blood flow. Unfortunately, this and many similar agents have shown great species specificity and have not produced adequate images in man. Nonetheless, an ongoing search is underway at many radiopharmaceutical companies as well as university centers to provide a technetium labeled alternative to thallium-201.

Conclusion

The field of nuclear cardiology is rapidly changing. Steadily increasing clinical reliance has been placed on the standard imaging techniques of gated blood pool ventriculography and thallium-201 perfusion imaging. Blood pool imaging has been broadened and expanded into detailed analysis of diastolic function and regional ventricular function. It has also proved useful in determining ventricular volumes and cardiac outputs. New short-lived tracers such as gold-198 and Krypton-81, while still quite experimental, may permit gated imaging of the right ventricle in isolation without requiring special multicrystal cameras. Perfusion imaging is undergoing a new renaissance with many advances in quantitative analysis and background subtraction as well as tomographic imaging.

The past decade has been an exciting one for nuclear cardiology. The next decade promises to be even more exciting with a consolidation of the ground already gained and a more wide-spread application of the many alternative techniques recently explored.

Acknowledgements

Preparation of this manuscript was supported in part by NIH grant HL 29716.

References

1. Richardson RL: Anger scintillation camera: fundamentals of the scintillation camera. In: Rollo FD (ed.), nuclear medicine physics, instrumentation and agents. CV Mosby Company, St Louis, 1977, pp 233–268.
2. White W: Resolution, sensitivity, and contrast in gamma camera design: a critical review. Radiology 132: 179–187, 1979.
3. Bacharach SL, Green MV, Borer JS: Instrumentation and data processing in cardiovascular nuclear medicine: evaluation of ventricular function. Semin Nucl Med 9 (4): 257–274, 1979.
4. Johnson RF Jr: Operation and quality control of the recilinear scanner. In: Rollo FD (ed.), Nuclear medicine physics, instrumentation, and agents. CV Mosby Company, St Louis, 1977, pp 361–366.
5. Graham LS, Perez-Mendez V: Special imaging devices. In: Rollo FD (ed.), Nuclear medicine physics, instrumentation, and agents. CV Mosby Company, St Louis, 1977, pp 280–286.

234

6. Strauss HW, McKusick KA, Boucher CA, Bingham JB, Pohost GM: Of linens and laces – the eighth anniversary of the gated blood pool scan. Semin Nucl Med 9 (4): 296–309, 1979.
7. Thrall JH, Pitt B, Brady TH: Radionuclide wall motion study and ejection fraction in clinical practice. Med Clin North Am 64 (1): 99–117, 1980.
8. Berger *et al.*: Nuclear cardiology. New Engl J Med 10: 70–93, 1981.
9. Chervu LR: radiopharmaceuticals in cardiovascular nuclear medicine. Semin Nucl Med 9 (4): 241–256, 1979.
10. Thrall JH, Freitas JE, Swanson D, Rogers WL, Clare JM, Brown ML, Pitt B: Clinical comparison of cardiac blood pool visualization with technetium-99m red blood cells labeled *in vivo* and with technetium-99m human serum albumin. J Nucl Med 19: 797–803, 1978.
11. Liu XJ, Harrison KS, Douglass KH, Camargo EE, Wagner HN Jr: A simplified method for background correction in measurement of left ventricular ejection fraction. J Nucl Med 23 (5): 81, 1982.
12. Brady TJ, Thrall JH, Keyes JW Jr, Brymer JF, Walton JA, Pitt B: Segmental wall-motion analysis in the right anterior oblique projection: comparison of exercise equilibrium radionuclide ventriculography and exercise contrast ventriculography. J Nucl Med 21 (7): 617–621, 1980.
13. Groch MW, Lewis GK, Murphy PH *et al.*: Radionuclide kymography for the assessment of regional myocardial wall motion. J Nucl Med 19: 1131–1137, 1978.
14. Bacharach SL, Green MV, Borer JS, Ostrow HG, Bonow RO, Farkas SP, Johnston GS: Beat-by-beat validation of ECG gating. J Nucl Med 21: 307–313, 1980.
15. Douglas MA, Ostrow HG, Green MV *et al.*: A computer processing system for ECG-gated radioisotope angiography of the human heart. Comput Biomed Res 9: 133–142, 1976.
16. Green MV, Brody WR, Douglas MA *et al.*: Ejection fraction by count rate from gated images. J Nucl Med 19: 880–883, 1978.
17. Burow RD, Strauss HW, Singleton R *et al.*: Analysis of left ventricular function from multiple gated acquisition cardiac blood pool imaging: comparison to contrast angiography. Circulation 56: 1024–1028, 1977.
18. Brady TJ, Lo K, Thrall JH, Walton JA, Bryner JF, Pitt B: Exercise radionuclide ejection fraction: correlation with exercise contrast ventriculography. Radiology 132: 703–705, 1979.
19. Borer JS, Kent KM, Bacharach SL, Green MV, Rosing DR, Seides SF, Epstein SE, Johnston GS: Sensitivity, specificity and predictive accuracy of radionuclide cineangiography during exercise in patients with coronary artery disease. Circulation 60: 572, 1979.
20. Brady TJ, Thrall JH, Clare JM, Rogers WL, Lo K, Pitt B: Exercise radionuclide ventriculography: practical considerations and sensitivity of coronary artery disease detection. Radiology 132: 697–702, 1979.
21. Manyari DE, Kostuk WJ, Purves PP: Left and right ventricular function at rest and during bicycle exercise in the supine and sitting positions in normal subjects and patients with coronary artery disease: assessment by radionuclide ventriculography. Am J Cardiol 51: 36–42, 1983.
22. Sorensen SG, Caldwell J, Ritchie J, Hamilton G: 'Abnormal' responses of ejection fraction to exercise, in healthy subjects, caused by region-of-interest selection. J Nucl Med 22: 1–7, 1981.
23. Slutsky R, Battler A, Karliner JS, Froelicher V, Ashburn W: First-third ejection fraction at rest compared with exercise radionuclide angiography in assessing patients with coronary artery disease. Radiology 136: 197–201, 1980.
24. Yamashina A, Roistacher N, Friedman MI, Pierson RN Jr: First-third ejection fraction: are radionuclide measurements accurate? J Nucl Med 22 (6): 9, 1981.
25. Osbakken MD, Boucher CA, Okada RD, Bingham JB, Strauss W, Pohost GM: Spectrum of global left ventricular responses to supine exercise: limitation in the use of ejection fraction in identifying patients with coronary artery disease. Am J Cardiol 51: 28–35, 1983.
26. Okada RD, Boucher CA, Strauss HW, Pohost GM: Exercise radionuclide imaging approaches to coronary artery disease. Am J Cardiol 46: 1188–1204, 1980.

27. Currie PJ, Kelly MJ, Harper RW, Federman J, Kalff V, Anderson ST, Pitt A: Incremental value of clinical assessment, supine exercise electrocardiography, and biplane exercise radionuclide ventriculography in the prediction of coronary artery disease in men with chest pain. Am J Cardiol 52: 927–935, 1983.

28. Battler A, Slutsky R, Karliner J, Froelicher V, Ashburn W, Ross J Jr: Left ventricular ejection fraction and first-third ejection fraction early after acute myocardial infarction: value for predicting mortality and morbidity. Am J Cardiol 45 (2): 197–202, 1980.

29. Qureshi S, Wagner HN Jr, Alderson PO, Housholder DF, Douglass KH, Lotter MG, Nickoloff EL, Tanabe M, Knowles LG: Evaluation of left ventricular function in normal persons and patients with heart disease. J Nucl Med 19: 135–141, 1978.

30. Bonow RO, Bacharach SL, Green MV, Kent KM, Rosing DR, Lipson LC, Leon MB, Epstein SE: Impaired left ventricular diastolic filling in patients with coronary artery disease: assessment with radionuclide angiography. Circulation 64 (2): 315–323, 1981.

31. Reduto LA, Wickmeyer WJ, Young JB, DelVentura LA, Reid JW, Glaeser DH, Quinones MA, Miller RR: Left ventricular diastolic performance at rest and during exercise in patients with coronary artery disease. Circulation 63 (6): 1228–1237, 1981.

32. Polak JF, Kemper AJ, Bianco JA, Parisi AF, Tow DE: Resting early peak diastolic filling rate: a sensitive index of myocardial dysfunction in patients with coronary artery disease. J Nucl Med 23: 471–478, 1982.

33. Miller TR, Goldman KJ, Sampathkumaran KS, Biello DR, Ludbrook PA, Sobel BE: Analysis of cardiac diastolic function: application in coronary artery disease. J Nucl Med 24: 2–7, 1983.

34. Mancini GBJ, Slutsky RA, Norris SL, Bhargava V, Ashburn WL, Higgins CG: Radionuclide analysis of peak filling rate, filling fraction, and time to peak filling rate: response to supine bicycle exercise in normal subjects and patients with coronary disease. Am J Cardiol 51: 43–51, 1983.

35. Juni JE, Green MV, Goose PW, Bacharach SL, Bonow RO: Flow-volume loops in the evaluation of global ventricular function. J Nucl Med 23 (5): 67, 1982.

36. Bacharach SL, Green MV: Data processing in nuclear cardiology: measurement of ventricular function. IEEE Trans Nucl Sci NS 29 (4): 1343–1354, 1982.

37. Green MV, Juni JE, Goose PA, Bacharach SL: A method for surveying patient populations for differences in global left ventricular function. Proc of the 9th Intern Conf on Computers in Cardiol, 1982.

38. Green MV, Findley SL, Bonow RO, Bacharach SL, Juni JE: Left ventricular flow-volume relations in normal subjects and patients with heart disease. Proc of the 10th Intern Conf on Computers in Cardiol, 1983.

39. Maddox DE, Wynne J, Uren R et al.: Regional ejection fraction: a quantitative radionuclide index of regional left ventricular performance. Circulation 59: 1001–1009, 1979.

40. Bodenheimer MM, Banka VS, Fooshee CM et al.: Detection of coronary heart disease using radionuclide determined regional ejection fraction at rest and during handgrip exercise: correlation with coronary anteriography. Circulation 58: 640–647, 1978.

41. Papapietro SE, Yester MV, Logic JR et al.: Method for quantitative analysis of regional left ventricular function with first-pass and gated blood pool scintigraphy. Am J Cardiol 47: 618–625, 1981.

42. Vitale DF, Green MV, Bacharach SL, Bonow RO, Watson RM, Findley SL, Jones AE: Assessment of regional left ventricular function by sector analysis: a method for objective evaluation of radionuclide blood pool studies. Am J Cardiol 52: 1112–1119, 1983.

43. Machac J, Horowitz SF, Miceli K, Pollack B, Lee K, Goldman ME, Goldsmith SJ, Teichholz LE: Quantification of cardiac conduction abnormalities using segmental vector Fourier analysis of radionuclide gated blood pool scans. J Am Coll Cardiol 2 (6): 1099–1106, 1983.

44. Adam WE, Tarkowska A, Bitter F, Stauch M, Geffers H: Equilibrium (gated) radionuclide ventriculography. Cardiovasc Radiol 2: 161–173, 1979.

236

45. Botvinick E, Dunn R, Frais M, O'Connel W, Shosa D, Herkens R, Scheinman M: The phase image: its relationship to patterns of contraction and conduction. Circulation 65 (3): 551–560, 1982.

46. Cardot JC, Berthout P, Verdenet J, Bidet A, Faivre R, Bassand JP, Bidet R, Maurat JP: Temporal Fourier analysis applied to equilibrium radionuclide cineangiography: importance in the study of global and regional left ventricular wall motion. Eur J Nucl Med 7: 353–358, 1982.

47. Links JM, Douglass H, Wagner HN Jr: Patterns of ventricular emptying by Fourier analysis of gated blood pool studies. J Nucl Med 21: 978–982, 1980.

48. Frais MA, Botvinick EH, Shosa DW, O'Connell WJ, Schenman MM, Hattner RS, Morady F: Phase image characterization of ventricular contraction in left and right bundle branch block. Am J Cardiol 50: 95–105, 1982.

49. Chan WC, Kalff V, Dick M, Rabinovitch MA, Jenkins J, Thrall JH, Pitt B: Topography of pre-emptying ventricular segments in patients with Wolff-Parkinson-White syndrome using scintigraphic phase mapping and esophageal pacing. Circulation 67: 1145–1146, 1983.

50. Botvinick EH, Frais MA, Shosa DW, O'Connell JW, Pacheco-Alvarez JA, Scheinman M, Hattner RS, Morady F, Faulkner DB: An accurate means of detecting and characterizing abnormal patterns of ventricular activation by phase image analysis. Am J Cardiol 50: 289–298, 1982.

51. Turner DA, VonBehren PL, Ruggie NT, Hauser RG, Denes P, Ali A, Messer JV, Fordham EW, Groch MW: Non-invasive identification of initial site of abnormal ventricular activation by leastsquare phase analysis of radionuclide cineangiograms. Circulation 65 (7): 1511–1518, 1982.

52. Ratib O, Henze E, Schön H, Schelbert HR: Phase analysis of radionuclide ventriculograms for the detection of coronary artery disease. Am Heart J 104 (1): 1–12, 1982.

53. Swiryn S, Pavel D, Byrom E, Bauerfeind RA, Strasberg B, Palileo E, Lam W, Wyndham CRC, Rosen KM: Sequential regional phase mapping of radionuclide gated biventriculograms in patients with sustained ventricular tachycardia: close correlation with electrophysiologic characteristics. Am Heart J 103 (3): 319–332, 1982.

54. Schultz DA, Wahl RL, Juni JE, Buda AJ, McMeekin JD, Struble LR, Tuscan M: Diagnosis of exercise-induced left bundle branch block at rest by scintigraphic phase analysis. (In preparation)

55. Pavel DG, Byron E, Lam W, Meyer-Pavel C, Swiryn S, Pietras R: Detection and quantification of regional wall motion abnormalities using phase analysis of equilibrium gated cardiac studies. Clin Nucl Med 8: 315–321, 1983.

56. Turner DA, Shima MA, Ruggie N, VonBehren PL, Jarosky MJ, Ali A, Groch MW, Messer JV, Fordham EW: Coronary artery disease: detection by phase analysis of rest/exercise radionuclide angiocardiograms. Radiology 148: 539–545, 1983.

57. Bacharach SL, Green MV, Bonow RO, De Graaf CN, Johnston GS: A method for objective evaluation of functional images. J Nucl Med 23: 285–290, 1982.

58. King MA, Doherty PW: Color-coded ejection fraction images for following regional function throughout the cardiac cycle. In: Esser PD (ed.), Functional mapping of organ systems and other computer topics, Symposium Proceedings. The Society of Nuclear Medicine, New York, 1981, pp 119–128.

59. Nakajima K, Bunko H, Tada A, Taki J, Tonami N, Hisada K, Misaki T, Iwa T: Phase analysis in the Wolff-Parkinson-White syndrome with surgically proven accessory conduction pathways: concise communication. J Nucl Med 25: 7–13, 1984.

60. Bacharach SL, Green MV, De Graaf CN, Van Rijk PT, Bonow RO, Johnston GS: Fourier phase distribution maps in the left ventricle: toward an understanding of what they mean. In: Esser PD (ed.), Functional mapping of organ systems and other computer topics. The Society of Nuclear Medicine, New York, 1981, pp 139–148.

61. Wendt RE, III, Murphy PH, Clark JW Jr, Burdine JA: Interpretation of multigated Fourier functional images. J Nucl Med 23: 715–724, 1982.

62. Bacharach SL, Green MV, Vitale D, White G, Douglas MA, Bonow RO, Larson SM: Optimum Fourier filtering of cardiac data: a minimum-error method. J Nucl Med 24: 1176–1184, 1983.

63. Mukai T, Tamaki N, Yonekura Y, Minato K, Morita R, Torizuka K: Optimum order harmonics of Fourier analysis in multigated blood pool studies. J Nucl Med 24 (5): 17, 1983.

64. Juni JE, Froelich J, McMeekin J, Bourdillon P, Rocchini A, Botti J, Buda A, Pitt B: Effects of heart rate variability on scintigraphic measurement of diastolic function. Circulation: III–246, 1983.

65. Botti J, Juni JE, Froelich J, Clare J: Approaches to arrythmia filtration in gated radionuclide ventriculograms. J Nucl Med Technol 11 (2): 90, 1983.

66. Adams R, Hine GJ, Zimmerman CD: Deadtime measurements in scintillation cameras under scatter conditions simulating quantitative nuclear cardiography. J Nucl Med 19: 538–544, 1978.

67. Sorenson JA: Deadtime characteristics of anger cameras. J Nucl Med 16: 284–288, 1975.

68. Sorenson JA, Phelps ME: Radionuclide imaging: other techniques and instruments. In: Physics in nuclear medicine. Grune & Stratton, Inc, New York, 1980, pp 313–315.

69. Kawana M, Krizek H, Porter J et al.: Use of [199]Tl as a potassium analog in scanning. J Nucl Med 11: 333, 1977.

70. Pitt B, Strauss HW: Clinical application of myocardial imaging with thallium-201. In: Strauss HW, Pitt B, James AE (ed.), Cardiovascular nuclear medicine. CV Mosby Company, St Louis, MO, 1979, pp 125–136.

71. Chu A, Murdock RH Jr, Cobb FR: Relation between regional distribution of thallium-201 and myocardial blood flow in normal, acutely ischemic, and infarcted myocardium. Am J Cardiol 50: 1141–1144, 1982.

72. Nielsen AP, Morris KG, Murdock R, Bruno FP, Cobb FR: Linear relationship between the distribution of thallium-201 and blood flow in ischemic and non-ischemic myocardium during exercise. Circulation 61 (4): 797–801, 1980.

73. Weich HF, Strauss HW, Pitt B: The extraction of thallium-201 by the myocardium. Circulation 56 (2): 188–191, 1977.

74. Grunwald AM, Watson DD, Holzgrefe HH Jr, Irving JF, Beller GA: Myocardial thallium-201 kinetics in normal and ischemic myocardium. Circulation 64 (3): 610–617, 1981.

75. Bergmann SR, Hack SN, Sobel BE: 'Redistribution' of myocardial thallium-201 without reperfusion: implications regarding absolute quantification of perfusion. Am J Cardiol 49: 1691–1698, 1982.

76. Sklar J, Kirch D, Johnson T, Hasegawa B, Peck S, Steele P: Slow late myocardial clearance of thallium: a characteristic phenomenon in coronary artery disease. Circulation 64 (7): 1504–1510, 1982.

77. Pohost GM, Alpert NM, Ingwall JS, Strauss HW: Thallium redistribution: mechanisms and clinical utility. Sem Nucl Med 10 (1): 70–93, 1980.

78. Okada RD, Boucher CA, Strauss HW, Pohost GM: Exercise radionuclide imaging approaches to coronary artery disease. Am J Cardiol 46: 1188–1204, 1980.

79. Kline RC: Myocardial perfusion imaging. In: Carey JE Jr, Kline RC, Keyes JW Jr (eds.), CRC Manual of nuclear medicine procedures, 4th edition. CRC Press, Inc, Boca Raton, FL, 1983, pp 22–23.

80. Goris ML, Daspit SG, McLaughlin P, Kriss JP: Interpolative background subtraction. J Nucl Med 17: 744, 1976.

81. Watson DD, Beller GA, Berger BC, Teates CD: Notes on the quantitation of sequential Tl-201 images. Software 6: 4, 1979.

82. Berger BC, Watson DD, Taylor GJ et al.: Quantitative thallium-201 exercise scintigraphy for detection of coronary artery disease. J Nucl Med 22: 585–593, 1981.

83. Meade RC, Bamrah VS, Horgan JD, Ruetz PP, Kronenwetter C, Yeh EL: Quantitative methods in the evaluation of thallium-201 myocardial perfusion images. J Nucl Med 19: 1175–1178, 1978.

238

84. Garcia E, Maddahi J, Berman D, Waxman A: Space/time quantitation of thallium-201 myocardial scintigraphy. J Nucl Med 22: 309–317, 1981.

85. VanTrain K, Garcia E, Berman D *et al.*: Normal limits for the quantitative analysis of stress thallium-201 myocardial scintigrams. J Nucl Med 24: 451, 1983.

86. Vogel RA: Quantitative aspects of myocardial perfusion imaging. Sem Nucl Med 10 (2): 146–156, 1980.

87. Maddahi J, Garcia EV, Berman DS, Waxman A, Swan HJC, Forrester J: Improved non-invasive assessment of coronary artery disease by quantitative analysis of regional stress myocardial distribution and washout of thallium-201. Circulation 64 (5): 924–935, 1981.

88. LeFree MT, Kirch VD, Steele PP: Seven-pinhole tomography – a technical description. J Nucl Med 22: 48–54, 1981.

89. Vogel RA, Kirch D, LeFree MT *et al.*: A new method of miltiplanar emission tomography using a seven-pinhole collimator and an anger scintillation camera. J Nucl Med 19: 648–654, 1978.

90. Rizi HR, Kline RC, Thrall JH *et al.*: Thallium-201 myocardial scintigraphy: a critical comparison of seven-pinhole tomography and conventional planar imaging. J Nucl Med 22: 493–499, 1981.

91. Gindi GR, Arendt J, Barrett HH, Chiu MY, Ervin A, Giles CL, Kujoory MA, Miller EL, Simpson RG: Thallium imaging with rotating slit apertures and rotating collimators. Med Phys 9 (3): 324–339, 1982.

92. Holman BL, Hill TC, Wynne J *et al.*: Single-photon transaxial emission computed tomography of the heart in normal subjects and in patients with infarction. J Nucl Med 20: 736–740, 1979.

93. Tamaki N, Mukai T, Ishii Y, Yonekura Y, Kambara H, Kawai C, Torizuka K: Clinical evaluation of thallium-201 emission myocardial tomography using a rotating gamma camera: comparison with seven-pinhole tomography. J Nucl Med 22: 849–855, 1981.

94. Kirsch CM, Doliwa R, Buell U, Roedler D: Detection of severe coronary heart disease with Tl-201: comparison of resting single photon emission tomography with invasive anteriography. J Nucl Med 24: 761–767, 1983.

95. Tamaki N, Yanekura Y, Minato K: Evaluation of non-transmural myocardial infarction by thallium single-photon emission CT. J Nucl Med 24: 18, 1983.

96. Tamaki N, Mukai T, Ishii Y, Yonekura Y, Yamamoto K, Kadota K, Kambara H, Kawai C, Torizuka K: Multiaxial tomography of heart chambers by gated blood pool emission computed tomography using a rotating gamma camera. Radiology 147: 547–554, 1983.

97. Burdine JA, Murphy PA, DePuey EG: Radionuclide computed tomography of the body using routine radiopharmaceuticals. II. Clinical applications. J Nucl Med 20: 108–114, 1979.

98. Keyes JW Jr, Brady TJ, Leonard PF, Svetkoff DB, Winter SM, Rogers WL, Rose EA: Calculation of viable and infarcted myocardial mass from thallium-201 tomograms. J Nucl Med 22: 339–343, 1981.

99. Weiss RJ, Buda AJ, Pasyk S, O'Neill WW, Keyes JW Jr, Pitt B: Non-invasive quantification of jeopardized myocardial mass in dogs using two-dimensional echocardiography and thallium-201 tomography. Am J Cardiol 52 (10): 1340–1344, 1983.

100. Galen RS: Predictive value of laboratory tests. Am J Cardiol 36: 536, 1975.

101. Karliner JS, Bouchard RJ, Gault JH: Hemodynamic effects of angiographic contrast material in man. Brit Heart J 34: 347–352, 1972.

102. Schelbert HR, Verba JW, Johnson AD, Brock GW, Alazraki NP, Rose FJ, Ashburn WL: Non-traumatic determination of left ventricular ejection fraction by radionuclide angiocardiography. Circulation 51: 902, 1975.

103. Massie BM, Kramer BL, Gertz EW, Henderson SG: Radionuclide measurement of left ventricular volume: comparison of geometric and count-based methods. Circulation 65 (4): 725–730, 1982.

104. Sandler H, Doge HT: The use of single plane angiocardiograms for the calculation of left ventricular volume in man. Am Heart J 75 (3): 325–334, 1968.

105. Dodge HT, Sandler H, Ballew DW, Lord JD Jr: The use of biplane angiocardiography for the measurement of left ventricular volume in man. Am Heart J 69 (5): 762–776, 1960.

106. Dumesnil JG, Shoucri RM: Effect of the geometry of the left ventricle on the calculation of ejection fraction. Circulation 65 (1): 91–98, 1982.

107. Slutsky R, Karliner J, Ricci D, Kaiser R, Pfisterer M, Gordon D, Peterson K, Ashburn W: Left ventricular volumes by gated equilibrium radionuclide angiography: a new method. Circulation 60: 293, 1980.

108. Dehmer GJ, Lewis SE, Hillis LD, Twieg D, Falkooff M, Parkey RW, Willerson JT: Non-geometric determination of left ventricular volumes from equilibrium blood pool scans. Am J Cardiol 45: 293, 1980.

109. Links JM, Becker LC, Shindledecker G, Guzman P, Burow RD, Nickoloff EL, Alderson PO, Wagner HN: Measurement of absolute left ventricular volume from gated blood pool studies. Circulation 65 (1): 82–90, 1982.

110. Rabinovitch MA, Kalff V, Koral K, Chan W, Juni JE, Lerman B, Lampman R, Walton J, Grassley D, Vogel RA, Pitt B, Thrall JH: Count-based left ventricular volume determination utilizing a left posterior oblique view for attenuation correction. Radiology 150 (3): 813–818, 1984.

111. Starling MR, Dell'Italia LJ, Walsh RA, Little WC, Benedetto Ar, Nusynowitz ML, Heyl B: Accurate estimates of absolute left ventricular volumes from equilibrium radionuclide angiographic count data using a simple geometric attenuation correction. J Am Coll Cardiol 3 (3): 789–798, 1984.

112. Nickoloff EL, Pherman WH, Esser PD, Bashist B, Alderson PO: Physical basis for attenuation corrections in radionuclide determination of left ventricular volume. Radiology (in press).

113. Harp G, Williams D, Ritchie JL: Left ventricular volume determination utilizing gated blood pool tomography. J Am Coll Cardiol 3 (2): 589, 1984.

114. Corbett JR, Jansen DE, Lewis SE, Wolfe C, Nicod P, Redish GR, Gabilani G, Filipchuk N, Willerson JT: Gated blood pool transaxial tomography: left ventricular volumes and ejection fraction. J Am Coll Cardiol 3 (2): 590, 1984.

115. Ackermann R, Tuscan M, Juni JE, Bean LC, McMeekin J, Wahl R: Technical considerations for gated tomographic blood pool imaging. J Nucl Med Technol 12 (2): 97, 1984.

14. Positron emission computed tomography

MALEAH GROVER and HEINRICH R. SCHELBERT

Introduction

Regional myocardial blood flow and substrate metabolism can be non-invasively evaluated and quantified with positron emission computed tomography (Positron-CT). Tracers of exogenous glucose utilization and fatty acid metabolism are available and have been extensively tested. Specific tracer kinetic models have been developed or are being tested so that glucose and fatty acid metabolism can be measured quantitatively by Positron-CT [1, 2]. Tracers of amino acid and oxygen metabolism are utilized in Positron-CT studies of the brain [3] and development of such tracers for cardiac studies are in progress [4]. Methods to quantify regional myocardial blood flow are also being developed [5]. Previous studies have demonstrated the ability of Positron-CT to document myocardial infarction [6, 7]. Experimental and clinical studies have begun to identify metabolic markers of reversibly ischemic myocardium [8, 9]. The potential of Positron-CT to reliably detect potentially salvageable myocardium and, hence, to identify appropriate therapeutic interventions is one of the most exciting applications of the technique.

Brief review of instrumentation and radiopharmaceuticals

Instrumentation

The physics and instrumentation of conventional nuclear medicine have been described in chapter 13. A brief review of the physics and instrumentation of Positron-CT will be presented here. In-depth discussions of these topics have been published previously [10–12]. Positron emitting isotopes are produced with a cyclotron which accelerates positive ions, usually protons or deuterons, to bombard a non-radioactive target. The positive ion combines with the target and a neutron is usually emitted leaving residual proton-rich unstable nuclei. These nuclei can return to stability by emitting an energetic positive electron or positron. The positron is slowed by collisions with electrons and will finally combine with an electron converting its mass into electromagnetic energy in a process called annihilation. The energy is emitted in the form of two gamma rays, each with an energy of 511 keV which leave the site of interaction at 180 degrees from each other. This annihilation event can be identified by the simultaneous or coincidence detection of the two photons in two separate detectors. In the actual imaging system, many coincidence detectors are placed in a ring about the patient providing a data set consisting of a large number of views as a function of angle about the patient (Figure 1). The data are processed mathematically to solve for the amount of positron emitters at each position in the cross-section being viewed by the tomograph and the result is displayed as an image. This process is similar to that of conventional radiographic computed tomography except instead of using an external source of radiation, the source is internal from the injected positron-emitting isotope. Thus, a Positron-CT image represents the cross-sectional distribution of tracer concentration and thereby enables non-invasive analysis of local biochemical reaction rates and substrate fluxes rather than simply delineating anatomy.

Radiopharmaceuticals

The most important positron-emitting radioisotopes used in biologic studies are Rb-82 (halflife 75 s), O-15 (halflife 2 min), N-13 (halflife 10 min), C-11 (halflife 20 min) and F-18 (halflife 110 min) [13] (Table 1). Rubidium-82, which unlike the other positron-emitting radioisotopes mentioned is obtained by continuous elution from a Sr-82/Rb-82 generator, has been used to measure regional myocardial blood flow (RMBF) [14, 15]. Water which has been labeled with O-15 and ammonia which has been labeled with N-13 have also been used to measure RMBF. Palmitic acid has been labeled with C-11 (CPA) and utilized to investigate free fatty acid (FFA) metabolism. Deoxyglucose has been labeled with F-18 (FDG) and utilized to investigate exogenous glucose uptake. A tracer kinetic model for FDG has been developed [1, 16, 17] and validated [18–20]. An initial tracer kinetic model has been developed for CPA but awaits further validation [2].

Measurement of regional myocardial blood flow

N-13 ammonia

N-13 ammonia was initially used with Positron-CT by Phelps *et al.* [21] to image cerebral and myocardial blood flow. Rapid clearance of the tracer from the blood and high myocardial extraction (nearly 100%) and retention (82%) [22] result in

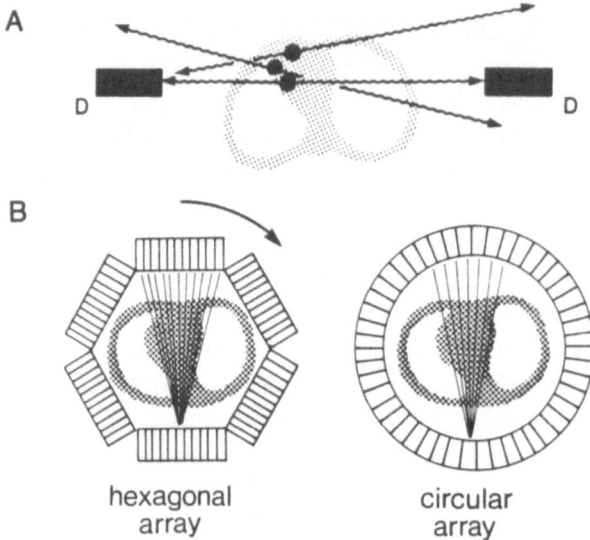

Figure 1. (A) Schematic representation of annihilation coincidence detection. When a positron interacts with an electron, the combined mass is converted into two 511 keV gamma rays which leave the site of interaction at an angle of 180°. If two opposing scintillation detectors, D, record coincident events, this is regarded as a true event. If only one of a pair of detectors records an event, this is regarded as being a random event. (B) In order to record all true events, opposing banks of detectors are placed in 360° around the object to be imaged. Every detector has a fan beam response as shown.

Table 1. List of positron-emitting radioisotopes discussed

Name	Halflife	Administered dose (mCi)[a]	Maximum absorbed dose (rads)[b]	
Blood flow				
Rubidium-82	75 s	120	Whole body	0.15
			Kidneys	2.16
O-15 Water	2 min	30	Whole body	0.05
			Lung	0.28
N-13 ammonia	10 min	20	Whole body	0.02
			Lung	1.67
Fatty acid metabolism				
C-11 palmitic acid	20 min	20	Whole body	0.24
			Liver	1.10
Glucose metabolism				
F-18 deoxyglucose	110 min	10	Whole body	0.06
			Heart	1.98

[a] This is the maximum dose allowed; usually the dose is smaller.
[b] This is calculated for the maximum allowable dose and represents the dose to the whole body and critical organ.

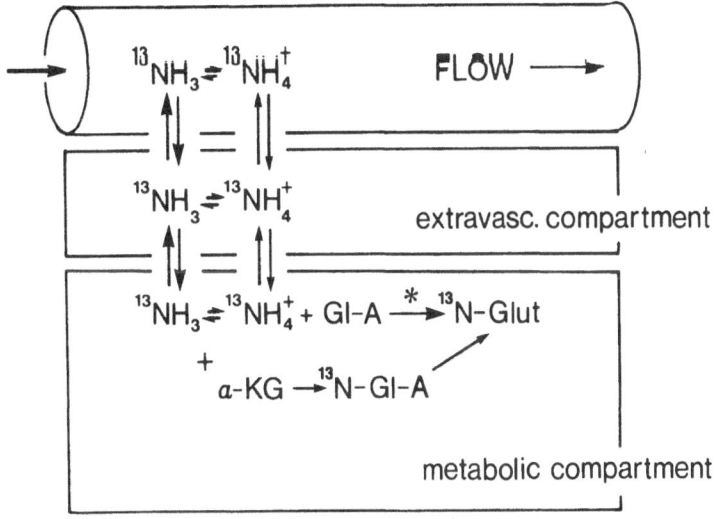

Figure 2. Proposed model for the uptake and retention of N-13 ammonia in myocardial cells. Nearly 100% of the tracer is extracted and back diffusion competes with metabolic trapping. The glutamic acid-glutamine and to a lesser extent, the ketoglutamate-glutamic acid reactions appear to be the primary trapping mechanisms. Gl-A = glutamic acid; Glut = glutamine; a-KG = a-ketoglutarate. (From Schelbert *et al.* [22], Figure 12, p 1268.)

high contrast cross-sectional images of the heart. Retention of N-13 ammonia in myocardium is reduced by inhibition of glutamate synthetase which implicates the glutamic acid-glutamine reaction as the primary mechanism for metabolic trapping of N-13 ammonia in cardiac muscle (Figure 2) [22–24]. Acute hemodynamic and metabolic interventions in experimental preparations have little effect on the initial myocardial extraction with the exception of low plasma pH and acute myocardial ischemia. Whether chronic alterations such as ischemia and myopathic diseases in patients will affect the relationship between myocardial N-13 ammonia extraction and regional blood flow awaits further investigation.

Rubidium-82 (Rb-82)

The single capillary transit extraction fraction of rubidium-82 exceeds 50% [25]. The tracer distributes in myocardium in proportion to blood flow. Rb-82 has two advantages over other positron-emiting tracers of blood flow. First, it is obtained from a Sr-82/Rb-82 generator, which obviates the need for an on-site cyclotron. Second, its short halflife (75 s) permits serial studies at short time intervals. For example, after obtaining a baseline flow study, an intervention to alter blood flow such as exercise or administration of a drug can be made and a second study done within 10 min. The disadvantage of the short physical halflife is that high efficiency tomographs are needed for obtaining statistically adequate images.

Initial measurements of net regional tissue uptake of Rb-82 for a given blood flow in relation to the total amount of Rb-82 (infused at a constant rate until equilibrium is achieved [14] reflect directional changes in regional myocardial blood flow as measured by microspheres [15]. Another approach for determining the 'extraction fraction' at a given flow and a tracer kinetic model for external measurement of regional myocardial blood flow with intravenous bolus administration of Rb-82 and beta probe imaging have been proposed by Mullani *et al.* [26–28].

Normal myocardial metabolism

Human myocardium prefers free fatty acids (FFA) over other substrates, a widely accepted notion previously established in human volunteers [29, 30]. However, myocardial substrate utilization at any given time largely depends upon substrate concentrations in arterial blood [31, 32]. Plasma substrate concentrations are highly variable and are affected by diet, physical activity and the endocrine state. For example, after moderate fasting, plasma FFA levels are high and the heart primarily relies on FFA for meeting its energy requirements. The fact that the heart's substrate metabolism was studied in human volunteers during cardiac catheterization which is usually performed after an overnight fast, when plasma FFA levels are high, may have lead to the notion of the human heart's preference for FFA over other substrates.

Positron-CT allows the non-invasive study of regional myocardial substrate metabolism without stringent dietary requirements. Studies can be performed after an overnight fast as well as after specific dietary interventions in order to examine their effects on the heart's substrate metabolism. An initial Positron-CT study in dogs demonstrated the dependence of myocardial substrate metabolism on plasma substrate concentrations [33]. Utilization of glucose and FFA was markedly altered when plasma substrate concentrations were changed in spite of similar myocardial oxygen consumption. These observations were also confirmed in healthy volunteers and in patients [34–36]. In the fasted state, preferential use of FFA was demonstrated with C-11 palmitic acid while oral glucose administration markedly altered plasma substrate concentrations and shifted the heart's substrate metabolism from FFA to glucose. As indicated in Figure 3, these changes were demonstrated non-invasively with Positron-CT using C-11 palmitic acid and FDG as tracers of myocardial FFA metabolism and exogenous glucose utilization, respectively.

Free fatty acid metabolism C-11 palmitic acid and the tracer kinetic model

Under most normal conditions the human heart uses several substrates simultaneously but preferentially metabolizes free fatty acids (FFA) [29, 30, 37, 38]. In fasting humans, the steady state extraction fraction for all FFA is 28% [39].

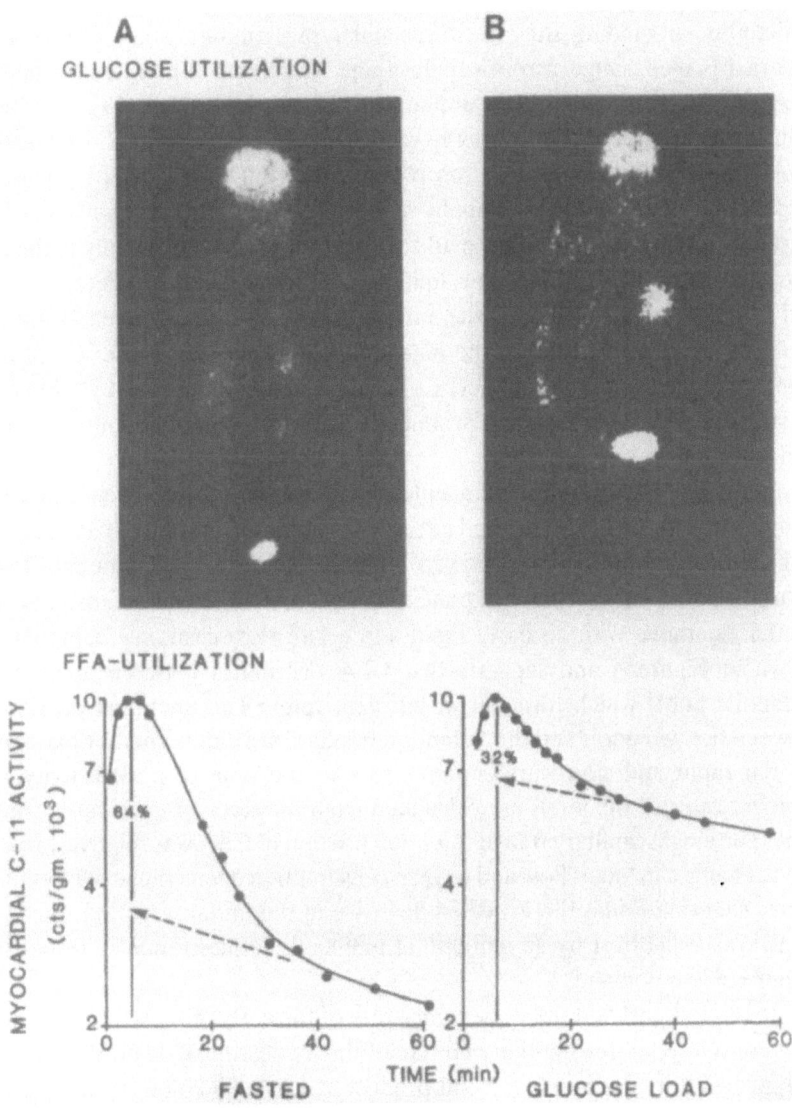

Figure 3. Myocardial C-11 tissue clearance curves obtained after serial PCT imaging following intravenous administration of C-11 palmitic acid. The curve on the left was obtained after an overnight fast and exhibits the typical biphasic clearance pattern with 64% entering the pool which is immediately oxidized and 39% entering the pool which is stored as endogenous lipids. The curve on the right was obtained after the oral ingestion of glucose. The early rapid clearance phase is decreased to 32% despite a similar heart rate and blood pressure indicating a change in myocardial substrate utilization.

Individual FFA have different extraction fractions with long-chain fatty acids having higher extraction fractions than short-chain fatty acids [40, 41]. The concentration gradient of FFA between plasma and cytosol appears to be a primary determinant of myocardial FFA uptake. Albumin concentration and the availability of binding sites on intracellular proteins are other factors which govern FFA exchange across capillary and sarcolemmal membranes because FFA are reversibly bound to albumin in plasma. In cytosol, FFA are metabolically 'sequestered' by the energy-requiring conversion to acyl CoA since acyl CoA cannot diffuse back into the plasma from the myocyte [42] (Figure 4). Depending on myocardial metabolic requirements, FFA then enters one of two metabolic pathways. It is either oxidized or stored in the cell, mainly in the form of triglycerides in the endogenous lipid pool. Acyl CoA is immediately oxidized and combines with carnitine at the outer mitochondrial membrane to form acyl-carnitine which is shuttled to the inner mitochondrial membrane. Carnitine is then exchanged for CoA and acyl-CoA subsequently enters the beta oxidation spiral. Acetyl CoA, a 2-carbon product of beta oxidation, then enters the citric acid cycle.

Myocardial C-11 palmitic acid uptake and turnover have been extensively studied [43–48]. Intravascular and intracoronary administration of CPA results in high myocardial extraction followed immediately by a small amount of back diffusion and a subsequent biexponential clearance. The characteristic biexponential clearance with an early rapid and a late slow clearance component is shown in Figure 4 and suggests that CPA distributes between at least two metabolic pools which turnover at different rates. The fractional distribution between the two pools and the 'retention fraction' are determined by extrapolating the rapid and slow curve components to the time of peak activity. The turnover rates of the pools are calculated from the slope of each curve component. The single capillary transit retention fraction of CPA was relatively insensitive to changes in blood flow and oxygen consumption over a range of physiologic values suggesting that the expected decrease in the initial retention fraction at high flows was offset by an increase in metabolic sequestration in response to higher oxygen demands.

The relative size and tissue clearance rate of the early rapid clearance component are related to the amount and rate of the myocardial C-11 production. C-11 CO_2 production represents the end product of CPA oxidation, thus suggesting that the early rapid curve component corresponds to an oxidation pool which turns over rapidly, whereas the later slow curve component corresponds to incorporation of the labeled carbon into triglycerides in the endogenous lipid pool with subsequent slow metabolism. An initial tracer kinetic model has been established by Huang *et al.* [2] and accurately predicts directional changes in myocardial FFA consumption.

The myocardial extraction fraction, E, and the tissue kinetics of CPA have been investigated in dogs and humans with slightly different results, perhaps in

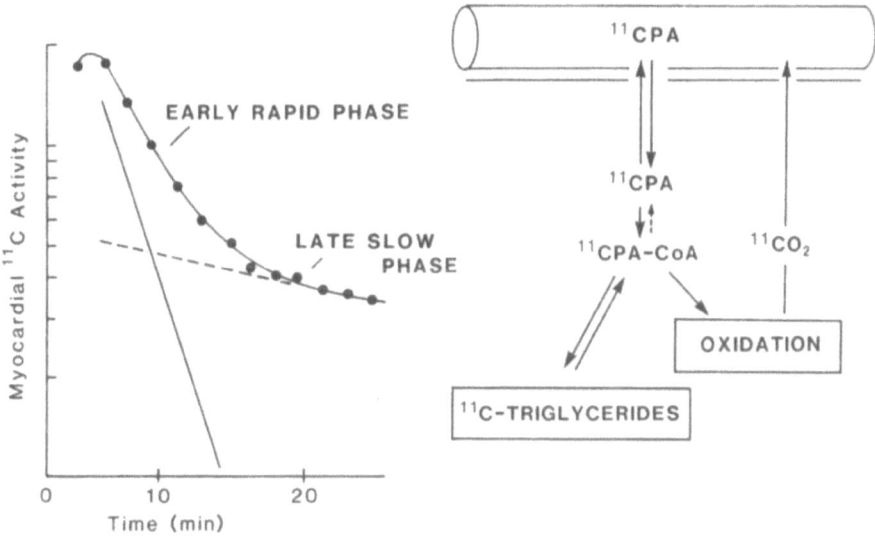

Figure 4. On the left is a schematic drawing of tissue clearance of C-11 activity from the myocardium following intravenous C-11 palmitic acid administration and serial PCT imaging. The time-activity curves were obtained from regions of interest assigned to the left ventricular myocardium and the left ventricular blood pool on the serial images. The data are corrected for partial volume effect and cross-contamination of activity between the blood pool and the myocardium. On the right is a schematic representation of the kinetics of C-11 palmitic acid in myocardium describing the exchange between plasma and the different tissue pools. The forward exchange from the cellular CPA to the CPA-CoA pool is virtually unidirectional. The CPA-CoA then enters oxidative and/or slow turnover pools. For details see text.

part due to differences in MVO_2 and its determinants such as heart rate and blood pressure during the experiments. In dogs studied after an overnight fast, E was calculated by the following equation:

$$E = \frac{[^{11}C_m]}{\int_0^t {}^{11}C_a \ t/dt \times F}$$

where $[^{11}C_m]$ is the peak myocardial C-11 concentration, $^{11}C_a$ the arterial C-11 concentration and F is the myocardial blood flow determined with radioactive gamma emitting microspheres by the arterial reference method [49]. Myocardial tissue clearance rates and fractional distribution of CPA were determined by exponential least square fitting of the myocardial C-11 time activity curves. E was 0.54 ± 0.25 SD with an average of 46.4% entering the rapid and 54.6% entering the slow turnover pool. The clearance halftimes were 3.0 ± 1.2 min for the rapid and 49.8 ± 25.9 min for the slow turnover phase.

In humans, blood C-11 activity curves were derived together with myocardial tissue clearance curves from serial images by assigning regions of interest to the left ventricular blood pool and myocardium. The characteristic biexponential clearance pattern of C-11 activity from myocardium was observed although the clearance halftimes were slower than in dogs as discussed above. Fifty percent of the extracted CPA entered the rapid turnover pool. If this pool reflects CPA oxidation, then these findings are similar to those of Most *et al.* [50] who studied fasted humans and recovered approximately 50% of C-14 palmitic acid as $^{14}CO_2$ in the coronary sinus blood which suggested immediate oxidation of this amount of the tracer. The 20 min physical halflife of C-11, the dose of radioactivity permissable in patients, and the efficiency of existing instrumentation limits the time for serial image acquisition. In humans the early rapid phase may not be completed until 20–25 min after tracer administration and the count rates during the late slow phase may be low so that biexponential curve fitting may be difficult. However, an index of the fraction of tracer undergoing immediate oxidation and its rate of oxidation can be obtained by dividing the product of the curve size and duration by the clearance halftime [35], an approach that allows assessment of the fractional tracer distribution in tissue and the relative size and halftime of the early rapid clearance phase.

Glucose metabolism, F-18 fluoro-2-deoxyglucose and the tracer kinetic model

Exogenous glucose utilization by the myocardium can be studied with F-18 2-fluoro 2-deoxyglucose (FDG). FDG competes with glucose for facilitated transport sites and for phosphorylation by hexokinase. After phosphorylation, the resultant compound, FDG-6-phosphate, is trapped in the myocardial cell because it is not a substrate for glycolysis or glycogen synthesis, dephosphorylation occurs slowly, and it has low membrane permeability (Figure 5).

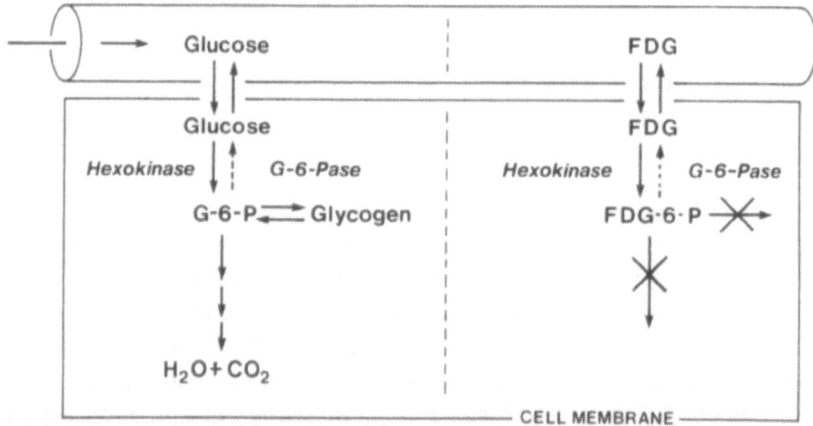

Figure 5. Comparison of plasma and tissue exchange and the initial metabolic step for glucose and FDG. G-6-P = glucose-6-phosphate; G-6-Pase = glucose-6-phosphatase. See text for details. (From Schelbert HR: 'The heart'. In: Bell PJ, Hollman BL (eds.), Computed emission tomography. Oxford University Press, New York, 1982, pp 91–133; Figure 3.7, p 155.)

A model was developed for estimating the rate of phosphorylation of exogenous glucose to FDG-6-phosphate [1, 16, 17]. External quantification of a single metabolic step which is representative for the substrate flux through a given pathway should allow measurement of the substrate flux. The model for FDG entails three compartments: a plasma compartment, a tissue compartment for glucose and FDG and a tissue compartment for FDG-6-phosphate. The model has been validated in the isolated arterially perfused rabbit septum [18] in isolated rabbit hearts perfused with blood [51] and in open chest dogs [20]. Further investigation is necessary to determine whether the model is applicable during clinically relevant conditions such as ischemia and in patients with metabolic derangements such as those present in diabetes and chronic renal failure.

Detection of coronary artery disease

Current non-invasive diagnostic techniques are limited in reliably detecting mild coronary stenoses (i.e. detection of disease prior to symptoms). Regional myocardial blood flow is often normal even when severe coronary stenoses are present. Interventions for testing the coronary flow reserve or provoking maldistribution of blood flow (e.g. exercise, atrial pacing, coronary vasodilation) are often required for diagnosis. Gould *et al.* [51] demonstrated that resting coronary blood flow did not decline until luminal narrowing of the coronary artery was more than 85% although the coronary flow reserve was attenuated with 50% luminal narrowing. The same investigators demonstrated that under highly idealized conditions, a 40% luminal stenosis could be detected if an optimum tracer of blood flow and an optimum imaging system were available. Detection of this degree of stenosis was almost achieved in chronically instrumented intact dogs; dipyridamole-induced coronary hyperemia, intravenous N-13 ammonia and Positron-CT cross-sectional imaging non-invasively identified a 47% stenosis [53].

Thirty-two patients with coronary artery disease documented by coronary arteriography and 13 healthy subjects were subsequently studied using the same protocol. A baseline Positron-CT study was obtained after intravenous injection of N-13 ammonia. A second Positron-CT study using N-13 ammonia was obtained after induction of coronary vasodilation with intravenous dipyridamole [54] (Figure 6). All 13 healthy subjects had homogeneous myocardial uptake of N-13 ammonia during basal conditions and after intravenous dipyridamole. During basal conditions in the patients with coronary artery disease, three patients demonstrated segmental reduction in N-13 ammonia uptake. One of these patients had a prior subendocardial myocardial infarction and the other two had high-grade coronary artery stenoses. After intravenous dipyridamole, 31 of the 32 patients developed new perfusion abnormalities (sensitivity 97%) resulting in the correct identification of 52 of the 58 (90%) stenosed vessels. The sensitivity of this technique was not significantly greater than stress thallium-201 scintigraphy in

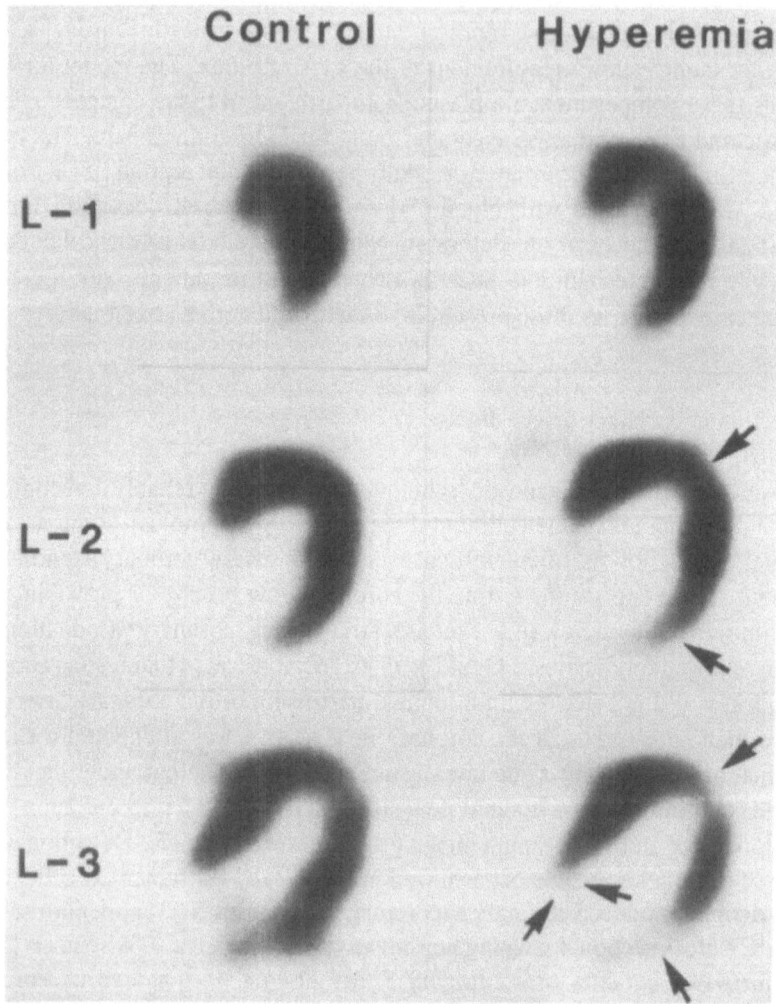

Control   Hyperemia

L-1

L-2

L-3

Figure 6. Control and hyperemic cross-sectional positron computed tomographic images of the myocardial N-13 ammonia distribution in a 67 year old woman with 100% stenosis of the proximal left anterior descending coronary artery. Level 1 (L-1) is recorded through the high anterior and lateral wall, level 2 (L-2) through the mid-left ventricle and level 3 (L-3) through the mid to lower left ventricle. The control images reveal uniform N-13 activity throughout the left ventricular myocardium suggesting adequate collateral blood flow to the anterior wall at rest. However, in the hyperemic images, N-13 activity was greatly reduced in the anterior wall. N-13 activity increased from rest to hyperemia by 32% in the lateral wall and by 40% in the interventricular septum but by only 13% in the anterior wall. The appearance of a defect in the hyperemic images therefore does not indicate a decrease in blood flow from the control state to hyperemia but an attenuated response to pharmacologic coronary vasodilation. (From Schelbert *et al.* [54].)

detecting the presence of coronary artery disease in patients but it was more accurate in identifying the number of stenosed coronary arteries. In fact, in three patients segmental perfusion defects were documented in regions supplied by coronary arteries with less than 50% cross-sectional narrowing. Therefore, this technique enhances the detection of the extent and functional significance of coronary artery stenoses.

Regional myocardial blood flow in myocardial ischemia

Selwyn *et al.* [15] examined regional myocardial blood flow with Rb-82 during supine exercise using the equilibrium infusion technique. Segments of decreased tracer uptake coincided with the site of ischemic electrocardiographic abnormalities. Interestingly, segmental reductions in Rb-82 uptake persisted even after symptoms and ECG abnormalities had resolved. However, no data were obtained about the presence or absence of wall motion abnormalities at the time of reduced Rb-82 uptake. Therefore, it is not certain whether the reduction in Rb-82 uptake is due to a reduction in blood flow or to a possible wall motion abnormality (partial volume effect) [55]. Transient segmental reductions in Rb-82 uptake also occurred spontaneously even in the absence of symptoms or ECG abnormalities [56]. Segmental defects in tracer uptake could also be induced in 10 of 14 patients by mental stress (the subjects were asked to perform simple arithemetic) in the same areas as the exercise-induced defects [57]. The regional abnormalities in tracer uptake could be abolished with nitrates.

These observations have several important clinical implications. Recovery of RMBF and/or regional wall motion abnormalities from transient regional ischemic episodes may be slower than suggested by relief of symptoms and resolution of electrocardiographic changes, a finding already demonstrated experimentally for regional wall motion abnormalities. In addition, transient segmental abnormalities of myocardial blood flow and/or metabolism may occur entirely asymptomatically and/or without electrocardiographic correlates. If these episodes truly represent 'silent ischemia', then silent ischemia may be much more common than previously suspected. Finally, the fact that uptake of Rb-82, which appears to represent blood flow, was decreased by the stress of mental arithmetic has profound implications on the potential effects of mental stress on regional myocardial blood flow. Whether segmental reductions in cation uptake (Rb is considered a potassium analog) may be responsible for these findings, as postulated by the investigators, needs further confirmation. When cross-sectional imaging is performed without ECG gated acquisition of data, regional wall motion abnormalities (i.e. absent or reduced systolic thickening) can cause artifactual segmental decreases in tissue tracer concentrations on tomographic images as a consequence of the partial volume effect [55, 58]. Therefore, prolonged recovery in segmental tracer uptake might represent a combination of reduced blood flow and abnormal wall motion rather than a primary defect in transmembraneous ion exchange.

Metabolic consequences of acute myocardial ischemia

Glucose metabolism during ischemia

The heart's ability to utilize different substrates as their levels change in plasma appears to be impaired during myocardial ischemia. Liedtke [59] defined beta oxidation as the locus most sensitive to oxgyen deprivation. In dog experiments, Opie *et al.* [60] have shown a decline in beta oxidation of FFA associated with an increase in glycolysis. Limited oxygen availability interferes with citric acid cycle activity and the electron transport chain. Pyruvate produced by anaerobic glycolysis is then unable to enter the citric acid cycle and is either converted to alanine or released as lactic acid. At this point, anaerobic glycolysis remains one of the few sources of ATP production. The hypothesis that Positron-CT could non-invasively demonstrate that acute myocardial ischemia resulted in an increase in exogenous glucose utilization associated with a decline in FFA oxidation was initially tested in dogs with a fixed LAD stenosis during rapid atrial pacing [61]. These studies demonstrated segmentally increased FDG uptake (either relative to the segmental decline in blood flow or in absolute terms), and for C-11 palmitate a decline in the size of the early rapid phase with delayed tracer clearance from tissue, observations consistent with impaired FFA oxidation and increased glycolytic flux.

Camici *et al.* [61] subsequently tested these findings in humans with coronary artery disease during and after exercise-induced ischemia. In seven patients with exercise-induced ECG abnormalities and/or angina, FDG uptake was increased in segments with reduced blood flow as demonstrated by Rb-82 imaging. The observation of increased FDG uptake and the presence of segmental defects in blood flow was subsequently defined as 'mismatch', a pattern that had also been noted earlier by Marshall *et al.* [19] in 15 patients with recent myocardial infarction (Figure 7). In Marshall's study, regions of 'mismatch' were more prevalent in patients with recurrent chest pain or transient electrocardiographic abnormalities than in patients with completed myocardial infarction in whom chest pain or electrocardiographic abnormalities no longer occurred. The mechanism(s) causing this 'mismatch' still need further elucidation. One possible explanation is that the area of 'mismatch' might represent demand-induced ischemia caused by a compensatory increase in function in segments supplied by diseased coronary arteries, while another explanation is that the 'mismatch' might reflect ischemia induced by a decrease in blood flow. In either case, the ischemic segment would only maintain metabolism by primarily using exogenous glucose. The observation that anaerobic metabolism of glucose is accelerated by coronary artery ligation has been demonstrated in dogs by Opie *et al.* [60].

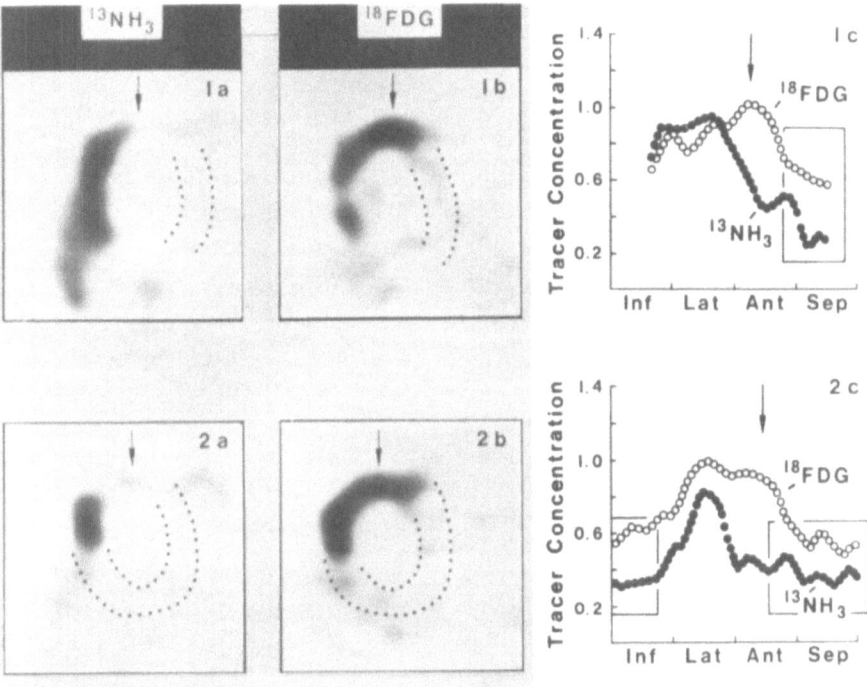

Figure 7. Positron computed tomography evaluation of regional perfusion (1a, 2a) and exogenous glucose utilization (1b, 2b) in a patient with a recent anterior and remote inferior infarction, refractory postinfarction angina and severe proximal three-vessel coronary artery disease. The first pair of cross-sectional images is through the body of the left ventricle and the second is through the apex. On the right are normalized FDG and N-13 ammonia tissue concentration curves generated from contiguous regions of interest with open and closed circles, respectively. Evaluation of regional perfusion alone in the N-13 ammonia image suggests that the entire anterior wall of the ventricle is infarcted. Evaluation of regional glucose utilization suggests that only the septum is infarcted (dotted lines in the first image) and that the anterior wall of the myocardium is ischemic (arrows). (From Marshall *et al.* [19].)

In patients with ischemic heart disease, Tillisch *et al.* [9] observed a similar pattern of 'mismatch'. In ten patients without angina at the time of the Positron-CT study, 23 segments demonstrated impaired wall motion. 'Mismatch' was present in 14 of these segments whereas blood flow and exogenous glucose utilization were both decreased in 9 segments (Figure 8). Interestingly, in 9 segments with electrocardiographic Q-waves and akinesis, 'mismatch' was noted in 4 segments while a concordant decrease in N-13 ammonia and FDG uptake was noted in 5 segments. These observations suggested the presence of a 'mismatch' between regional exogenous glucose uptake and blood flow. They implied the persistence of residual metabolic activity in myocardium with impaired function. This finding may aid in distinguishing ischemic but potentially salvageable myo-

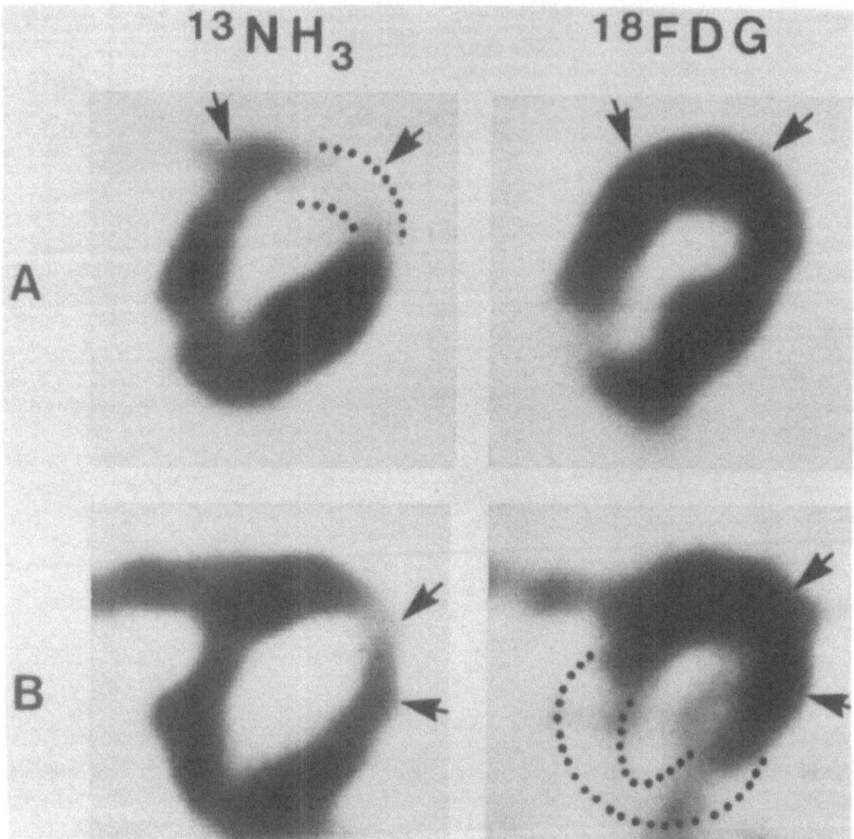

Figure 8. N-13 ammonia and PCT images obtained in two patients with ischemic heart disease who did *not* have angina during the Positron-CT study. (A) This patient had a normal ejection fraction. Increased FDG uptake relative to blood flow as demonstrated by ^{13}NH$_3$, i.e. 'mismatch' is seen in the distal septum and apex (arrows). (B) This patient had an ejection fraction of 20%. An area of 'mismatch' is seen in the apex and lateral wall (arrows).

cardium from irreversibly injured myocardium. The ability to document the presence or absence of salvageable myocardium will help tremendously in deciding on an appropriate therapeutic regimen and in assessing the results of therapy.

Free fatty acid metabolism during ischemia

During acute myocardial ischemia, myocardial uptake of C-11 palmitic acid (Figure 9) as well as its fractional distribution and clearance in tissue are altered (Figure 10). Blood flow is a major determinant of the net uptake of C-11 palmitic acid. In addition, during ischemia disproportionately more C-11 palmitic acid diffuses back into the vascular space [33, 48, 62] suggesting impairment of the

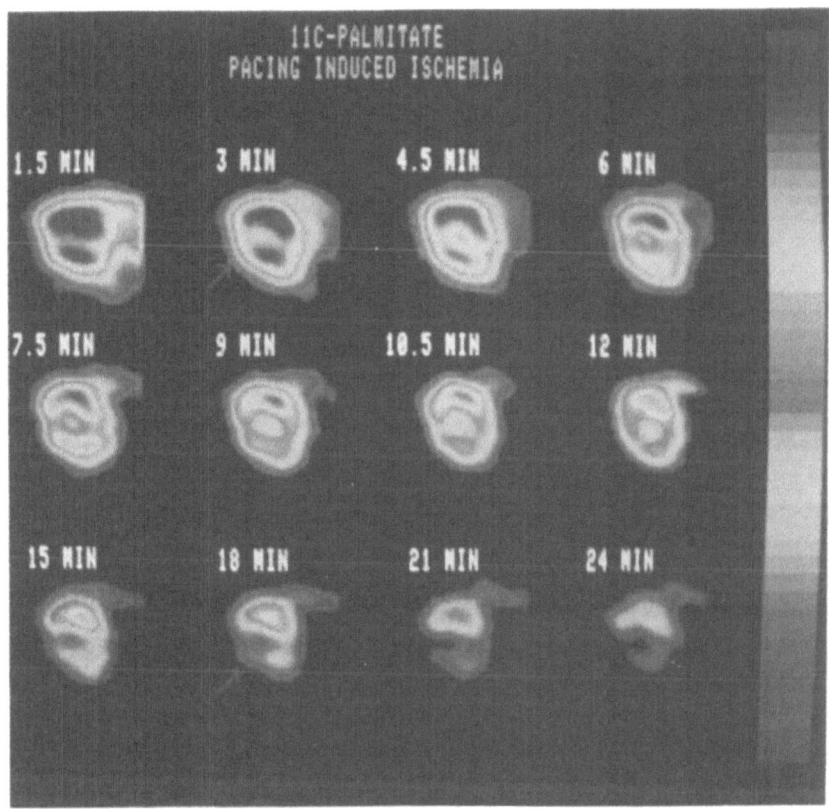

Figure 9. FFA metabolism during pacing-induced ischemia. These cross-sectional sequential images were obtained by rapid serial PCT imaging after C-11 palmitic acid injection during pacing-induced ischemia. The initial C-11 images show most of the activity in the blood pool. After C-11 activity has cleared from blood, the myocardium is visualized and depicts the decrease in C-11 activity in the anterior wall which closely correlates with the reduction in flow. While C-11 concentrations in the ischemic segment change little in time, there is rapid clearance of C-11 activity from normal myocardium. (From Schelbert HR: 'The heart'. In: Ell PJ, Holman BL (eds.), Computed emission tomography. Oxford University Press, New York, 1982, pp 91–133.)

initial metabolic sequestration by the energy-requiring activation of palmitate to palmitate CoA. Both factors account for the reduced net extraction of C-11 palmitic acid in acutely ischemic segments. Further, less C-11 palmitic acid is immediately oxidized while more C-11 palmitic acid is deposited in the endogenous lipid pool.

Changes in FFA metabolism during ischemia were investigated in dogs by Lerch *et al.* [46]. They found that regional clearance of C-11 palmitic acid was more heterogeneous in myocardium supplied by a vessel with a stenosis of greater

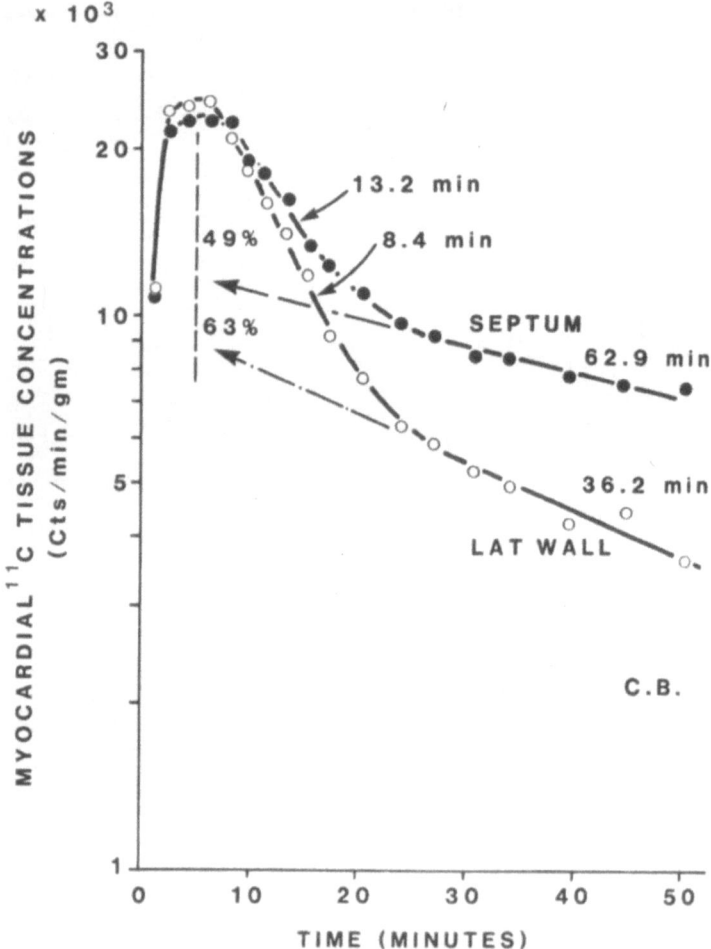

Figure 10. Time-activity curves obtained during pacing-induced ischemia derived from a region of interest over the non-ischemic lateral wall and the ischemic septum. C-11 activity increases in both normal (open circles) and ischemic (solid circles) myocardium. Subsequent clearance of C-11 activity from ischemic and normal myocardium is biexponential. By back extrapolation of the slow clearance phase, the relative sizes of the early rapid components can be estimated. In ischemic compared with normal myocardium the relative size of the early curve component is smaller (49% vs. 63%) and the halftime of the early clearance phase is slower (8.4 min vs. 13.2 min).

than 70%. This heterogeneity was due to reduced clearance of C-11 palmitic acid in regions supplied by the stenotic vessel. This difference in C-11 palmitic acid clearance in normal versus ischemic myocardium was even greater during pacing.

Henze *et al.* [36] investigated the effect of increasing the heart rate in 15 patients with rate programmable pacemakers, most of whom had coronary artery disease as evidenced by coronary arteriography, a typical history of effort-induced angina and/or ischemic electrocardiographic changes. An initial study was performed after an overnight fast with the pacemaker rate set as low as possible. After C-11 palmitic acid was injected intravenously, serial Positron-CT images were obtained to evaluate tracer turnover. The pacemaker rate was then increased and maintained just below the anginal threshold. After a second injection of C-11 palmitic acid, serial Positron-CT imaging was repeated. In patients without coronary artery disease, the fractional distribution of C-11 palmitic acid in tissue changed with the higher workload, that is, a disproportionately greater fraction entered the rapid oxidation turnover pool, yet the initial tracer uptake and subsequent clearance from tissue remained homogeneous. However, in patients with coronary artery disease, initial tracer uptake became more heterogeneous with pacing. In ischemic segments, the fraction of C-11 palmitic acid entering the initial pool decreased and its tissue clearance became slower, indicating a decline in oxidation of FFA in acutely ischemic segments.

Myocardial infarction

Segmental decreases in or absence of C-11 palmitic acid uptake have been shown to correlate with the site and extent of infarcted myocardium [6, 7, 63, 64]. The reproducibility of estimating the infarct size was tested in four patients and was within 10%. Positron-CT is able to detect and discriminate between non-transmural and transmural myocardial infarctions [7]. All 22 transmural infarctions were imaged as confluent regions of homogeneously decreased C-11 activity. In 23 of 24 patients with non-transmural infarcts, two observations were made. First, the area of diminished C-11 activity was often non-transmural and a thin area of normal C-11 uptake was present. Second, heterogeneity of C-11 uptake was present in myocardium not directly affected by the infarction. The authors ascribed this latter observation to an admixture of normal and infarcted cells in myocardium adjacent to the infarcted segment.

In the study by Marshall *et al.* [19], only 2 of 19 areas of infarction were not detected by Positron-CT. Of particular interest is a patient who, early after infarction, had increased glucose utilization in a myocardial segment with decreased blood flow and absent function. When restudied six weeks later, blood flow and glucose utilization had reverted to normal while segmental function was normal 10 days after the acute event (Figures 11, 12). These findings are encouraging as they support the hypothesis that Positron-CT can identify injured yet viable myocardium that has the potential to recover normal function.

Using Positron-CT and C-11 palmitic acid, Billadello *et al.* [65] examined 'reciprocal' ST segment depression in 20 patients with acute myocardial infarction. Nine of 13 (69%) patients with inferior infarctions had ST depression in the anterior precordial leads. These patients with anterior ST depression had more inferior ST elevation (0.48 ± 0.35 SD versus 0.07 ± 0.19, p<0.05), higher peak plasma MB creatine kinase levels (354 ± 134 versus 80 ± 34 IU/liter) and larger

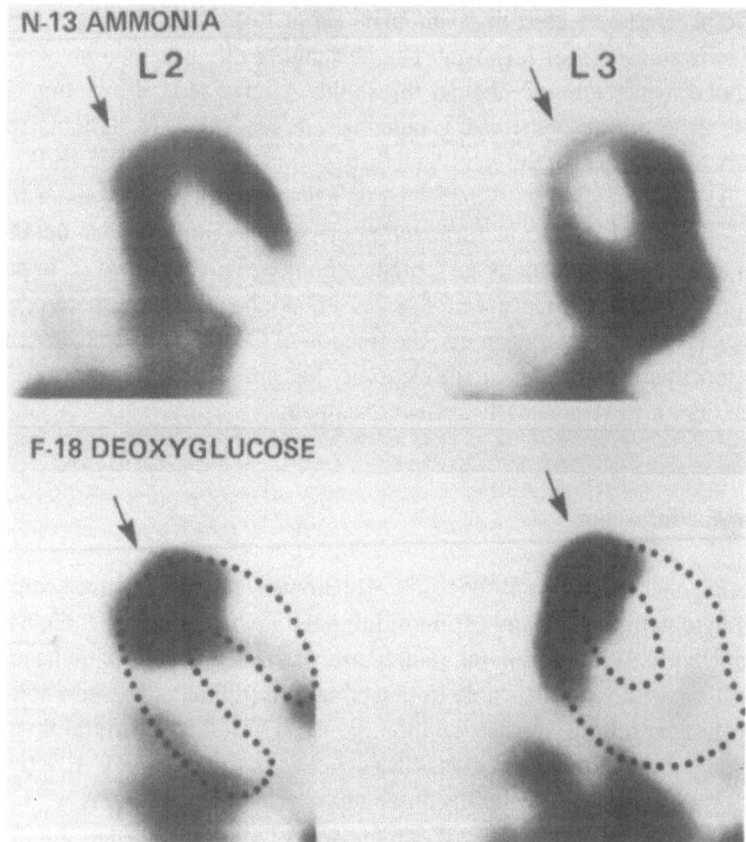

Figure 11. N-13 ammonia and FDG scans at two levels through the left ventricle. A large apical area of increased FDG uptake compared with N-13 ammonia uptake is seen (arrows). This finding has been designated as 'mismatch'.

infarct size as estimated by Positron-CT (58 ± 13 versus 33 ± 10 PET-g-eq) compared with the patients who did not have anterior ST depression. Three of these nine patients had anterior defects on the early Positron-CT study, two of which resolved on a later study. All three had wall motion abnormalities which may have caused artifactual segmental defects in tracer uptake as discussed above. The patient with a persistent defect in C-11 palmitic acid uptake anteriorly had an anteroseptal wall motion abnormality with 100% occlusion of the left anterior descending coronary artery and a 75 to 99% occlusion of the circumflex coronary artery.

None of the patients with anterior infarction had inferior ST depression and of the patients with inferior infarction who did not have precordial ST depression, one had a small anterior area of depressed C-11 palmitic acid uptake that was no longer present on the later study. Cardiac catheterization in that patient demon-

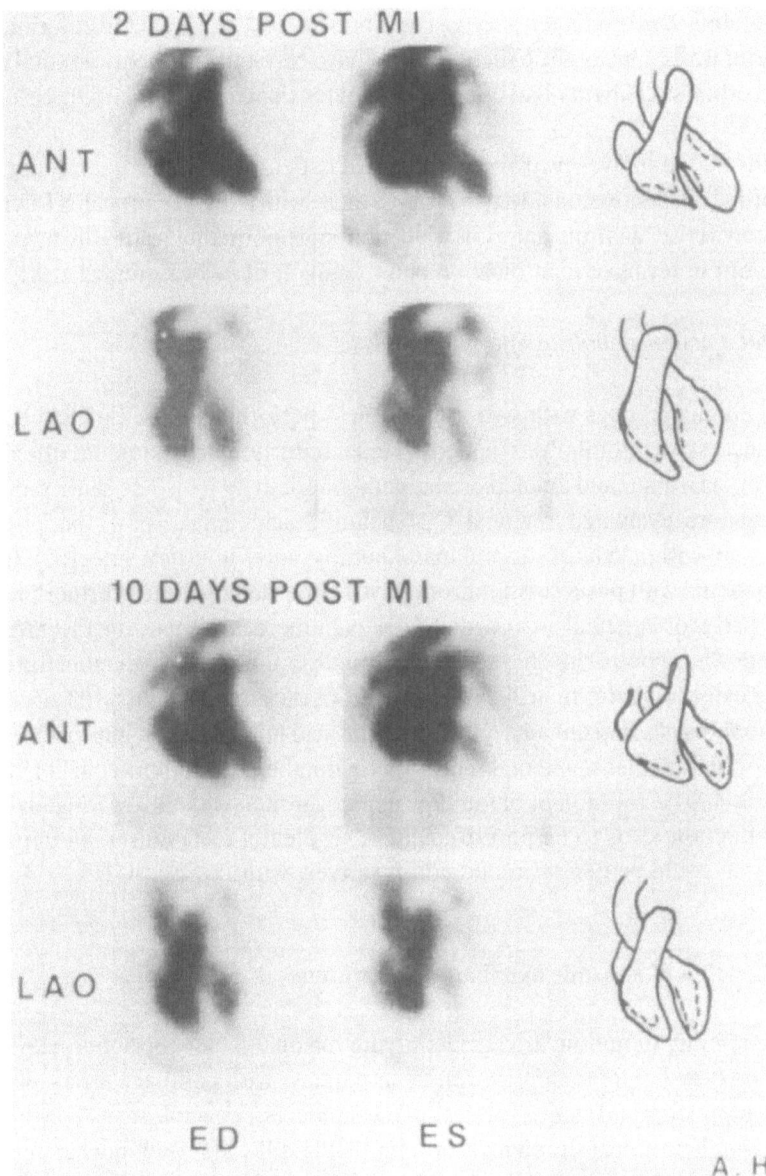

Figure 12. MUGA study of the patient with a large apical region of 'mismatch' presented in Figure 9. Two days after a clinical subendocardial myocardial infarction, an area of apical akinesis is seen in the anterior (ANT) and LAO projections (upper four pictures and two line drawings; end-diastole (solid lines) is depicted on the left and end-systole (dotted lines) on the right.) Ten days after the myocardial infarction, the apical wall motion has returned to normal (lower for pictures and line drawings). ED = end-diastole; ES = end-systole.

strated less than 25% obstruction of the LAD and normal anterior wall motion. All patients had homogeneous C-11 palmitic acid uptake in the inferior and posterior walls. One of the patients did not have coronary arteriography and none of the other six patients had a lesion of greater than 75% in the right coronary artery.

In the above study, Positron-CT separated patients with inferior infarction and precordial ST depression into two groups: those with truly 'reciprocal' ST depression and those with an anterior wall motion abnormality. This distinction is important in terms of identification and treatment of myocardium at risk.

Free fatty acid metabolism after thrombolysis

Initial studies in dogs with C-11 palmitic acid performed approximately 60 min after successful thrombolysis demonstrated a reduction in the amount of jeopardized myocardium and an increase in metabolic activity [66]. The same group of investigators evaluated regional C-11 palmitic acid uptake in 17 patients on admission, within 18 hr of streptokinase therapy, and 7 to 10 days later [67]. In the nine patients with unsuccessful thrombolysis, four demonstrated further impairment (4%) of regional myocardial C-11 palmitic acid uptake in the affected segment when comparing the late and early images and only two demonstrated an improvement (greater than 20%). However, of the eight patients with successful thrombolysis, six had enhanced C-11 palmitic acid uptake (mean improvement of 28%) or had smaller segmental reductions in uptake. The authors concluded that clot lysis and restoration of blood flow in myocardium with an evolving myocardial infarction leads to an improvement in segmental metabolism, an improvement that could be demonstrated non-invasively with Positron-CT.

Identification of ischemic but viable myocardium

The possibility of non-invasively identifying regional metabolic abnormalities in acute myocardial infarction as well as in patients with coronary artery disease raises interesting and clinically relevant questions. For example, can Positron-CT identify ischemically injured myocardium that is still viable and, hence, likely to benefit from therapeutic interventions such as intracoronary or intravenous thrombolysis, angioplasty or coronary artery bypass grafting? Both C-11 palmitic acid and FDG in conjunction with a blood flow tracer may be suitable for identifying reversibly injured ischemic myocardium.

As mentioned earlier, the 'mismatch' observed in patients with stress-induced ischemia was also seen in patients with recent myocardial infarction and in patients with ischemic heart disease who had regional wall motion abnormalities but did not have symptoms or clinical evidence of acute ischemia at the time of the Positron-CT study. These observations raise several questions. While the 'mismatch' observed by Camici *et al.* [61] was consistent with known metabolic changes induced by exercise-induced ischemia, findings made by our group in asymptomatic patients who had not been exercised were less clear. Did this 'mismatch' reflect a metabolic alteration in tissue that was recovering from a single ischemic event or from many recurrent and perhaps silent ischemic events, thus representing the metabolic correlate to what recently has been referred to as 'stunned myocardium' [68]? Did this pattern reflect chronic ischemia or a chronic adaptation in regional metabolism to a low oxygen state? Regardless of the underlying mechanism, this pattern is clinically relevant because it could identify the presence of tissue that has undergone ischemic injury but is still metabolically active and hence, potentially salvageable.

Schwaiger *et al.* [8] in our laboratory pursued this question in chronic dog experiments. After a 3 hr balloon occlusion of the left anterior descending coronary artery and subsequent reperfusion, regional metabolism and function were studied over a 4-week period. A 'mismatch' in the reperfused segment at 24 hr after reperfusion was consistent with enhanced regional glucose utilization and lactic acid production deteremined by the Fick method and invariably predicted subsequent recovery of regional function and absence of scar tissue at 4 weeks. Regional function, monitored by ultrasonic crystals, always improved when FDG uptake was increased regardless of whether function initially deteriorated within the first 24 to 48 hr of reperfusion. Functional recovery was usually observed at 1 week and was either complete or slightly less than control at 4 weeks.

Effects of bypass surgery and prediction of functional recovery

Tillisch *et al.* [9] studied ten patients with resting wall motion abnormality in 23 regions. In 14 of the 23 regions, Positron-CT disclosed increased or normal FDG uptake while in 9 regions, both FDG and N-13 ammonia uptake were proportionately decreased. After coronary artery bypass grafting, 13 of the 14 regions with increased preoperative FDG uptake showed an improvement in wall motion, whereas none of the regions without FDG uptake showed improvement. These findings again support the hypothesis that the Positron-CT technique can distinguish irreversibly infarcted from abnormally contracting but viable myocardium.

Patients with congestive heart failure

In a heterogeneous group of patients with congestive heart failure, Henze *et al.* [35, 36] tested the hypothesis that the ability of the myocardium to alternate among substrates in response to changes in plasma levels of those substrates may be impaired in intrinsic myocardial disease. C-11 palmitic acid uptake and clearance were measured after an overnight fast when plasma FFA levels were in the upper range of normal and plasma glucose levels were low, and were measured again 2 hr after oral glucose administration when the converse was true. The results obtained in normal volunteers were compared with those of the patients with congestive failure. In the fasting normal volunteers, approximately 50% of the C-11 palmitic acid extracted by myocardium was rapidly oxidized whereas less entered the oxidation pool when the plasma glucose levels were high and plasma FFA levels were low. The same pattern was seen in seven of the fifteen patients with cardiomyopathy, whereas in the remaining eight patients, a reduction in the amount of C-11 palmitic acid undergoing immediate oxidation as well as in its clearance rate was observed. After glucose administration, the latter patients demonstrated a seemingly paradoxical increase in the amount of C-11 palmitic acid immediately oxidized as well as in its clearance rate. The mechanism(s) explaining these findings remain to be elucidated although several hypotheses exist and can be tested with Positron-CT. Preferential glucose utilization may represent the inability of abnormal myocardium to switch among substrates according to their availability. The response to glucose is even more intriguing. Perhaps the presence of glucose caused an increase in diffusion of [^{11}C] labeled compounds out of the myocardium. Another explanation is glucose was utilized to replenish metabolic intermediates in the citric acid cycle which facilitate entry of 2-carbon fragments provided by beta oxidation, hence the increase in FFA oxidation.

Cardiomyopathies

Cardiomyopathies, occurring in various forms such as dilated, obstructive and restrictive, have remained an enigma in cardiology. The hypothesis that metabolic derangements may underlie, result from, or contribute to the development of certain forms of cardiomyopathy can be tested using Positron-CT. If early metabolic abnormalities and/or specific metabolic derangements can be identified, then perhaps specific therapeutic regimens can be designed and implemented before irreversible myocardial damage occurs. Current treatment of idiopathic congestive cardiomyopathy is often frustrating, a sentiment expressed by Shabetai in a recent review: '... the true pathologic fault in idiopathic congestive cardiomyopathy remains elusive; individual prognosis is still little better than an intelligent guess, and treatment continues to be an empirical art instead of a precise science' [69]. Initial studies in ischemic, idiopathic and Duchenne's cardiomyopathy have demonstrated metabolic patterns different from those observed in normal volunteers. Whether the abnormal metabolic patterns can be utilized to guide therapeutic and prognostic decision making remains a future challenge for researchers utilizing Positron-CT.

Ischemic vs. non-ischemic cardiomyopathies

Positron-CT is able to distinguish ischemic from non-ischemic cardiomyopathy [70, 71]. Patients with ischemic cardiomyopathy had at least one region of homogeneously decreased C-11 palmitic acid uptake whereas patients with non-ischemic dilated cardiomyopathy had a more heterogeneous pattern of C-11 palmitic acid uptake. The inhomogeneous pattern did not correlate with abnormalities of myocardial blood flow or of wall motion. To explain the heterogeneous pattern, the authors postulated patchy myocardial involvement by the disease process with resultant impairment of FFA metabolism. If these findings prove to be sufficiently sensitive and specific, it may be possible to make earlier diagnoses in some forms of cardiomyopathy with Positron-CT and perhaps to choose appropriate therapeutic regimens based on given metabolic abnormalities.

Duchenne's muscular dystrophy

The posterobasal segment of the left ventricle is selectively involved with replacement of myocardium by connective tissue in the sex-linked disease, Duchenne's muscular dystrophy [72, 73]. Ultrastructural abnormalities have been shown to precede gross histological changes. The question was posed whether a metabolic abnormality could be detected with the Positron-CT technique in the specific region of myocardial involvement. Fifteen infant and adolescent males with documented Duchenne's muscular dystrophy, including the ECG abnormality of decreased posterobasal forces were studied [74]. Ventricular function was evaluated with echocardiography and equilibrium radionuclide ventriculography, and myocardial blood flow was assessed with Tl-201 scintigraphy. The Positron-CT study was performed using N-13 ammonia to evaluate blood flow and FDG to evaluate utilization of exogenous glucose. In 14 patients, decreased N-13 ammonia uptake was present in the left ventricular myocardium in the basal, lateral, or inferior portion and in some patients in the entire free wall of the left ventricle. Technically adequate and interpretable FDG images were obtained in 12 patients, 11 of whom had increased FDG uptake in areas of decreased N-13 ammonia uptake (Figure 13); this is the concept of 'mismatch' discussed above although the mechanisms for the existence of 'mismatch' in patients with Duchenne's muscular dystrophy may be different from those in patients with ischemic cardiac disease. These areas of 'mismatch' did not seem to correlate with areas of wall motion or blood flow abnormalities. Questions which still remain to be answered include whether the metabolic processes responsible for the 'mismatch' are causative or compensatory in nature and whether they precede the clinical manifestation of the myocardial involvement.

The similarity of the metabolic pattern seen in this particular disease to that seen in ischemic heart disease is intriguing. Does it reflect a metabolic abnor-

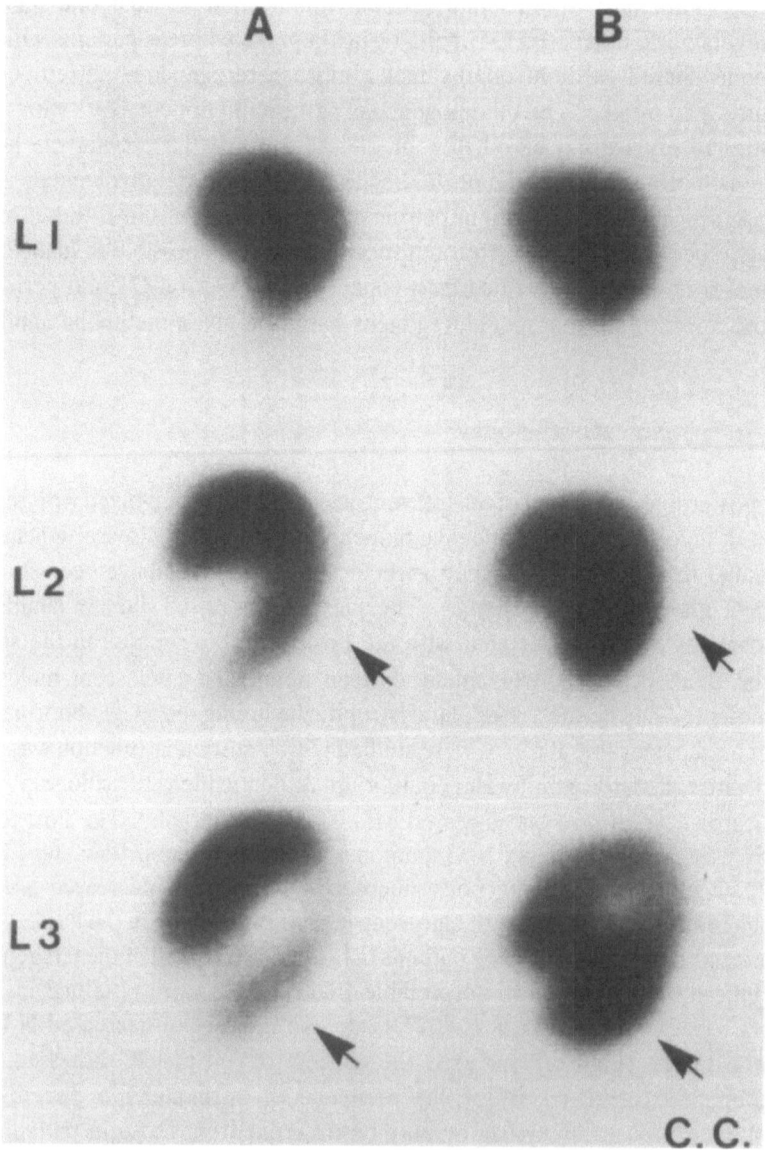

Figure 13. N-13 ammonia images (A) from apex to base (L1–L3) in a patient with Duchenne's muscular dystrophy demonstrating an area of decreased uptake in the lateral wall (arrows). FDG images (B) demonstrate 'mismatch', i.e. increased FDG uptake relative to N-13 ammonia uptake (arrows).

mality or is it a response to another underlying metabolic defect? For example, regardless of the initial defect, oxidation of FFA is most vulnerable and declines while substrate metabolism shifts to glucose for production of high energy phosphates in order to maintain function. Thus, it is possible to ascribe the absence of regional dysfunction in the affected segment to a compensatory adjustment. Once this compensatory mechanism becomes inadequate or impaired, regional mechanical dysfunction ensues. Along the same line of thought, it would appear that such regional metabolic abnormalities would antedate clinically apparent regional dysfunction or clinically manifest disease. Obviously, such a hypothesis needs further documentation.

Summary

Although the first Positron-CT imaging devices were completed more than 10 years ago, application of this new technology to the non-invasive study of the human heart has been slow. Considerable investigative efforts were devoted to designing techniques for retrieval of true indicator tissue concentrations from the cross-sectional images of the heart, to define in isolated heart preparations and in animal experiments the relationship of the uptake and subsequent turnover of positron-emitting tracers in myocardial tissue to known biochemical information and, lastly to develop techniques for the in vivo quantification of regional metabolic rates and substrate fluxes. These efforts will undoubtedly continue, although the past several years have seen testing and implementation of techniques developed in the animal experimental setting to the human heart for investigation of human cardiovascular disease. Results of the clinical investigations, for example the studies with N-13 ammonia and drug-induced coronary hyperemia for the detection of coronary artery disease and the studies with C-11 palmitic acid for the detection of myocardial infarction, are similar to observations made with other approaches which confirms the validity and accuracy of Positron-CT for the non-invasive study of human cardiac disease. Other data obtained using Positron-CT have provided new and unique insights into human cardiac disease which also attests to a gain in diagnostic accuracy and new possibilities with Positron-CT. Of great interest have been the effect of mental stress on regional myocardial blood flow and/or function in ischemic heart disease and the delayed recovery of regional blood flow and function after transient ischemia. Studies with tracers of blood flow and metabolism have provided indirect evidence for the possible existence of silent ischemia and its metabolic correlates. Investigation of dilated myocardiopathies suggests it may be possible to separate the ischemic from the idiopathic type and has presented evidence for a disturbance in substrate metabolism. Investigation of the abnormal metabolism may ultimately provide some understanding of this disease process and may lead to an improvement in therapy. Similarily, findings in the regional myocardiopathy of Duchenne's muscular dystrophy have provided initial evidence for bio-chemical abnormalities even in the absence of functional or blood flow correlates thus suggesting the possibility of early disease detection. Other segmental bio-chemical abnormalities in ischemic heart disease observed with Positron-CT may in fact represent the metabolic counterpart to 'stunned' myocardium or an adaptation to chronic oxygen deprivation. They may also reliably identify ischem-ically injured but potentially viable myocardium and thus profoundly affect clinical management of patients with ischemic heart disease including acute myocardial infarction.

The above findings demonstrate the utility and versatility of the Positron-CT technique. This technique provides a unique tool to non-invasively investigate regional myocardial metabolism in an attempt to detect cardiac disease prior to irreversible damage and to more precisely design therapeutic regimens. These goals are within the realm of the possible in the near future.

Acknowledgements

Work was supported in part by DOE Contract #DE-AM03-76-SF00012, by The American Heart Association, Los Angeles, Affilitate #617 IG4, and National Institutes of Health, Grant #4-447150-31826 in Bethesda Maryland.

References

1. Huang SC, Phelps ME, Hoffman EJ, Sideris K, Selin CJ, Kuhl DE: Non-invasive determintion of local cerebral metabolicrate of glucose in man. Am J Physiol 238: E69–E82, 1980.
2. Huang SC, Schwaiger M, Selin C, Phelps ME, Schelbert HR: Tracer kinetic model of C-11 palmitate for estimating regional free fatty acid utilization in myocardium. J Nucl Med 24: P12, 1983.
3. Phelps ME, Mazziotta JC, Huang SC: Study of cerebral function with positron computed tomography. J Cerebral Blood Flow and Metab 2: 113–162, 1982.
4. Henze E, Schelbert HR, Barrio JR, Egbert JE, Hansen HW, MacDonald NS, Phelps ME: Evaluation of myocardial metabolism with N-13 and C-11 labeled amino acids and positron computed tomography. J Nucl Med 23: 671–681, 1982.
5. Huang SC, Schwaiger M, Carson RE, Henze E, Hoffman EJ, Phelps ME, Schelbert HR: An 0-15 water clearance method for quantitative regional myocardial blood flow measurements. J Nucl Med 23: P69, 1982.
6. Sobel BE, Weiss ES, Welch MJ, Siegel BA, Ter-Pogossian MM: Detection of remote myocardial infarction in patients with positron emission transaxial tomography and intravenous ^{11}C-palmi-tate. Circulation 55: 853, 1977.
7. Geltman EM, Biello D, Welch MJ, Ter-Pogossian MM, Roberts R, Sobel BE: Characterization of non-transmural myocardial infarction by positron-emission tomography. Circulation 65: 747–755, 1982.
8. Schwaiger M, Ellison D, Johanson-Vinten J, Hansen H, Yeatman L, Schelbert HR: Sustained regional abnormalities in cardiac metabolism after transient ischemia in the chronic dog model. 1983 (In preparation).

9. Tillisch J, Marshall R, Schelbert H, Huang SC, Phelps ME: Reversibility of wall motion abnormalities; preoperative determination using positron tomography, ^{18}fluorodeoxyglucose and ^{13}NH$_3$. Circulation 68: III-387, 1983.

10. Phelps ME: Emission computed tomography. Semin Nucl Med 7: 337-365, 1977.

11. Zielonka JS: Cardiac tomography. In: Holman BL, Parker JA (eds.), Computer-assisted cardiac nuclear medicine. Little, Brown & Co, Boston, 1981, pp 445-477.

12. Muehllehner G, Colsher JG: Instrumentation. In: Ell PJ, Holman BL (eds.), Computed emission tomography. Oxford University Press, New York, 1982, pp 3-41.

13. Comar D, Berridge M, Maziere B, Crouzel C: Radiopharmaceuticals labeled with positron-emitting radioisotopes. In: Ell PH, Holman BL (eds.), Computed emission tomography. Oxford University Press, New York, 1982, pp 42-90.

14. Budinger TF, Derenzo SE, Huesman RH, Sherman LG, Moyer BR, Yano Y: Quantitative myocardial flow extraction data using gated ECT. J Nucl Med 21: P16, 1981.

15. Selwyn AP, Allan RM, L'Abbate A, Horlock P, Camici P, Clark J, O'Brien HA, Grant PM: Relation between regional myocardial uptake of rubidium-82 and perfusion: absolute reduction of cation uptake in ischemia. Am J Cardiol 50: 112-121, 1982.

16. Sokoloff L, Reivich M, Kennedy C, Des Rosiers MH, Patlak CS, Pettigrew KD, Sakuradao O, Shinohara M: The [^{14}C]-deoxyglucose method for the measurement of local cerebral glucose utilization: theory, procedure and normal values in the conscious and anesthetized albino rat. J Neurochem 28: 897-916, 1977.

17. Phelps ME, Huang SC, Hoffman EJ, Selin C, Sokoloff L, Kuhl DE: Tomographic measurement of local cerebral glucose metabolicrate in humans with (F-18) 2-fluoro-2-deoxy-D-glucose: validation of method. Ann Neurol 6: 371-388, 1979.

18. Krivokapich J, Huang SC, Phelps ME, Barrio JR, Wantanabe CR, Selin CE, Shine KI: Estimation of rabbit myocardial metabolic rate for glucose using fluorodeoxyglucose. Am J Physiol 243: H884-895, 1982.

19. Marshall RC, Tillisch JH, Phelps ME, Huang SC, Carson RC, Henze E, Schelbert HR: Identification and differentiation of myocardial ischemia and infarction in man with positron computed tomography ^{18}F-labeled fluorodeoxyglucose and N-13 ammonia. Circulation 64: 766-778, 1983.

20. Ratib O, Phelps ME, Huang SC, Henze E, Sellin CE, Schelbert HR: Positron tomography with deoxyglucose for estimating local myocardial metabolism. J Nucl Med 23: 577-586, 1982.

21. Phelps ME, Hoffman EJ, Coleman RE, Welch MJ, Raichle ME, Weiss FS, Sobel BE, Ter-Pogossian MM: Tomographic images of blood pool and perfusion in brain and heart. J Nucl Med 17: 603-612, 1976.

22. Schelbert HR, Phelps ME, Huang SC, MacDonald NS, Hansen H, Selin C, Kuhl DE: N-13 ammonia as an indicator of myocardial blood flow. Circulation 63: 1259-1272, 1981.

23. Bergmann ST, Hack S, Tewson T, Welch MJ, Sobel BE: The dependence of accumulation of ^{13}NH$_3$ by myocardium on metabolic factors and its implications for the quantitative assessment of perfusion. Circulation 61: 34-43, 1980.

24. Krivokapich J, Huang SC, Phelps ME, MacDonald NS, Shine KI: Dependence of ^{13}NH$_3$ myocardial extraction and clearance on flow and metabolism. Am J Physiol 242 (Heart Circ Physiol II): H536-H542, 1982.

25. Ziegler HW, Goreski CA: Kinetics of rubidium uptake in the working dog heart. Circ Res 29: 208-220, 1971.

26. Mullani NA, Gould KL: First-pass measurements of regional blood flow with external detectors. J Nucl Med 24: 577-581, 1983.

27. Mullani NA, Goldstein RA, Gould KL, Marani SK, Fisher DJ, O'Brien HA Jr, Loberg MD: Myocardial perfusion with rubidium-82. I. Measurement of extraction fraction and flow with external detectors. J Nucl Med 898-906, 1983.

28. Goldstein RA, Mullani NA, Marani SK, Fisher DJ, Gould KL, O'Brien HA: Myocardial perfusion with Rb-82. II. Effects of metabolic and pharmacologic interventions. J Nucl Med 24: 907-915, 1983.

29. Carlsten A, Hallgren B, Jagenburg R, Svansborg A, Werko L: Myocardial metabolism of glucose, lactic acid, amino acids, and fatty acids in healthy human individuals at rest and at different work loads. Scand J Clin Labs Invest 13: 418–428, 1961.

30. Wahlquist ML, Kaijer L, Lassers W, Carlson LA: Fatty acid as a determinant of myocardial substrate and oxygen metabolism in man at rest and during prolonged exercise. Acta Med Scan 193: 89–96, 1973.

31. Schlant RC: Metabolism of the heart. In: Hurst JW, Schlant RC, Wenger NR (eds.), The heart, 4th ed. McGraw-Hill Book Co, Inc, New York, 1978, p 107.

32. Randle PJ, Tubbs PK: Carbohydrate and fatty acid metabolism. In: Berne RM, Sperelakis N, Geiger SR (eds), Handbook of physiology. Section 2: The cardiovascular system. Vol I: The heart. The American Physiological Society, Bethesda, MD, 1979, p 805.

33. Schelbert HR, Henze E, Schon HR, Keen R, Hansen H, Selin C, Huang SC, Barrio JR, Phelps ME: C-11 palmitate for the non-invasive evaluation of regional myocardial fatty acid metabolism with positron computed tomography. III. In vivo demonstration of the effects of substrate availability on myocardial metabolism. Am Heart J 105: 492–504, 1983.

34. Schelbert HR, unpublished.

35. Henze E, Grossman RG, Najafi A et al.: Measurement of C-11 palmitate kinetics after metabolic interventions in normals and patients with cardiomyopathy using positron emission computed tomography. Am J Cardiol 49: 1023, 1982.

36. Henze E, Grossman EJ, Huang SC, Barrio JR, Phelps ME, Schelbert HR: Myocardial uptake and clearance of C-11 palmitic acid in man: effects of substrate availability and cardiac work. J Nucl Med 23: P12, 1982.

37. Keul J, Doll E, Steim H, Homburger H, Kern H, Reindell H: Uber den Stoffwechsel des menschlichen Herzens. I. Substratversorgung des gesunden Herzens in Ruthe wahrend und nach korperlicher Arbeit. Pfluegers Archiv 282: 1–27, 1965.

38. Neely JR, Rovetto MJ, Oram JF: Myocardial utilization of carbohydrate and lipid. Prog Cardiovasc Dis 15: 289–329, 1972.

39. Ballard F, Danforth W, Nagel S, Bing R: Myocardial metabolism of fatty acids. J Clin Invest 39: 717–723, 1960.

40. Evans JR: Cellular transport of long chain fatty acids. Can J Biochem 42: 955–969, 1964.

41. Rothlin ME, Bing BJ: Extraction and release of individual free fatty acids by the heart and fat depots. J Clin Invest 40: 1380–1386, 1961.

42. Rose CP, Goresky CA: Constraints on the uptake of labeled palmitate by the heart. Circ Res 41 (4): 534–545, 1977.

43. Hoffman EJ, Phelps ME, Weiss ES et al.: Transaxial tomographic imaging of canine myocardium with ¹¹C-palmitic acid. J Nucl Med 18: 57–61, 1977.

44. Klein MS, Goldstein RA, Welch MJ, Sobel BE: External assessment of myocardial metabolism with ¹¹C-palmitate in rabbit hearts. Am J Physiol (Heart Circ Physiol) 6: H51–H58, 1979.

45. Goldstein RA, Klein MS, Welch MJ, Sobel BE: External assessment of myocardial metabolism with C-11 palmitate in vivo. J Nucl Med 21: 342–348, 1980.

46. Lerch RA, Ambos HD, Bergmann SR, Welch MJ, Ter-Pogossian MM, Sobel BE: Localization of viable, ischemic myocardium by positron-emission tomography with ¹¹C-palmitate. Circulation 64: 689–699, 1981.

47. Schon HR, Schelbert HR, Robinson G, Najafi A, Huang SC, Hansen H, Barrio J, Kuhl DE, Phelps ME: C-11 labeled palmitic acid for the non-invasive evaluation of regional myocardial fatty acid metabolism with positron computed tomography. I. Kinetics of C-11 palmitic acid in normal myocardium. Am Heart J 103: 532–47, 1982.

48. Schon HR, Schelbert HR, Najafi A, Hansen H, Robinson GR, Huang SC, Barrio J, Phelps ME: C-11 labeled palmitic acid for the non-invasive evaluation of regional myocardial fatty acid metabolism with positron computed tomography. II. Kinetics of C-11 palmitic acid in acutely ischemic myocardium. Am Heart J 103: 548–561, 1982.

49. Heymann MA, Payne BD, Hoffman JIE *et al.*: Blood flow measurements with radionuclide-labeled particles. Prog Cardiovasc Dis 20: 55–79, 1977.

50. Most AS, Brachfield N, Gorlin R, Wahren J: Free fatty acid metabolism of the human heart at rest. J Clin Invest 48: 1177–1188, 1969.

51. Marshall RC, Huang SC, Nash WW, Schelbert HR, Phelps ME: Tracer kinetic analysis of 2-^{3}H-glucose to measure myocardial glucose transport and phosphorylation. Circulation 68: III–67, 1983.

52. Gould KL: Assessment of coronary stenosis with myocardial perfusion imaging during pharmacologic coronary vasodilation. IV. Limits of detection of stenosis with idealized experimental cross-sectional myocardial imaging. Am J Cardiol 42: 761–8, 1978.

53. Gould KL, Schelbert HR, Phelps ME, Hoffman EJ: Non-invasive assessment of coronary stenoses with myocardial perfusion imaging during pharmacologic coronary vasodilation. V. Detection of 47 percent diameter coronary stenosis with intravenous nitrogen-13 ammonia and emission-computed tomography in intact dogs. Am J Cardiol 43: 200–208, 1979.

54. Schelbert HR, Wisenberg G, Phelps ME, Gould KL, Henze E, Hoffman EJ, Gomes A, Kuhl DE: Non-invasive assessment of coronary stenoses by myocardial imaging during pharmacologic coronary vasodilation. VI. Detection of coronary artery disease in human beings with intravenous N-13 ammonia and positron computed tomography. Am J Cardiol 49: 1197–1207, 1982.

55. Hoffman EJ, Huang SC, Phelps ME: Quantitation in positron emission computed tomography. 1. Effect of object size. J Comp Assist Tomogr 3 (3): 299–308, 1979.

56. Deanfield JE, Selwyn AP, Chierchia S, Maseri A, Ribeiro P, Krikler S, Morgan M: Myocardial ischemia during daily life in patients with stable angina: its relation to symptoms and heart rate changes. Lancet 2: 753–758, 1983.

57. Deanfield J, Shea M, Wilson R, Horlock P, Selwyn A: Mental stress and ischemia in patients with coronary disease. Circulation 68: III–258, 1983.

58. Parodi O, Schelbert HR, Schwaiger M, Hansen H, Selin C, Hoffman EJ: Artifactual reductions of segmental indicator tissue concentrations on tomographic images of the heart caused by regional wall motion abnormalities. 1984 (in preparation).

59. Liedtke AJ: Alterations of carbohydrate and lipid metabolism in the acutely ischemic heart. Prog in Cardiovas Dis 23 (5): 321–336, 1981.

60. Opie LH, Owen P, Riemersma RA: Relative rates of oxidation of glucose and free fatty acids by ischemic and non-ischemic myocardium after coronary ligation in the dog. Eur J Clin Invest 3: 419, 1973.

61. Schelbert HR, Henze E, Keen R, Schon HR, Hansen H, Selin C, Huang SC, Barrio JR, Phelps ME: C-11 palmitate for the non-invasive evaluation of regional myocardial fatty acid metabolism with positron computed tomography. IV. In vivo evaluation of acute, experimentally induced myocardial ischemia. Am Heart J 106 (4): 736–750, 1983.

61. Camici P, Kaskl JC, Shea MS, Selwyn AP, Jones T, Maseri A: Increased myocardial glucose utilization in exertional angina. Circulation 68: III–324, 1983.

62. Schelbert HR, Henze E, Guzy PM, Don-Michael TA, Schwaiger M, Barrio JR: Non-invasive evaluation of regional myocardial fatty acid metabolism in man with C-11 palmitic acid and Positron-CT. J Nucl Med 24: P12, 1983.

63. Weiss ES, Ahmed SA, Welch MS, Williamson JR, Ter-Pogossian MM, Sobel BE: Quantification of infarction in cross-sections of canine myocardium in vivo with positron-emission transaxial tomography and ^{11}C-palmitate. Circulation 55: 66–73, 1977.

64. Ter-Pogossian MM, Klein MS, Markham J, Roberts R, Sobel BE: Regional assessment of myocardial metabolic integrety in vivo by positron-emission tomography with ^{11}C-labeled palmitate. Circulation 61: 242–255, 1980.

65. Billadello JJ, Smith JL, Ludbrook PA, Tiefenbrunn AJ, Jaffee AS, Sobel BE, Geltman EM: Implications of 'reciprocal' ST segment depression associated with acute myocardial infarction identified by positron tomography. J Amer Col Cardiol 2 (4): 616–624, 1983.

66. Bergmann SR, Lerch RA, Fox KA, Ludbrook PA, Welch MJ, Ter-Pogossian MM, Sobel BE: Temporal dependence of beneficial effects of coronary thrombolysis characterized by positron tomography. Am J Med 73: 573–581, 1982.

67. Ludbrook PA, Geltman EM, Tiefenbrunn AJ, Jaffe AS, Sobel BE: Restoration of regional myocardial metabolism by coronary thrombolysis in patients. Circulation 68: III–325, 1983.

68. Braunwald E, Kloner RA: The stunned myocardium: prolonged postischemic ventricular dysfunction. Circulation 66 (6): 1146–1149, 1982.

69. Shabetai R: Cardiomyopathy: How far have we come in years, how far yet to go? J Amer Coll Cardiol 1: 252–263, 1983.

70. Geltman EM, Smith JL, Beecher D, Ludbrook PA, Ter-Pogossian MM, Sobel BE: Altered regional myocardial metabolism in congestive cardiomyopathy detected by positron tomography. Am J Med 74: 773–785, 1983.

71. Eisenberg JD, Smith JL, Sobel BE, Geltman EM: Differentiation of ischemic from non-ischemic cardiomyopathy by positron emission tomography (PET). Circulation 68: III–386, 1983.

72. Brooke MH: A clinician's view of neuromuscular diseases. The Williams & Wilkins Co, Baltimore, 1979.

73. Perloff JK, DeLeon AC Jr, Doherty D: The cardiomyopathy of progressive muscular dystrophy. Circulation 33: 625–648, 1966.

74. Perloff JK, Henze E, Schelbert HR: Alterations in regional myocardial metabolism, perfusion and wall motion in Duchenne's muscular dystrophy studied by radionuclide imaging. Circulation 69: 33–42, 1983.

15. Magnetic resonance imaging of the heart

ALEX M. AISEN and ANDREW J. BUDA

Physical principles

Introduction

Atomic nuclei consist of protons and neutrons bound together, and thus possess a positive electrical charge. Those nuclei which contain an odd number of protons or neutrons also possess the property of spin; and, as moving electrical charges, they have magnetic moments. Such nuclei, which include those of the naturally abundant isotopes of hydrogen (^{1}H), sodium (^{23}Na), and phosphorus (^{31}P), as well as a non-radioactive but only one-percent abundent isotope of carbon (^{13}C), can experience the phenomenon of nuclear magnetic resonance (NMR).

NMR was discovered by groups lead by Felix Bloch at Stanford and Edward Purcell at Harvard during the late 1940's, for which they recieved the Nobel Prize in physics in 1952. The technique quickly became a powerful laboratory tool for studying small, uniform samples placed in small test-tubes. During the early 1970's, Paul Lauterbur at State University of New York, Stonybrook proposed the magnetic field gradient technique which is the basis of NMR imaging [1], now often termed simply magnetic resonance imaging (MRI). This development permitted the spatial localization of NMR signals from heterogenous objects, including human subjects. During the late 1970's prototype NMR imagers were developed at several centers in Great Britain. The technology quickly proved its clinical utility, and development proceeded at a rapid pace; today, perhaps a dozen or so companies offer NMR imaging devices, and clinical and laboratory trials are underway at numerous research centers. This chapter will briefly review the physical principals of NMR imaging, followed by a review of its cardiac applications.

Quantum mechanical background

As noted above, nuclei of isotopes containing an odd number of protons or neutrons have two physical properties which together make nuclear magnetic resonance possible, spin and magnetic moments. The spin behaves analogously to the spin of familiar macroscopic objects, such as a toy top or a gyroscope. However, as a consequence of quantum mechanics, nuclear spin can have only a small number of possible values (unlike the toy top, which can spin at any speed and in many directions); for hydrogen two spin states are allowed, with opposite orientations; these are sometimes called spin-up and spin-down. Since the nuclear magnetic fields are a consequence of the spin, the north-south orientation of the fields will also be oppositely directed.

If an external magnetic field is applied, for example by placing a sample in a laboratory magnet, these spin states tend to align themselves with the external magnetic field. The different spin states take on different energy levels. In this situation, the two spin states of hydrogen are often termed parallel and anti-parallel. Not surprisingly, there is a tendency for the nuclei to align themselves such that the nuclear south magnetic poles are aligned with the north pole of the external magnetic field; this is the lower energy or, by convention, parallel state. The behavior is analogous to a compass needle in the Earth's magnetic field. Unlike the compass needle, the nuclear magnetic moments are small enough to be affected by thermal motion, which tends to jumble the orientations. The degree of randomization is given by the Boltzmann equation, and is so great that for external magnetic fields of the size employed in medical applications, the ratio of parallel to anti-parallel nuclei is only about 1.0000001; thermal motion overcomes virtually all of magnetic alignment. As a result, the NMR signals are very low and sophisticated equipment is required to detect them. These thermal effects become less pronounced as the magnetic field strength increases, one reason why there is a tendency to use stronger magnets in MRI scanners.

There is another of the behavior of spinning objects in external force fields that must now be considered, and that is the phenomenon of precession. Spinning objects have angular momentum; in the presence of an external force, the resulting torque causes their spin axis to itself take on a circular motion, above and beyond the spin motion. This behavior is familiar to those who have observed a spinning toy top in the Earth's gravity; the precessional motion results in the top tracing out a cone, with its apex corresponding to the point of the top. This is shown in Figure 1. Hence, when an ensemble of appropriate atomic nuclei (such as a tube of water, or H_2O) is placed in an external magnetic field, there is a tendency for the nuclei to align themselves with the field, and for the aligned spins to precess. This is shown in simplified form in Figure 2. At this point it is appropriate to introduce a simplification made possible because actual macroscopic samples consist of very, very many nuclei. As noted above, individual nuclei take on only a small number of possible spin orientations, for hydrogen parallel and anti-parallel. When dealing with a large number of nuclei, the average orientation of the ensemble can be considered; this average can take on essentially any orientation, rather than just up and down. This simplification

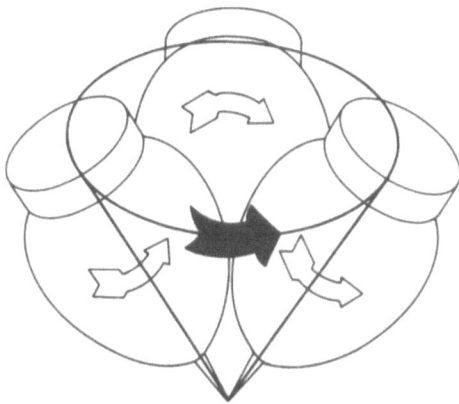

Figure 1. Spinning toy top in vertically oriented gravitational field precessing in a circle (dark arrow). (Reprinted by permission of the publisher from: Nuclear magnetic resonance: physical principles and instrumentation. In: Amendola B, Amendola M (eds.), Recent trends in radiation oncology and related fields. Elsevier Science Publishing Co, Inc, 1983.)

makes it possible to study the behavior of spinning nuclei using the simpler rules of classical physics, rather than those of quantum mechanics. This convention will be used in the discussion which follows, and we will be speaking of large numbers of nuclei, or ensembles, rather than individual spinning nuclei. The orientation of the ensemble spin axes can take on arbitrary directions; in the presence of an external magnetic field, the low energy or ground state is parallel to the magnetic field, and referred to as 0°.

Finally, it is worth noting that in the context of NMR imaging, one is never concerned with the spin frequency; that is a quantity with little physical meaning. Rather, it is the precessional frequency that is of great interest.

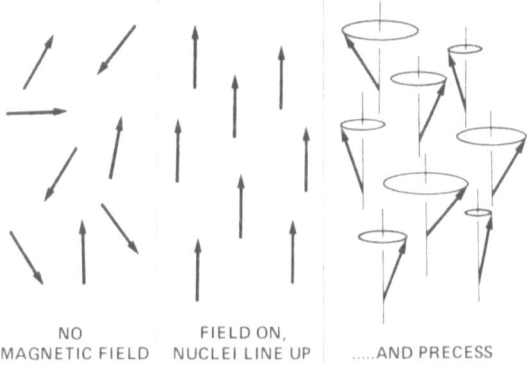

NO
MAGNETIC FIELD

FIELD ON,
NUCLEI LINE UP

.....AND PRECESS

Figure 2. Spinning atomic nuclei (represented by the arrows) lining up and precessing in a vertically oriented magnetic field. (Reprinted by permission of the publisher from: Nuclear magnetic resonance: physical principles and instrumentation. In: Amendola B, Amendola M (eds.), Recent trends in radiation oncology and related fields. Elsevier Science Publishing Co, Inc, 1983.)

Nuclear magnetic resonance

The nuclear precessional frequency will have a precise value dependent on only two factors: the type of nuclei (e.g. ^1H) and the strength of the magnetic field; this is given by the Larmor equation:

$$\omega = \gamma H$$

where ω is the precessional frequency, γ is a proportionality constant termed the gyromagnetic ratio which is different for each NMR isotope, and H is the strength of the magnetic field. For nuclei in a practical laboratory magnet, the precessional or Larmor frequency will be on the order of megahertz, which is in the radio frequency (RF) range.

If an electromagnetic or RF signal is applied to an ensemble of NMR nuclei in a magnetic field, and the frequency of the signal is the Larmor frequency, the phenomenon of resonance will occur. Nuclei in the ensemble will absorb small amounts of energy from the RF signal. This absorption is manifest not by a change in the precessional or Larmor frequency (since the value of the static external field , H_0, is not changing) but rather by a flipping of the magnetic nuclei from the lower energy parallel spin state to the higher energy anti-parallel state; this is manifest by a change in the precessional angle of the ensemble away from the lowest energy, $0°$, ground state. The amount of energy absorbed is proportional to both the strength of the RF field and the length of time it is left on; as more energy is absorbed, the precessional angle increases from $0°$ through $90°$ and on to $180°$, in which more nuclei are in the higher energy anti-parallel state than the lower energy parallel state. A pulse of RF signal just long enough to move the spin direction $90°$ is termed a $90°$ pulse, as diagrammed in Figure 3; a pulse twice as long would be a $180°$ pulse.

Immediately after an excitatory RF pulse is turned off, the spin ensemble will begin to return to the low energy or ground state, this process is called relaxation (Figure 4). The speed with which the nuclei relax is described by an exponential time constant (similar to the familiar half-life of radioactive decay), called T_1. The magnitude of T_1 is related to the chemical environment of the nuclei in complex ways, many not well understood; suffice it to say that a given species of nucleus will have a relaxation time that varies with its chemical and physical state.

Consider an ensemble of nuclei after the $90°$ pulse shown in Figure 3; in this diagram the external, static magnetic field is in the 'z' direction. Immediately after the pulse, two processes occur simultaneously. The first is relaxation back to the ground energy state, as described above, and with time constant T_1. The second process is spin dephasing. Immediately after the excitatory pulse, the spin systems are all pointing in the same direction (to the right in Figure 3) and are said to be in-phase. When the pulse is over, they begin spreading out, or going out of phase, in the x-y plane. This dephasing occurs concurrently with their motion

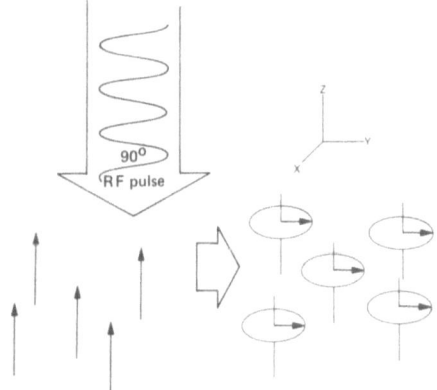

Figure 3. Effect of a 90° RF pulse on the nuclear spin ensembles. The external magnetic field is in the vertical, or z, direction. The axes move 90° away from the unexcited ground (vertical) direction. The external magnetic field is in the vertical, or z, direction. (Reprinted by permission of the publisher from: Nuclear magnetic resonance: physical principles and instrumentation. In: Amendola B, Amendola M (eds.), Recent trends in radiation oncology and related fields. Elsevier Science Publishing Co, Inc, 1983.)

away from the x-y plane (T_1 relaxation), and with a time constant called T2. For biological systems, T_2 is usually much shorter than T_1; it can never be greater than T_1. Like T_1, T_2 varies with the chemical environment of a sample. Figure 5 shows T_1 relaxation (also called spin-lattice relaxation), Figure 6 shows T_2 relaxation (also called spin-spin relaxation), and Figure 7 demonstrates what actually happens, a combination of the two processes occurring simultaneously.

Hence, immediately after a 90° pulse, an ensemble of spins will be in a higher

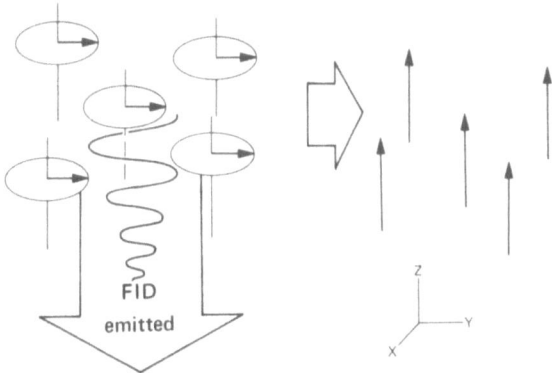

Figure 4. The 'excited' nuclear spin ensembles emit a radiofrequency signal termed an FID (free induction decay) as they 'relax' back to the ground state. (Reprinted by permission of the publisher from: Nuclear magnetic resonance: physical principles and instrumentation. In: Amendola B, Amendola M (eds.), Recent trends in radiation oncology and related fields. Elsevier Science Publishing Co, Inc, 1983.)

276

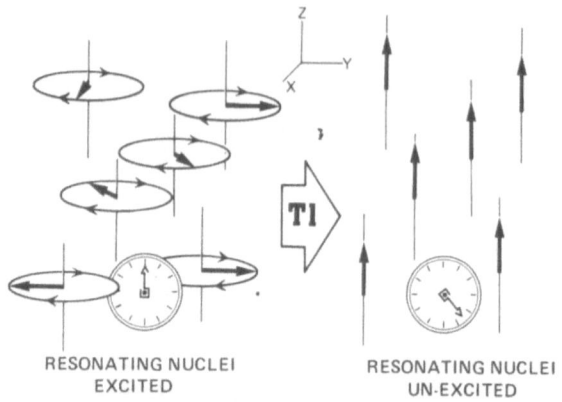

RESONATING NUCLEI
EXCITED

RESONATING NUCLEI
UN-EXCITED

Figure 5. T_1 relaxation time: the rate at which the excited nuclear ensembles return to the ground state. In this case, the left-hand diagram shows the nuclear spin ensembles previously excited by a 90° RF pulse, in an out-of-phase state, i.e. after T_2 relaxation has already occurred. (Reprinted by permission of the publisher from: Nuclear magnetic resonance: physical principles and instrumentation. In: Amendola B, Amendola M (eds.), Recent trends in radiation oncology and related fields. Elsevier Science Publishing Co, Inc, 1983.)

energy or excited state. It will instantly begin to relax towards its ground state, and as it does so, a RF signal will be emitted. The magnitude of this signal, termed a free induction decay or FID, will depend on at least three properties of the sample being measured: the concentration of the NMR nuclei, and the T_1 and T_2 relaxation times. It will also depend on certain properties of the instrument used to make the measurement, including unavoidable inhomogeneities in the external magnetic field. In order to measure just the intrinsic properties of the sample, rather more complex sequences of RF pulses must be used; a description of these

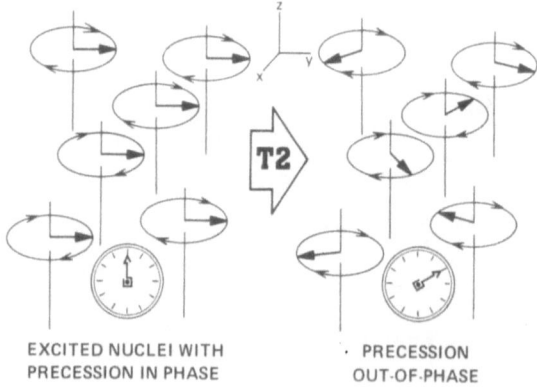

EXCITED NUCLEI WITH
PRECESSION IN PHASE

· PRECESSION
OUT-OF-PHASE

Figure 6. The nuclear spin ensembles, shown on the left immediately after a 90° excitatory pulse, lose phase coherence; the rate at which they do so is given by T_2. (Reprinted by permission of the publisher from: Nuclear magnetic resonance: physical principles and instrumentation. In: Amendola B, Amendola M (eds.), Recent trends in radiation oncology and related fields. Elsevier Science Publishing Co, Inc, 1983.)

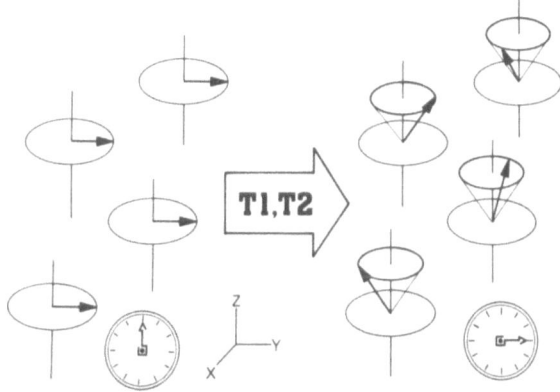

Figure 7. In actuality, T_1 and T_2 relaxation occur concurrently. The figure on the left illustrates the nuclear spin ensembles immediately after a 90° excitatory pulse; the diagram on the right shows them after partial T_1 and complete T_2 relaxation have occurred. (Reprinted by permission of the publisher from: Nuclear magnetic resonance: physical principles and instrumentation. In: Amendola B, Amendola M (eds.), Recent trends in radiation oncology and related fields. Elsevier Science Publishing Co, Inc, 1983.)

is beyond the scope of this chapter, and the reader is referred elsewhere [2, 3]. Suffice it to say such measurements are possible.

As noted above, the Larmor or precessional frequency is dependent on the external magnetic field experienced by a nucleus. In an NMR device, the bulk of this field in contributed by an external magnet that is part of the instrument. However, the microscopic field felt by the nucleus will be modified slightly by the electrical charges of its atomic neighbors in a characteristic manner. This modification (sometimes called shielding) is termed the chemical shift, and can be extremely useful in identifying the chemical species (i.e. the molecule) a resonating nucleus belongs to. The variation in Larmor frequency is extremely small, on the order of parts per million. Though it is potentially one of the most useful measurements one can make using NMR methods, the technical difficulties are great, particularly when NMR instruments are scaled up to accommodate human beings. Most NMR imagers measure the hydrogen density and the relaxation times, but are unable to discern chemical shift; more advanced instruments, generally operating at higher magnetic fields, are now being developed which have this additional capability.

In summary, if a sample containing a suitable isotope such as common hydrogen is placed in a static external magnetic field, there will be a tendency for the hydrogen nuclei to align themselves with the external field, and to precess at a characteristic frequency which will vary linearly with the strength of the external field. If an RF pulse at the precessional or Larmor frequency is applied, the nuclei will absorb a small amount of energy, and become excited. Immediately after the excitatory pulse is concluded, the nuclei will relax back to their ground state; analysis of this process permits measurement of at least four sample properties: the hydrogen density; two relaxation times, T_1 and T_2; and the chemical shift.

278

Pulse sequences

Different sequences of precisely timed RF pulses of well defined intensities are used to generate NMR images; different sequences produce images with varying intensity dependencies on the magnetic parameters. For example, the commonly used spin-echo sequence consists of, in simplest form, a 90° RF pulse, a pause of a fraction of a second customarily termed TE/2 (typically TE/2 is 10–30 ms), followed by a 180° pulse. After an interval, termed TR, following the initial 90° pulse (typically ~1 s) , the sequence repeats (Figure 8). The NMR signal will be emitted at TE milliseconds and its intensity given by:

$$I = f p \, (1\text{-}exp \, [TR/T_1]) \, exp \, (\text{-}TE/T_2)$$

where f is related to any fluid flow which might be present, p is the sample or pixel hydrogen density, TR and TE are the intervals mentioned above, and T_1 and T_2 are the sample relaxation times. Many other pulse sequences have been developed with different function forms. The pulse sequence and timing intervals used in the double spin-echo approach used by one manufacturer are shown in Figure 8.

The choice of pulse sequence will thus have a major effect on the appearance of the MR image, much like varying the X-ray tube current ('ma'), timing ('ms'), or kilovoltage ('kvp') will influence the appearance of a conventional X-ray, only much more so. The relative intensities of different tissues and structures, their contrast, and indeed the ability to discriminate between normal and pathologic tissues is highly dependent on the pulse sequences and timing intervals employed. Optimal use of MRI requires a thorough understanding of the underlying physical principles as well as their clinical application, so that imaging parameters which optimize signal to noise ratios and lesion visibility can be chosen in each diagnostic situation.

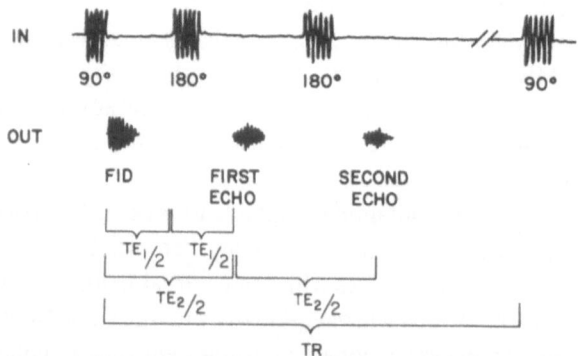

Figure 8. Schematic drawing showing the RF pulses comprising a dual spin-echo pulse sequence (top line); initial spin excitation is produced by a 90° RF pulse; 'spin-echos' (bottom line) are signals produced by the sample or patient in response to the two 180° RF pulses. The initial FID is ignored by the imager.

Magnetic resonance imaging

Thus far the question of spatial localization has not been raised in this discussion; acheiving such localization is fundamental to generating an image, or map, of NMR parameters in space in a complex 'sample' such as a human being. The wavelength of the RF signals is on the order of tens of meters, so that determination of the origin of the RF signal cannot be easily employed to achieve spatial localization; some devices do use small RF antennac (called surface coils) having limited range and placed around or over the tissue of interest to achieve localization, but this method is not applicable to imaging. The approach used in virtually all MRI devices is based on the deliberate introduction of known variation in the large external magnetic field using field gradient coils. Since the Larmor frequency is proportional to this external magnetic field, spatial variation in the magnetic field is translated into frequency variation in the Larmor frequency. This is illustrated in Figure 9. Here, a linear gradient is applied; the field is stronger near the patient's head than feet, and thus the corresponding Larmor frequency is higher.

Though the applied gradient need not be linear and can be applied along any arbitrary axis, it is apparent that a given gradient can only yield spatial information along one of the three dimensions. Hence, more complex variations on this theme must be used to generate high resolution images of three-dimensional objects. The gradient can be applied either during the excitatory pulse or during receipt of the relaxation signal; indeed, both approaches can be used simultaneously, and the gradient can be changed between the two phases of the experiment. If a gradient is applied during excitation, and a narrow band RF signal is employed, only a portion of the sample will be excited, and even in the absence of a gradient during the read-out phase, only that portion of the sample initially excited can contribute to the perceived signal; this is termed selective excitation.

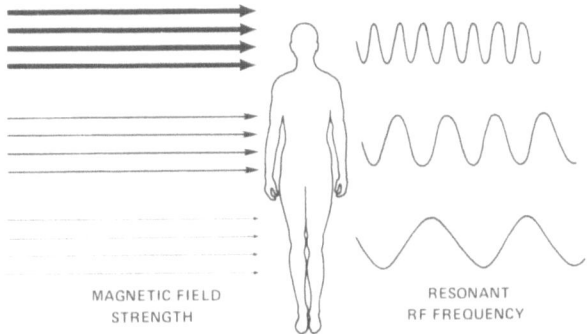

MAGNETIC FIELD
STRENGTH

RESONANT
RF FREQUENCY

Figure 9. The effects of a spatially varying magnetic field on the resonant Larmor frequency are illustrated. (Note: The amount of variation shown in this figure is very much greater than would be used in an actual imager.) (Reprinted by permission of the publisher from: Nuclear magnetic resonance: physical principles and instrumentation. In: Amendola B, Amendola M (eds.), Recent trends in radiation oncology and related fields. Elsevier Science Publishing Co, Inc, 1983.)

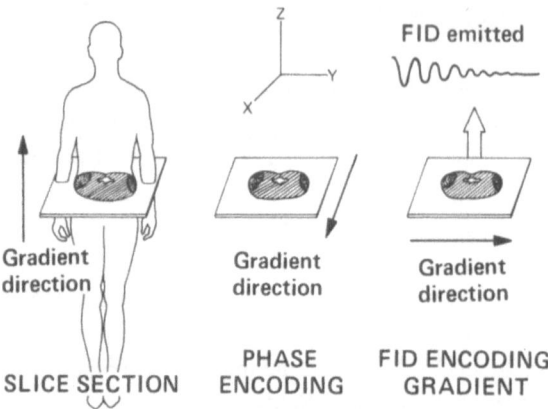

Figure 10. A scheme for imaging is illustrated; refer to the text for details. (Reprinted by permission of the publisher from: Nuclear magnetic resonance: physical principles and instrumentation. In: Amendola B, Amendola M (eds.), Recent trends in radiation oncology and related fields. Elsevier Science Publishing Co, Inc, 1983.)

If a gradient is applied during the read-out phase, frequency (Fourier) analysis of the signal will yield spatial information along the axis of the gradient. To obtain enough signal information to calculate spatial information along more than one axis, necessary to produce an image, multiple experiments or measurements must be performed, and the data combined. Several approaches have been successfully used to generate images. If the gradient direction is rotated between experiments, back-projection algorithms analogous to those used in X-ray computed tomography can be employed to reconstruct the image. Alternatively, phase-encoding gradients can be added, and a two-dimensional Fourier transform used to reconstruct an image [4]; the latter approach is probably more commonly used, and is illustrated in Figure 10.

In general, a combination of selective excitation and read-out gradients are used to produce NMR images. It is a consequence of the need to make multiple measurements that NMR imaging time is on the order of several minutes, a limitation unlikely to change substantially. Hence, the minimum amount of time necessary to perform hydrogen imaging is likely to remain at several minutes; it is, however, possible to generate multiple tomograohic slices concurrently in one several minute period, by selectively exciting multiple planes.

NMR images are intrinsically motion sensitive; if the object being imaged moves between excitation and read-out, this will be reflected in the image. This phenomenon is potentially quite useful in quantitating the flow of fluids such as blood. Various techniques have been suggested to measure blood flow, and pulse sequences have been developed which produce images in which flow is quantitated [5].

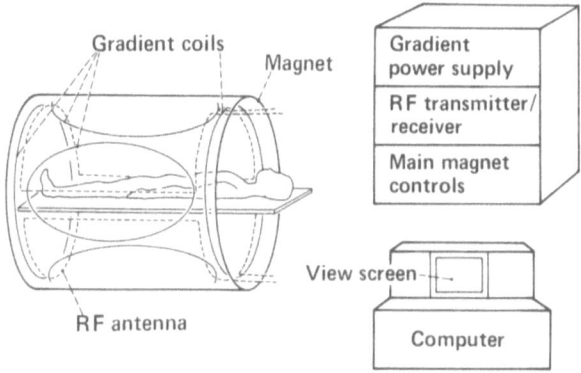

Figure 11. The components of a 'typical' NMR imager. (Reprinted by permission of the publisher from: Nuclear magnetic resonance: physical principles and instrumentation. In: Amendola B, Amendola M (eds.), Recent trends in radiation oncology and related fields. Elsevier Science Publishing Co, Inc, 1983.)

Instrumentation

The components of an MRI device are shown schematically in Figure 11. The largest, most expensive, and indeed the component unique to MRI is the magnet. The magnet must produce a field of between about 1 and 20 kilogauss (for comparison, the Earth's field is about 0.5 gauss, and the field of a household magnet perhaps 500 gauss near its surface) uniform over the imaging volume to at least 100 parts per million; if spectroscopic (chemical shift) or non-hydrogen (e.g. phosphorus or sodium) imaging is to be performed, fields at the high end of the range are necessary. Chemical shift imaging also requires much greater field homogeneity than density and relaxation time imaging. Higher field strengths have disadvantages as well. They are more expensive, and it is more difficult to find a suitable site for one in a hospital setting. In addition, though image noise generally decreases at higher fields, tissue contrast may diminish as well. The latter effect results from smaller intrinsic variation in tissue relaxation times at high magnetic fields. The issue of the 'optimal' field strength for medical applications is far from settled.

Several kinds of magnets are used: resistive, superconducting and permanent. Resistive magnets are scaled up electromagnets. They are relatively inexpensive to purchase, and straight-forward to operate. Field strengths are generally limited to about 1.5 kilogauss, though at least one recent design offers 2.4 kilogauss. Resistive systems are probably limited to hydrogen imaging, and image quality is often not as good as with superconducting designs.

Superconducting magnets are more expensive, and must be filled regularly with cyrogenic liquid helium and nitrogen. They offer much greater field strengths and homogeneity than resistive designs, and can be built with field strengths high enough to accomodate applications such as phosphorus imaging and spectroscopy.

Permanent magnets have very low operating costs, and generally have lower fringe fields (the magnetic field away from the magnet) than current resistive or superconducting systems. Some designs are quite heavy.

Siting an MRI magnet can be difficult, as both the effects of the environment on the system and the effects of the magnetic field on the environment must be taken into account. In general, large moving metal objects can interfere with the operation of a scanner, so parking lots and elevators must be at least about 50 feet from a system. Operation of the magnet poses certain safety considerations; ferromagnetic objects such as scissors or oxygen tanks can turn into hazardous projectiles near a magnet. Patients with pacemakers containing magnetic switches must be kept well away from the magnet; current guidelines use 5 gauss as the threshold, about 18–27 feet from the center of a 5 kilogauss magnet. These siting problems are less severe for permanent magnet systems, which have small or nearly absent fringe fields, and may become less onerous for other designs as well, as manufacturers solve the difficult engineering problems inherent in shielding MRI systems.

Other components of an MRI scanner include the gradient coils and control circuits, and the RF system. The latter consists of a coil which serves as the antenna (generally, the same coil is used for both transmission of the excitatory pulses and receipt of the signal), and a transmitter and receiver. Because the emitted signals are so small, special attention must be paid to keeping out interference. This normally requires placing the system in a specially constructed RF shielded room, termed a Faraday cage.

The display and photographic consoles are similar to those used in X-ray computed tomography and digital radiography.

Clinical applications

Introduction

NMR has numerous applications in both the laboratory and the clinical arena. The discussion which follows is largely limited to the latter.

As noted above, several biologically relevent nuclei can undergo nuclear magnetic resonance, including the naturally abundant isotopes of hydrogen, sodium, and phosphorus. Of these, hydrogen has by far the largest molar concentration in the body; it also has an intrinsic NMR sensitivity (at constant field) about 11 times greater than sodium and 15 times greater than phosphorus. As a result, hydrogen is the only element suitable for high resolution imaging. Hydrogen images are functions of the hydrogen density and the relaxation times; most of the signal comes from water. Chemical shift imaging of hydrogen at a resolution sufficient to separate water from fat has been demonstrated, and will be discussed further below. Phosphorus compounds are of course crucial in energy metabolism, and a great deal of attention has been directed at chemical shift imaging of phosphorus; such images take a long time to acquire and are of intrinsically poor resolution; this subject, too, is discussed more fully in the material which follows.

Hydrogen imaging of the heart

Hydrogen NMR images of the heart have a spatial resolution on the order of 1 to 2 mm; better resolution theoretically may be possible using 'zoom' imaging techniques (in which signal acquisition is limited to the heart, excluding the surrounding lungs), but it is doubtful that finer practical resolution will be possible because of the long imaging times and resultant motion blurring. Images can be acquired using either of two approaches: slice imaging and volume imaging. In the former, the heart is imaged as a series of contiguous or nearly contiguous tomographic planes. This is similar to X-ray computed tomography, except that with MRI, imaging can be in coronal or sagittal as well as transverse planes; it is possible that some manufacturers might implement oblique planar imaging, so that true cardiac long axis and short axis images can be obtained. Planar imaging generally yields the highest resolution in the tomographic section; resolution in the perpendicular direction is much poorer, on the order of 5 to 10 mm. Imaging times are on the order of 5 to 10 min for a series of slices which would encompass the heart; more time might be required if pulse sequences designed to optimize tissue characterization were employed. Direct volume imaging is also possible; here, a three-dimensional Fourier technique [4] is used, and data is acquired from the entire volume of the heart at once. Such techniques generally have acquisition times several times longer, but permit more versatile control over resolution, with finer resolution in the third dimension. Viewing of the volume data in oblique planes corresponding to the long and short axis projections often used in other imaging modalities is possible. A comparison of the two methods has been recently reported by Go *et al.* [6].

Magnetic resonance imaging of the thorax and the heart produces varying signal intensities from different tissues. Bone, calcified structures, flowing blood and air produce little or no signal intensity and appear as dark structures. Subcutaneous and epicardial fat produce high signal intensity, and vascular and myocardial tissues produce an intermediate signal intensity. The high contrast that results between myocardium and the blood filled cavity, and the myocardium and epicardial fat and surrounding lungs, leads to precise definition of endocardial and epicardial borders. Thus left ventricle wall thickness and thickening dynamics can be measured.

Because of the long time required to image, good depiction of cardiac anatomy requires the use of gated acquisition, generally performed using the electrical

ECG signal. This is more complex than it might at first seem, because the strong RF pulses present during imaging can interact with most conventional cardiac monitoring systems. However, the technical problems have now been largely overcome, and ECG-gated MRI is becoming available. The employment of such devices generally increases imaging times several-fold. Even greater anatomic detail is provided if respiratory gating is combined with cardiac gating, and as of this writing, devices with this capability are just coming into use.

At present, hydrogen magnetic resonance imaging of the heart is limited to mapping hydrogen density and the two relaxation times; chemical shift information is not available, and though blood flow through the heart is reflected in the images, this has not yet been done quantitatively. The images do demonstrate blood flow in vessels, but the appearance depends on a combination of effects including the imaging method used, the velocity of flow, and the direction of flow relative to the imaging device. In most circumstances, blood vessels appear dark, that is as areas of diminished or absent signal intensity. However, in some cases, paradoxical enhancement occurs, and bright areas appear in blood vessels; the appearance can be quite dramatic. Hydrogen MRI can be used for two purposes: the evaluation of cardiac and great vessel anatomy, and the assesment of global and regional LV function [6–10], and the use of the tissue characterization capabilities of MRI to assess the metabolic state of the myocardium [11–14]. These will be addressed in turn.

MRI offers a great advantage in studying the heart: there is great contrast on magnetic resonance images between myocardium and blood, since the latter is a flowing liquid. It was recognized early that the myocardium could be easily seen with good endocardial and epicadial detail, and separated from the chamber cavities. Great vessel anatomy is easily discerned on MR images (Figure 12). The superior vena cava, ascending and descending aorta, and pulmonary vessels are clearly visualized. This has provided recognition of aortic abnormalities such as aortic aneurysms and aortic dissections (Figure 13). The resolution of the images is great enough to visualize intimal flaps of dissections and mural thrombus, and sluggish flow within the false channel of the dissection. Further, particularly with the use of gated acquisition, significant internal structure in the heart can be seen (Figure 14), including the valve apparatus and papillary muscles. Clear visualization of the walls of all four chambers appears possible. Areas of post-infarction thinning of ventricular wall can be seen, and mural thrombus in areas of prior transmural myocardial infarction can be visualized. MRI is clearly useful in the diagnosis and/or follow-up of patients with anatomic cardiac abnormalities, including congenital heart disease and the hypertrophic cardiomyopathies. It is sometimes possible to visualize the coronary arteries and bypass grafts; it is not yet clear whether MRI will prove reliable enough for routine use in studying these vessels. The normal pericardium, composed primarily of fibrous tissue, produces little magnetic resonance signal, whereas surrounding epicardial fat produces regions of high intensity. Thus, it has been possible to detect thickened pericar-

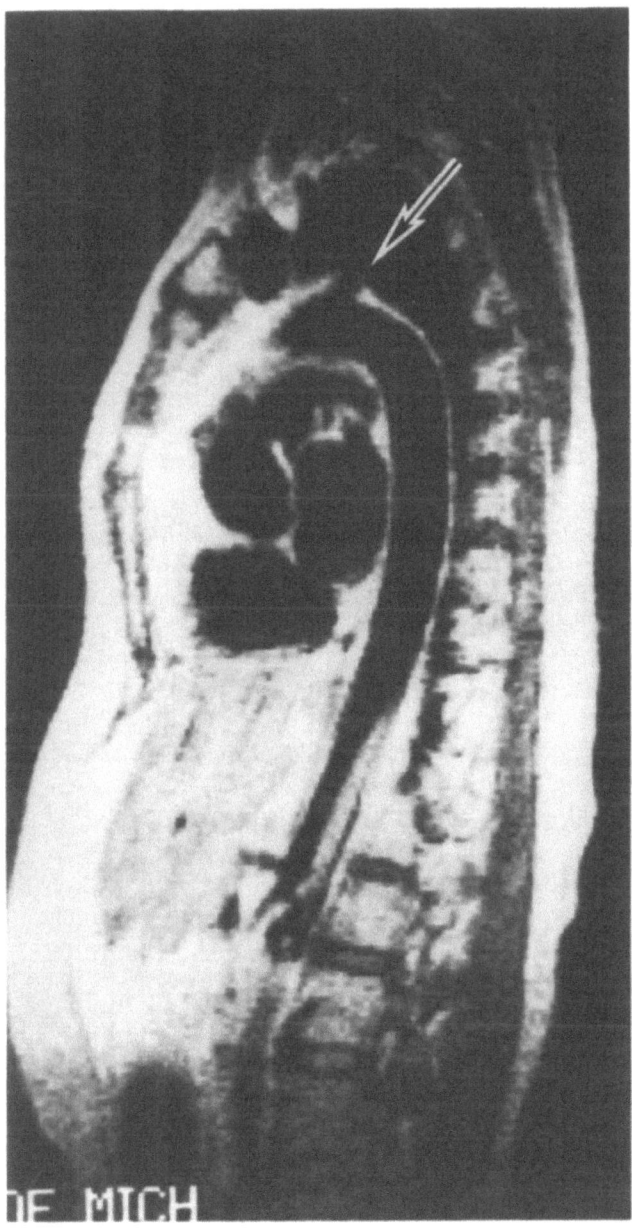

Figure 12. Gated sagittal image showing the heart and portions of the aortic arch; the orifice of the left carotid artery (arrow) is visible.

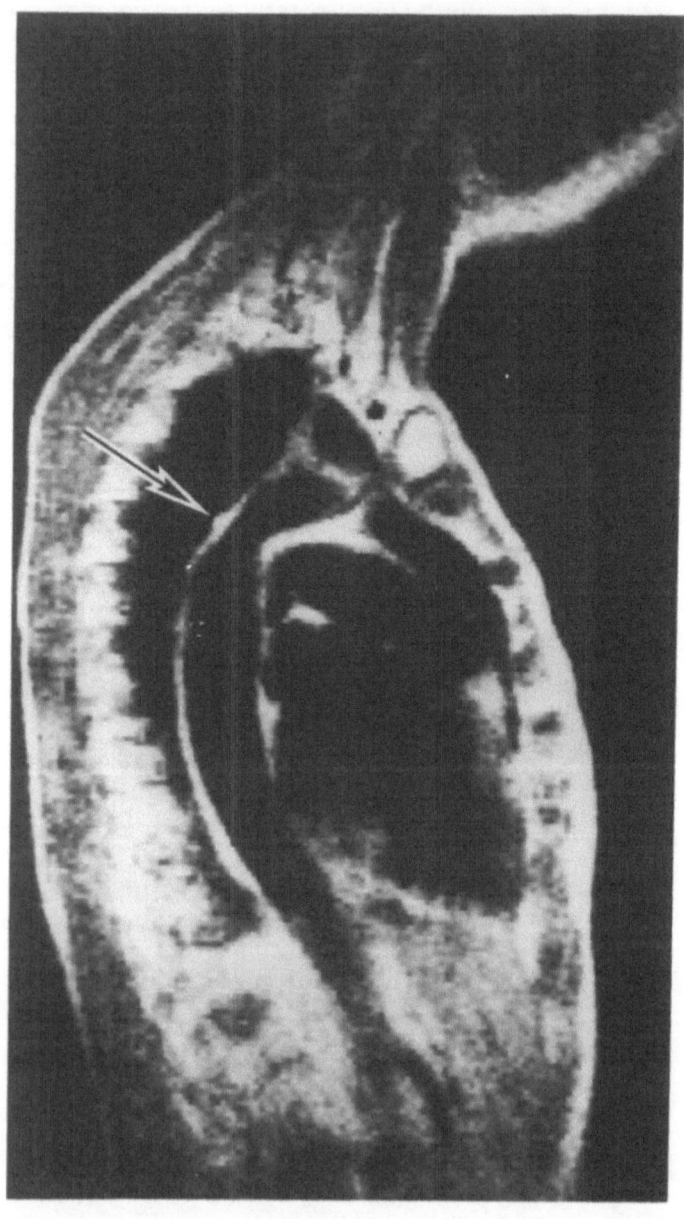

Figure 13. Ungated sagittal image of a patient with Takayasu's Arteritis, and an aortic stenosis (arrow).

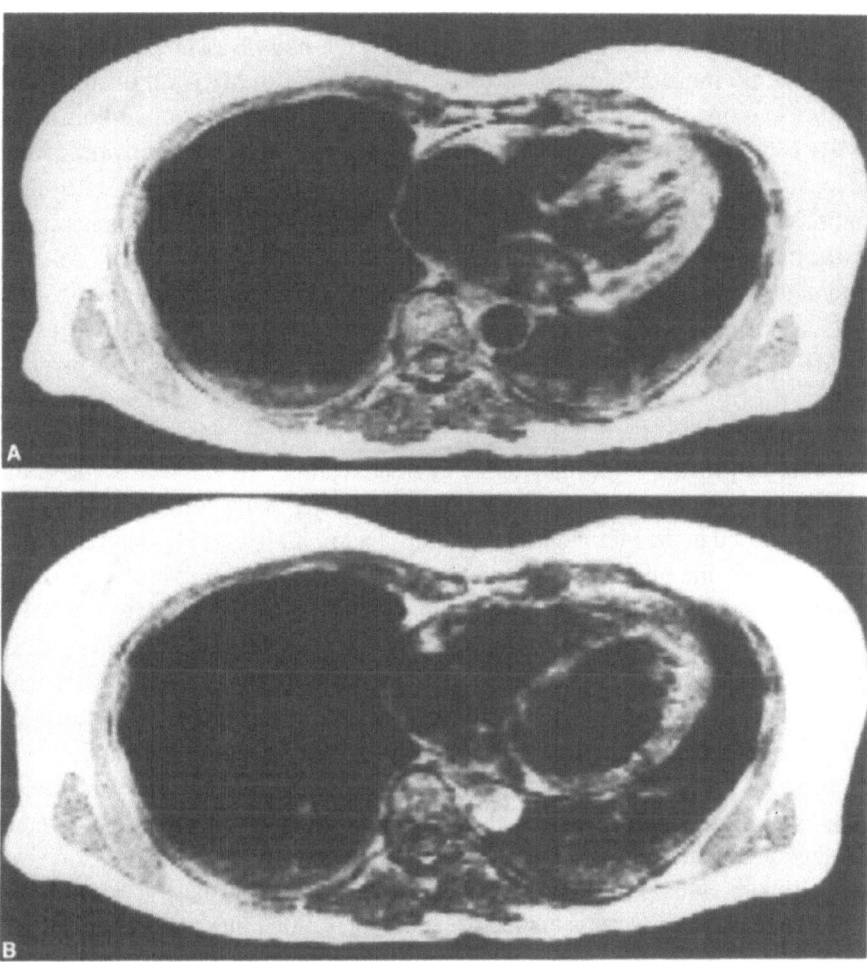

Figure 14. Gated Transverse images through an adult thorax, showing the heart at end-diastole (A) and end-systole (B).

dium as a dark rim around the myocardium in patients with constrictive pericarditis. Clearly the clinical experience with cardiac MRI is in its infancy and further clinical experience will better define the use and accuracy of MRI in the diagnosis of a variety of cardiac disease.

Another important application will be the use of MRI to evaluate left ventricular wall motion and thickening (Figure 14B). The three-dimensional shape and volume of the ventricle can be accurately measured, and the changes through the cardiac cycle determined. Further, the image contrast between blood and myocardium is great enough so that the development of semi-automated computer algorithms for accurate measurement of ejection fraction and related quantities should be feasible.

MRI offers various advantages over traditional methods for imaging the heart. In comparison with contrast ventriculography, it is non-invasive and far easier to perform; no ionizing radiation is used. The accuracy of MRI will likely exceed that of radionuclide studies, though clinical data are still lacking on this issue. MRI is more generally applicable than echocardiography, and provides better depiction of cardiac anatomy; it is, of course, far more expensive. MRI offers more versatile depiction of cardiac anatomy than X-ray computed tomography (which is limited to transverse planes), and does not require the large doses of iodinated contrast material to opacify the blood. While computed tomography attains less than 5% soft-tissue contrast, MRI achieves 20% to 25% contrast.

MRI offers great potential in characterizing the metabolic state of myocardium; it is not yet clear whether or not hydrogen imaging will live up to this promise. However, there is initial data which suggests that hydrogen imaging may be able to provide important tissue characterization. In excised canine heart tissues, prolongation of relaxation times following acute infarction has been demonstrated in the infarcted myocardium (Figure 15) [11, 13, 14]. A recent study of in vivo canine infarction using gated MRI has demonstrated increased signal intensity compared to normal myocardium. The T_2 relaxation time was $69 + 3\%$ longer in the infarcted myocardium compared to normal myocardium. Even greater image contrast can be obtained through the use of intravascular paramagnetic contrast agents, which serve to accentuate the appearance of perfusion abnormalities [12]. Currently, no such agents are approved for human use; such approval is probably several years away. However, the in vivo utility of MRI in this application has not yet been clearly demonstrated. There are often dramatic changes in the magnetic properties of tissues following excision, so direct in vivo/ in vitro correlations must be interpreted cautiously. Further, there is likely substantial loss of precision in measuring the relaxation times using a whole body sized imager as opposed to a smaller device. Finally, it must be pointed out that there are practial difficulties in imaging acutely ill patients; respirators, most monitoring devices, and infusion pumps cannot be brought near the imaging magnet.

In conclusion, it is evident that myocardial thinning and tissue changes in chronic myocardial infarction are visible on MRI images; whether or not the technique will be valuable in the more important assessment of ischemia and/or acute infarction has yet to be determined. Work is underway at several institutions on the development of MRI contrast agents, analogous to the iodinated agents used in X-ray studies but with the potential for far greater versatility [15, 16]. These will undoubtedly greatly expand the utility of MRI in the diagnosis of myocardial disease.

Non-hydrogen imaging

Two elements, phosphorus and sodium, may prove useful in MRI of the heart. As

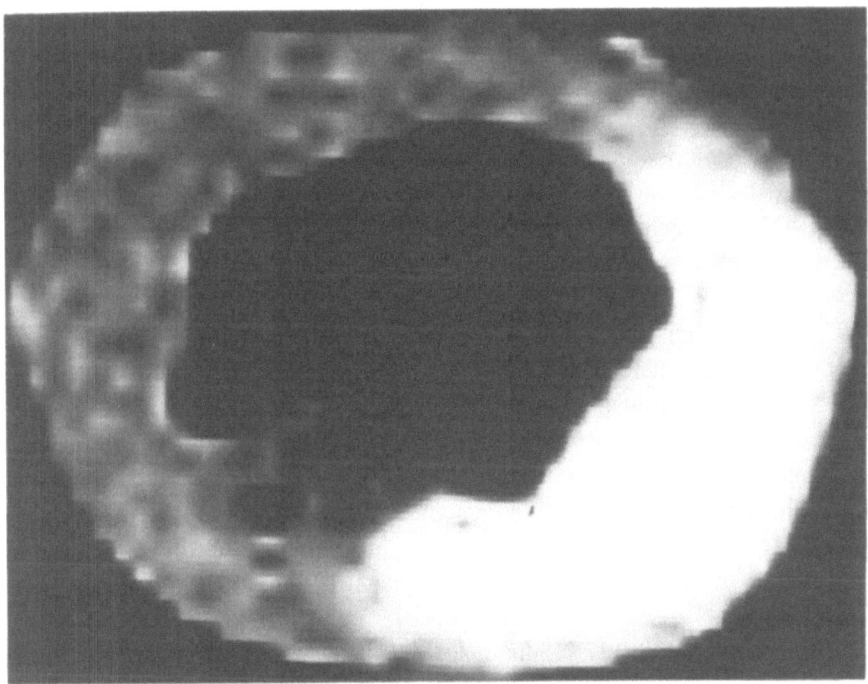

Figure 15. Transverse image through an intact, excised canine heart. Immediately prior to sacrifice, the animal experienced a one hour occlusion of the posterior circumflex coronary artery, followed by a two hour reperfusion period. The resulting infarct is seen as an area of increased intensity, largely because of a prolonged T_2 relaxation time.

noted previously, both produce far smaller signals than hydrogen, and are thus much more difficult to study. Imaging times are on the order of one to several hours, and resolution on the order of several centimeters. Some improvement is likely, but it will not be dramatic.

Phosphorus compounds are the energy sources of cells, and the in vivo measurement of their concentrations would be of very great diagnostic importance. Such measurements require that chemical shift imaging be performed, a technique much more demanding than the hydrogen imaging just discussed. In general, larger magnets with much more homogeneous fields must be used; superconducting magnets are likely necessary, and the fringe field will be larger than with smaller magnets.

In in-vitro work, NMR techniques have already found great use in the study of small tissue or cell samples. These techniques are now being applied to intact animals. Surface coils, small RF antennaes whose range is limited to on the order of several centimeters, and small magnets with limited homogeneous field volumes, have been used to achieve spatial localization; such methods generally work best when a coil can be surgically implanted on the organ of interest, reducing interference from subcutaneous tissues. Studies have been performed on numerous organs, including the heart. In humans, work on skeletal muscle and the brain has been reported. More recently, the field gradient methodolgy of MRI has been applied to phosphorus to achieve spatial localization, and it is this approach that is likely to prove clinically useful. Spatial resolution need not be great, but resolution in the 'chemical shift' dimension must be great enough to permit identification of the various phosphorus compounds of interest, including ATP, ADP, phosphocreatine and inorganic phosphates. Preliminary results have been reported in vivo, usually from measurements in the brain or skeletal muscle [17].

Changes in energy metabolism in exercise, as well as abnormalities in several inherited enzyme defects and infarction have been demonstrated. Using high-resolution but non-imaging apparatus, many interesting results have been reported including the measurement of cardiac phosphorus balance in normal and ischemic myocardium in intact hearts [18, 19], of phorphorus metabolism and intracelular pH in normal volunteers and a patient with McArdle's syndrome [20], and of cerebral phosphorus metabolism in infants [21]. In addition, the use of phosphorus spectroscopy in a large bore imaging system has been described [22, 23].

Also of some interest is sodium imaging. Chemical shift studies are not necessary, so the magnetic field homogeneity requirements are not as great as for phosphorus, but higher field strengths than for hydrogen imaging are needed. Sodium imaging is of interest because of the great difference in sodium concentration between intra- and extracellular fluid (0.012 M v. 0.145 M); a differential maintained by an energy dependent pump. Images demonstrating dramatic changes in cat brain sodium concentration following acute infarction have been published [24]. The change may be a result of an increase in intracellular sodium; an increased relative amount of extracellular fluid, and/or increased NMR visibility of sodium due to changes in the chemical milieu. The role of this methodolgy in studying the heart is not yet clear.

Conclusion

Magnetic resonance imaging is in its infancy, However, initial observations and clinical experience suggest that this imaging modality will play an important role in the evaluation of cardiac dynamics, coronary flow, myocardial tissue characterization, and myocardial metabolism. The full potential of cardiac magnetic resonance imaging will be established within the next decade. It should prove to be useful not only in the assessment of clinical problems, but also a very powerful research tool to explore fundamental questions in the pathophysiology of heart disease.

Acknowledgements

Preparation of this manuscript was supported in part by NIH grant HL 29716.

References

1. Lauterbur PC: Image formation by induced local interactions: examples employing nuclear magnetic resonance. Nature 242: 190–191, 1973.
2. Farrar TC, Becker ED: Pulse and fourier transform NMR: introduction to theory and methods. Academic Press, New York, 1971.
3. Fukushima E, Roeder SBW: Experimental pulse NMR: a nuts and bolts approach. Addison-Wesley Publishing Co, Reading, MA, 1981.
4. Kumar A, Welti D, Ernst RR: NMR fourier zeugmatography. J Magn Reson 18: 69–83, 1975.
5. Singer JR, Crooks LE: Nuclear magnetic resonance blood flow measurements in the human brain. Science 221: 654–656, 1983.
6. Go RT, MacIntyre WJ, Yeung HN, Kramer DM, Geisinger M, Chilcote W, George C, O'Donnell JK, Moodie DS, Meaney TF: Volume and planar gated cardiac magnetic resonance imaging: a correlative study of normal anatomy with thallium-201 SPECT and cadaver sections. Radiology 150: 129–135, 1984.
7. Hawkes RC, Holland GN, Moore WS, Roebuck EJ, Worthington BS: Nuclear magnetic resonance (NMR) tomography of the normal heart. J Comput Assist Tomogr 5: 605–612, 1981.
8. Herfkens RJ, Higgins CB, Hricak H, Lipton MJ, Crooks LE, Lanzer P, Botvinick E, Brundage B, Sheldon PE, Kaufman L: Nuclear magnetic resonance imaging of the cardiovascular system: normal and pathologic findings. Radiology 147: 749–759, 1983.
9. Fletcher BD, Jacobstein MD, Nelson AD, Riemenschneider TA, Alfidi RJ: Gated magnetic resonance imaging of congenital cardiac malformations. Radiology 150: 137–140, 1984.
10. Lanzer P, Botvinick EH, Schiller NB, Crooks LE, Arakawa M, Kaufman L, Davis PL, Herfkins R, Lipton MJ, Higgins CB: Cardiac imaging using gated magnetic resonance. Radiology 150: 121–127, 1984.
11. Williams ES, Kaplan JI, Thatcher F, Zimmerman G, Knoebel SB: Prolongation of proton spin lattice relaxation times in regionally ischemic tissue from dog hearts. J Nucl Med 21: 449–453, 1980.
12. Brady TJ, Goldman MR, Pykett IL, Buonanno FS, Kistler JP, Newhouse JH, Burt CT, Hinshaw WS, Pohost GM: Proton nuclear magnetic resonance imaging of regionally ischemic canine hearts: effect of paramagnetic proton signal enchancement. Radiology 144: 343–347, 1982.
13. Higgins CB, Herfkens R, Lipton MJ, Sievers R, Sheldon P, Kaufman L, Crooks LE: Nuclear magnetic resonance imaging of acute myocardial infarction in dogs: alterations in magnetic relaxation times. Am J Cardiol 52: 184–188, 1983.
14. Wesbey G, Higgins CB, Lanzer P, Botvinik E, Liptyon MJ: Imaging and characterization of acute myocardial infarction in vivo by gated nuclear magnetic resonance. Circulation 69: 125–130, 1984.
15. Brasch RC: Work in progress: methods of contrast enchancement of NMR imaging and potential applications. Radiology 147: 781–788, 1983.
16. Runge VM, Clanton JA, Lukehart CM, Partain CL, James AE: Paramagnetic agents for contrast-enchanced NMR imaging: a review. AJR 141: 1209–1215, 1983.
17. The reader is referred to several reports in the Scientific Program of the Society of Magnetic Resonance in Medicine, Second Annual Meeting, August 16–19, 1983, San Francisco, CA, available from the Society offices at P.O. Box 9750, Berkeley, CA, for $15.00.
18. Grove TH, Ackerman JJH, Radda GK, Bore PJ: Analysis of rat heart in vivo by phosphorus nuclear magnetic resonance. Proc Natl Acad Sci USA 77: 299–302, 1980.

19. Nunnally RL, Bottomley PA: Assessment of Pharmacological treatment of myocardial infarction by phosphorus-31. NMR 211: 177–180.

20. Ross BP, Radda GK, Gaddian DG, Rocker G, Esiri M, Falconer-Smith J: Examination of a case of suspected McArdle's syndrome by ^{31}P nuclear magnetic resonance. N Engl J Med 304: 1338–1342, 1981.

21. Cady EB, Dawson MJ, Hope PL, Tofts PS, Costello AMD, Delpy DT, Reynolds EOR, Wilkie DR: Non-invasive investigation of cerebral metabolism in newborn infants by phosphorus nuclear magnetic resonance spectroscopy. Lancet 1: 1059–1062, 1983.

22. Bottomley PA, Hart HR, Edelstein WA, Schenck JF, Smith LS, Leve WM, Mueller OM, Redington RW: Anatomy and metabolism of the normal human brain studied by magnetic resonance at 1.5 Tesla. Radiology 150: 441–446, 1984.

23. Maudsley AA, Hilal SK, Simon HE, Wittekoek S: Multinuclear applications of chemical shift imaging. Scientific Program: Society of Magnetic Resonance in Medicine Second Annual Meeting August 16–19, 1983, San Francisco, CA, pp 230–231.

24. Hilal SK, Maudsley AA, Simon HE, Perman WH, Bonn J, Mowad ME, Silver AJ, Ganti SR, Sane P, Chien IC: In vivo NMR imaging of tissue sodium in the intact cat before and after acute cerebral stroke. AJNR 4: 245–249, 1983.

16. Future directions and integrative approaches in digital cardiac imaging

ANDREW J. BUDA and G.B. JOHN MANCINI

Over the past decade, there has been a rapid development of new cardiac imaging technologies. This has led to new insights and better understanding of basic cardiac pathophysiology which has undoubtedly contributed to the impressive decline in cardiovascular mortality in recent years [1]. Precise anatomic diagnosis, physiologic assessment, and accurate prognosis have been made available by these new technologies.

Individual present strengths and weaknesses of each modality are summarized in Table 1. From this table, it is clear that many modalities are complementary in their information regarding cardiac structure and function, cardiac tissue characterization, coronary anatomy and blood flow, and myocardial metabolic activity.

The digital computer

The digital computer has become the main focus and theme in cardiac imaging. Despite many advances, medical image processing continues to lag behind other classical applications of image processing, but there is little doubt that this technology has incredible potential in studying the heart. There are several problems that need to be overcome including compatibility of computer systems, storage and archival needs, and ease of operation. Solutions to these and other technical problems should be forthcoming in the next few years. There will continue to be a natural reluctance to adopt these new technologies until there is evidence of practical advantages.

At the present time, each cardiac imaging system stands alone. Both acquisition and processing are performed on one system, and there is little or no communication among different systems. In the future, it is likely that there will be modality-specific acquisition systems with central multi-modality processing networks and individual processing stations. This will allow processing of digitally acquired data at independent work stations, provide sharing of developed image processing algorithms, and allow transfer of data from multiple modalities to

Table 1. Comparison of cardiac imaging modalities

	Echo/Doppler	Nuclear RNA	TL-201	Digital Radiography	Coronary Angiography	CT	PET	MRI
Ischemic heart disease	+	++	++	++	++	+	++	(++)?
Cardiac valves	++	–	–	–	–	–	–	(+)?
Cardiomyopathy	++	++	–	++	–	++	++	(++)?
Thrombi	++	–	+	+	–	+	–	(++)?
Tumors	++	–	–	++	–	++	–	(++)?
Calcification	++	–	–	++	++	++	–	(++)?
Coronary bypass grafts	–	–	–	+	++	+	–	(+)?
Pericardium	++	–	–	–	–	++	–	(++)?
Congenital abnormalities	++	+	–	+	–	+	–	(++)?
Great vessels	+	+	–	++	–	++	–	(++)?
Tissue characterization	++	–	–	–	–	+	–	(++)?
Metabolism	–	–	–	–	–	–	++	(++)?

CT = computed tomography; MRI = magnetic resonance imaging; PET = positron emission tomography; RNA = radionuclide angiography; TL-201 = thallium-201 scintigraphy.

multiple users. This will promote correlative and complementary studies of cardiac disease.

Cardiac imaging specialists

This integrative, cross-modality approach will require interdisciplinary and inter-departmental cooperation. Basic scientists with an interest in image processing will cross from modality to modality. The technologic transfer from one imaging modality to another should be great. The development of integrative cardiac imaging using a multi-modality approach will necessitate the training of cardiologists and cardiovascular radiologists with expertise in the understanding and interpretation of various imaging modalities. No longer will it be sufficient to be an 'echocardiographer', a 'nuclear cardiologist', or an 'angiographer'; the new breed of cardiac imaging specialist will be a physician with a sound knowledge of digital computing and image processing, three-dimensional cardiac anatomy, and cardiac physiology and metabolism. He will work with an interdisciplinary team consisting of engineers, physicists, and other basic scientists. Although such an individual may be primarily involved with one or two imaging modalities, he will coordinate the application and interpretation of multiple modalities. These trends are already obvious as physicians with nuclear or echo backgrounds become involved with other new modalities such as digital radiography, positron emission tomography, or magnetic resonance imaging.

Trends to non-invasive imaging

There have been increasing efforts towards non-invasive diagnosis of cardiac disease. This trend is to be encouraged with the goal being total cardiac assessment without invasive catheterization. There are increasing strides in this direction with the development of radionuclide angiography, two-dimensional echocardiography, and digital radiography to assess left ventricular function; two-dimensional and Doppler echocardiography to evaluate valvular disease; thallium-201 imaging and positron emission tomography to examine myocardial perfusion; and positron emission tomography to determine metabolic function. Indeed, these non-invasive techniques have obviated the necessity of cardiac catheterization in several types of valvular, congenital, or myopathic processes by providing adequate diagnostic information required for medical or surgical intervention [2]. However, the precise localization and characterization of coronary artery disease continues to elude non-invasive assessment and requires coronary angiography. Although there have been advances in the visualization of proximal coronary arteries by 2-D echo and by peripheral injection using digital radiography, there is little hope that a non-invasive technique will replace coronary angiography for anatomic assessment of coronary arteries within the next decade. More likely, regional three-dimensional mapping of the functional physiologic and metabolic effects of anatomic coronary disease will help guide the physician and surgeon in the future to specific sites for revascularization.

In the interval, coronary angiography will continue to provide precise anatomic information for spatial localization of coronary lesions. Increasing studies of correlates between precise anatomic grade of coronary lesions and physiologic and metabolic consequences may demonstrate that angiographic anatomy is not the best indicator of disease particularly in the range of intermediate lesions [3]. Further, the evaluation of collateral function has been notoriously difficult by standard angiographic techniques and this assessment should prove to be increasingly amenable to digital techniques.

In addition to these non-invasive approaches, the combination of digitally based modalities to invasive studies should expand our knowledge base of ischemic heart disease. Digital angiographic assessment of coronary perfusion and coronary flow reserve using contrast-induced hyperemia should become increasingly important following appropriate careful validation [4]. The use of other traditional non-invasive techniques, such as echocardiography, nuclear cardiology, and Doppler echocardiography during invasive procedures and surgery has increased the diagnostic utility of these techniques and has added to our understanding of cardiac pathophysiology. Esophageal two-dimensional echocardiography during surgery has produced more effective intraoperative monitoring techniques [5] and two-dimensional echocardiographic assessment of coronary vessels intraoperatively should provide more precise intraoperative coronary lesion localization [6]. Similarly, the use of a nuclear probe during anesthetic induction [7] and the development of small portable gamma detectors [8] should further facilitate hemodynamic monitoring intraoperatively or during high risk procedures.

Cardiac structure

There are several techniques at present which adequately assess cardiac structure. The best techniques in the future will be those with highest spatial and temporal resolution. Typically, two-dimensional echocardiography, computed tomography, and magnetic resonance imaging will provide the most detailed information concerning structural integrity of cardiac and intracardiac tissues. The emphasis at present and increasingly in the future will be on tomographic imaging so that understanding of tomographic and three-dimensional anatomy of the heart will be important. With sufficient tomographic sections and precise spatial registration, three-dimensional reconstruction of the heart [9] is now possible and should become increasingly feasible in the near future. The three-dimensional reconstructed heart should allow us to better study contour and shape which may prove to be an important physiologic parameter.

Because of the physical limitations of ultrasound which limits its diagnostic utility in approximately 10% of patients, it is likely that ultrafast dynamic computed tomography and magnetic resonance imaging will become the standards for precise evaluation of cardiac anatomic structure. However, these new expensive technologies cannot be justified for use in cardiac structural analysis alone and will be developed for other combined purposes such as myocardial function, perfusion, and tissue characterization. The ease, simplicity, and portability of two-dimensional echocardiography will nevertheless help maintain its important diagnostic position in future years.

Cardiac function

Although invasive contrast angiography has been the 'gold standard' of resting, global left ventricular volume and function for several years, it will be replaced by other techniques. For example, radionuclide ventriculography is increasingly being accepted as an accurate method for assessment of left ventricular volume and function. In addition, digital radiography using either left ventricular injection or peripheral injection has clear advantages to standard contrast ventriculography. Digital radiography with a peripheral injection is much less invasive; with a central injection, ventriculography requires significantly less contrast load. For all of these reasons, standard contrast ventriculography will gradually be replaced by digital radiographic and nuclear techniques in the assessment of left ventricular volumes and function.

There are several recent studies indicating that two-dimensional echocardiography will play a more important role in the quantitative analysis of left ventricular function. Present off-line systems for manual digitization of video images will be replaced by more automated techniques [10]. This will, by necessity, increase the complexity of computing capabilities of two-dimensional echocardiography and require a trade-off in terms of price and portability which may limit its general acceptance. Nevertheless, future quantitative enhancement of two-dimensional echocardiography will require further development of digital acquisition and image processing using larger computers than are presently interfaced to the echo unit. It is most likely that both portable and larger nonportable computer interfaced two-dimensional echo systems will be available for left ventricular functional analysis. More expensive technologies, such as ultrafast multi-slice computed tomography and magnetic resonance imaging, also promise to provide accurate assessment of global left ventricular volumes and function.

Although global left ventricular function provides important information concerning cardiac performance, there is increasing attention being paid to regional left ventricular function in the analysis of ischemic disease. Digital radiography is limited to planar long axis views which may limit careful and complete regional assessment. Tomographic approaches using radionuclide ventriculography, cardiac computed tomography, two-dimensional echocardiography, and magnetic resonance imaging will all provide more complete regional analysis by producing serial circumferential studies of all myocardial regions. The development of three-dimensional techniques using these tomographic approaches will provide topographic regional maps of the heart as important locators of underlying coronary disease.

Cardiac functional reserve

Functional reserve has traditionally been assessed with dynamic exercise during radionuclide ventriculography or, less frequently, during conventional left ventricular angiography. However, newer digital imaging modalities with high spatial resolution will be more sensitive to movement artifact which may limit the applicability of exercise during digital radiography and dynamic cardiac computed tomography. Respiratory artifacts and technical difficulties limit exercise two-dimensional echocardiographic studies. The long acquisition times necessary for cardiac assessment will limit the capability of exercise in combination with magnetic resonance imaging studies. As a result, alternative physiologic and pharmacologic stress interventions will become increasingly important in the future [11].

Cardiac pacing by intracardiac or esophageal routes combined with physiologic or pharmacologic increases in blood pressure may adequately increase rate-pressure product to mimic dynamic exercise. Similarly, other pharmacologic stress maneuvers [12] will be investigated to assess their applicability in combination with digital modalities when dynamic exercise is impractical or impossible.

Myocardial tissue characterization

Tissue characterization is defined as the assessment of the structure of tissue using imaging modalities. With echocardiography, the acoustic properties of tissue can provide information concerning alteration of normal histology and pathology [13]. Further technical improvements will make ultrasound tissue characterization increasingly important in the diagnosis of specific myocardial processes and ischemia and infarction in the future.

Limited tissue characterization of infarcted myocardium is now possible using radionuclide techniques and contrast enhanced computed tomographic scanning. This has resulted in more precise quantification of infarct size in man [14, 15].

The ability of magnetic resonance imaging to characterize myocardial tissue is largely unexplored and requires further investigation. There is recent evidence to suggest that magnetic resonance imaging may accurately detect and localize regionally ischemic and infarcted tissue [16], but its ability to characterize other pathologic states needs to be defined.

Coronary anatomy and blood flow

As discussed previously, selective coronary angiography will continue to be required to outline specific coronary lesions, but digital radiographic techniques will aid in automatic anatomic quantitation of these lesions [17]. Digital coronary radiographic techniques for assessment of coronary flow and flow reserve using wash-in [4] and wash-out [18] densitometric determination are in the early stages of development, and hold promise for the future. Clearly, further basic validation studies to clearly define potential limitations and misinterpretations are necessary. If these techniques withstand the test of careful scrutiny, it is likely that they will make a major contribution to the functional assessment of structural coronary disease.

Other tomographic methods to examine coronary flow and myocardial perfusion will also be more fully explored. At present, tomographic thallium-201 myocardial perfusion studies show promise as a method to better localize specific lesions of the coronary artery. Positron emission tomography using blood flow tracers is likely to allow non-invasive measurements of absolute regional blood flow in the human heart. For example, the net extraction of N-13 ammonia as the product of the extraction fraction and blood flow has been demonstrated to be proportional to myocardial blood flow in the dog. Similarily, studies using rubidium-82 indicate that measures of absolute regional blood flow measurements will be possible in man.

Ultrafast computed axial tomography with contrast may be able to examine aspects of myocardial perfusion, but this will require further exploration. Contrast two-dimensional echocardiography using a variety of contrast agents has proven useful in studying serial perfusion patterns in the laboratory animal [19]. The application of this technique to man is uncertain.

Finally, there is great excitment regarding the potential of magnetic resonance imaging (MRI) to assess myocardial blood flow. MRI studies will be difficult to combine with exercise so that pharmacologic stress procedures such as intravenous dipyridamole will be used to assess coronary reserve and perfusion inhomogeneities related to mild, subcritical lesions.

Metabolic activity

Positron emission tomography now permits assessment of metabolic activity of the myocardium using a variety of cyclotron produced tracers. Utilization of exogenous glucose by myocardium can be measured using F-18 2-fluro-2-deoxyglucose, regional myocardial fatty acid metabolism by C-11 palmitic acid, and regional blood flow using N-13 ammonia and rubidium-82. The development of new metabolic tracers should allow greater biochemical probing of the heart with positron tomography. The development of new radiopharmaceuticals, such as I[131]metaiodobenzylguanidine [13], will allow further metabolic studies using standard gamma cameras in both planar and tomographic views.

The introduction of sodium and phosphorus nuclear magnetic resonance units will allow greater study of metabolic processes of the normal and diseased heart. These approaches to metabolic imaging will allow a mechanism to assess cell viability independent of perfusion and function. This may have important implications in the assessment of therapeutic interventions which may produce metabolic changes before alterations in function or perfusion are apparent. Similarly, metabolic imaging may provide clues to the early stages of disease before structural, functional, or perfusion abnormalities are apparent. The study of alternate pathways of metabolic substrate utilization in congestive heart failure should provide further insight into the basic myocardial derangements leading to myocardial dysfunction.

Integrative approaches

Integrative approaches of function and perfusion in the animal model have produced a better understanding of normal and ischemic conditions. Non-uniformity of perfusion and function have demonstrated the complexity of flow-function relationships even in the normal heart. The development of ischemia has introduced further complexities in flow-function relationships.

The many imaging modalities discussed allow new integrative approaches to the study of structural-functional-perfusion-metabolic interactions. Many of these interactions have neither been explored in the animal laboratory nor in man. Differences in coupling mechanisms in ischemic and reperfusion states may shed light on several confusing observations. Clearly, future investigations in animal and man will explore in detail the metabolic axis of the flow-function-metabolic axis and probe further into cellular function.

Costs

Cardiac imaging is an expensive technology. However, there has been dramatic reduction of computer costs in recent years. For example, ten years ago, the manufacturers' cost for a 64 million bit memory would have been over $600 000 whereas it is approximately $3 000 today. This dramatic reduction in production costs have made powerful imaging technologies clinically practical.

With increasing emphasis on cost containment, there will be attempts by health care administrators to limit the redundancy of clinical assessment. This will lead to careful scrutiny of cost benefit issues related to cardiac digital techniques. The cardiologist will have to make more knowledgeable choices among the many modalities available according to the clinical situation. Given the several options presently available for analysis of cardiac structure and function, the appropriate test will depend on the individual clinical situation and the precision of the information required. By necessity, the physician will need to carefully formulate investigative algorithms of clinical care.

Conclusion

Digital cardiac imaging is quickly evolving as a multi-modality, interdisciplinary field that will attract increasing attention in future years. Integrative approaches will allow precise three-dimensional mapping of structural, functional, and metabolic activity of the heart. The promise of the future by these sophisticated technologies will be better understanding and the earlier detection of cardiac disease.

Acknowledgements

Preparation of this manuscript was supported in part by NIH grant HL 29716.

References

1. Braunwald E: The present state and future of academic cardiology. Circulation 66: 487–490, 1982.
2. St John Sutton MG, St John Sutton M, Oldershaw P, Sacchetti R, Paneth M, Lennox SC, Gibson RV, Gibson DG: Valve replacement without preoperative cardiac cathetherization. N Engl J Med 305: 1233–1238, 1981.
3. Wright CB, Doty DB, Easthan CL, Marcus ML: Measurement of coronary reactive hyperemia with a Doppler probe. Intraoperative guide to hemodynamically significant lesions. J Thorac Cardiovasc Surg 80: 888–897, 1980.
4. Vogel RA, LeFree M, Bates E, O'Neill W, Foster R, Kirlin P, Smith D, Pitt B: Application of digital techniques to selective coronary arteriography: use of myocardial contrast appearance time to measure coronary flow reserve. Am Heart J 107: 153–164, 1984.
5. Hanrath P, Schluter M, Thier W, Langestein BA, Bleifeld W: Clinical implications of transesophageal echocardiography: present status and future aspects. In: Meyer J, Schweizer P, Erbel R (eds.), Advances in Noninvasive Cardiology. Martinus Nijhoff, The Hague, 1983, pp 31–37.
6. Sahn DJ, Barratt-Boyes BG, Graham K, Kerr A, Roche A, Hill D, Brandt PWT, Copeland JG, Manunana R, Temkin LP, Glenn W: Ultrasonic imaging of the coronary arteries in open-chest humans: evaluation of coronary atherosclerotic lesions during cardiac surgery. Circulation 66: 1034–1044, 1982.

7. Wagner HN, Wake R, Nickloff E, Natarajan TK: The nuclear stethescope: a simple device for the generation of left ventricular function curves. Am J Cardiol 23: 747–750, 1976.

8. Wilson RA, Sullivan PA, Moore RH, Zielonka JS, Alpert NM, Boucher CA, McKusick KA, Strauss HW: An ambulatory ventricular function monitor: validation and preliminary clinical results. Am J Cardiol 52: 601–606, 1983.

9. Geiser EA, Ariet M, Conetta DA, Lupkiewicz SM, Christie LG Jr, Conti CR: Dynamic three-dimensional echocardiographic reconstruction of the intact human left ventricle: technique and initial observations in patients. Am Heart J 103: 1056–1065, 1982.

10. Buda AJ, Delp EJ, Meyer CR, Jenkins JM, Smith DN, Bookstein FL, Pitt B: Automatic computer processing of digital two-dimensional echocardiograms. Am J Cardiol 52: 384–389, 1983.

11. Buda AJ: Physiologic stress interventions in cardiac imaging. In: J. Thrall (ed.), Diagnostic interventions in nuclear medicine. Yearbook Medical, Chicago (in press).

12. Gould KL: Assessment of coronary stenosis with myocardial perfusion imaging during pharmacologic coronary vasodilation. IV. Limits of detection of stenosis with idealized experimental cross-sectional myocardial imaging. Am J Cardiol 42: 761–768, 1978.

13. Mimbs JW, Bauwens D, Cohen RD, O'Donnell M, Miller JG, Sobel BE: Effects of myocardial ischemia on quantitative ultrasonic backscatter and identification of responsible determinants. Circ Res 49: 89–96, 1981.

14. Holman BL, Goldhaber SZ, Kirsch C, Polak JF, Friedman BJ, English RJ, Wynne J: Measurement of infarct size using single photon emission computed tomography and technetium-99m pyrophosphate: a description of the method and comparison with patient prognosis. Am J Cardiol 50: 503–511, 1982.

15. Doherty PW, Lipton MJ, Berninger WH, Skioldebrand CG, Carlsson E, Redington RW: The defection and quantitation of myocardial infarction in-vivo using transmission computed tomography. Circulation 63: 597–606, 1981.

16. Wisbey G, Higgins CB, Lanzer P, Botvinik E, Lipton MJ: Imaging and characterization of acute myocardial infarction in-vivo by gated nuclear magnetic resonance. Circulation 69: 125–130, 1984.

17. Brown BG, Bolson E, Frimer M, Dodge HT: Quantitative coronary arteriography: estimation of dimensions, hemodynamic resistance, and atheroma mass of coronary artery lesions using the arteriogram and digital computation. Circulation 55: 329–337, 1977.

18. Nivatpumin T, Vas R, Pfaff, Whiting J, Forrester J: Changes in myocardial perfusion due to reactive hyperemia measured by digital angiography. Circulation (abstr) 68 (supp III): III–42, 1983.

19. Sakamaki T, Tei C, Meerbaum S, Shimoura K, Kondo S, Fishbein MC, Y-Rit J, Shah PM, Corday E: Verification of myocardial contrast two-dimensional echocardiographic assessment of perfusion defects in ischemic myocardium. J Am Coll Cardiol 3: 34–38, 1984.

Index